Providing Diabetes Care in General Practice

Fifth edition

Comments and reviews of this edition of
Providing Diabetes Care in General Practice:

'The best just got better. Treasure it.'
Eugene Hughes, Chairman,
Primary Care Diabetes Europe

'My overall impression of the book is hugely positive.
I think Gwen Hall has done a fine job of updating it and adding
the new information and developments.'
Rosie Walker, Health Education Specialist,
In Balance Healthcare UK

'I am sure that this new expanded edition will be widely
appreciated and used.'
Dr Roger Gadsby, Senior Clinical Lecturer,
University of Warwick

'I think this is a really good book and provides a vast amount
of detail and support to healthcare professionals who will
be reading it.'
Bridget Turner, Head of Healthcare and Policy,
Diabetes UK

'This book is an excellent practical guide for primary care
practitioners providing diabetes care.'
Dr Patricia Cremin, Lecturer,
National University of Ireland, Galway

Comments and reviews of earlier editions of
Providing Diabetes Care in General Practice:

'The complete guide for the primary health care team.'
Dr Michael Hall, Chairman,
Diabetes UK

'It is a real contribution to a modern understanding of so
many aspects of diabetes.'
Professor Harry Keen, former Vice President,
Diabetes UK

'An extremely useful text for primary healthcare teams in
improving the quality of care for people with diabetes.'
Dr John Toby, Chairman of Joint Committee,
Royal College of General Practitioners

'Anyone reading it will be in very safe hands and feel their
confidence in diabetes growing chapter by chapter.'
Dr Charles Fox, Consultant Physician,
Northampton General Hospital

'The book has been invaluable, specifically in helping us set up
our training practices in diabetes and the courses attached to
this scheme.'
Helma Grant, Practice Nurse,
Leicestershire

'I love the practical approach taken in the book . . . which I am
sure will help primary care practitioners save time and produce
a better service.'
Dr Charles Price, Consultant in Public Health Medicine,
Sheffield Health

'The book is an extraordinary and necessary piece
of information.'
Maria L de Alva, former President,
International Diabetes Federation

Providing Diabetes Care in General Practice

A Practical Guide to Integrated Care

Fifth edition

Gwen Hall RMN, RGN, BSc (Hons)

*Diabetes Specialist Nurse/Clinical Educator
  in Primary Care*

Visiting Fellow, University of Surrey

*Associate Clinical Teacher,
  University of Warwick Diabetes Care*

Vice Chair, Primary Care Diabetes Society

Associate Editor, Diabetes and Primary Care

Class Publishing ▪ London

Text © Mary MacKinnon 1993, 1995, 1998, 2002
Text © Gwen Hall 2007
Typography © Class Publishing (London) Ltd 1993, 1995, 1998, 2002, 2007

Printing history
First edition, 1993
Second edition, 1995
Third edition, 1998
Fourth edition, 2002
Fifth edition, 2007

The author and publishers welcome feedback from the users of this book. Please contact the publishers.

Class Publishing, Barb House, Barb Mews, London W6 7PA, UK
Telephone: 020 7371 2119
Fax: 020 7371 2878 [International +4420]
Email: post@class.co.uk
www.class.co.uk

The information presented in this book is accurate and current to the best of the author's knowledge. The author and publisher, however, make no guarantee as to, and assume no responsibility for, the correctness, sufficiency or completeness of such information or recommendation. The reader is advised to consult a doctor regarding all aspects of individual health care.

A CIP catalogue record for this book is available from the British Library

ISBN 13: 978 1 85959 154 3
ISBN 10: 1 85959 154 X

10 9 8 7 6 5 4 3 2 1

Edited by Carrie Walker

Designed and typeset by Martin Bristow

Artwork by David Woodroffe

Printed and bound: Korotan Ljubljana, Slovenia

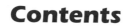

Contents

Part III About diabetes   **301**

Appendices   **357**

About the author

Gwen Hall is a Registered Mental Nurse and Registered General Nurse.

In 1986, she was appointed part-time Practice Nurse at Haslemere Health Centre in Surrey. It was 19 years before she was tempted away into diabetes specialism. During that time, she trained as a Nurse Practitioner and was team leader for the practice's integrated team of doctors and nurses, which was selected by the Audit Commission as an area of good practice.

While working in Haslemere, Gwen combined the part-time roles of Diabetes Facilitator and Practice Nurse Trainer for the Health Authority. She is an Advanced Leader for the University of Warwick Certificate in Diabetes Care and has been a British Heart Foundation trainer. When Primary Care Groups were being formed, Gwen undertook the role of Coronary Heart Disease facilitator before accepting PCT employment as a Diabetes Specialist Nurse in Primary Care in Guildford and Waverley.

She was elected to the Education Committee of Diabetes UK, has served on the Department of Health Clinical Outcomes Group and participated in the NHS Executive Nurse Leadership Project. She was a founder member and then elected representative of Primary Care Diabetes UK and is now Vice Chairman of the Primary Care Diabetes Society.

She is on the editorial board of *Practice Nurse* journal and is Associate Editor of *Diabetes and Primary Care*. She writes regularly for magazines and journals and has contributed chapters to several publications.

Gwen is a Visiting Fellow of the University of Surrey. In her spare time she does not watch soaps!

Dedication

To Kevin the kidney for his part in my family

Foreword

I first became interested in diabetes in 1993, when an audit of diabetes in my practice showed that care was, shall we say, 'suboptimal'. It was at this time that Mary MacKinnon's book first appeared on the bookshelves. *Providing Diabetes Care in General Practice* rapidly became reference, resource, tool, bible.

Some years later, I had the good fortune to work with Mary on a number of projects, even spouting Shakespeare at her inaugural Mary MacKinnon lecture! I found that her lucid writing style was underpinned by an immensely practical approach, a touching compassion and an unerring sense of humour.

The task of updating, and bringing to an eager public, the fifth edition of her book is unenviable. How can you preserve the underlying structure and principles of a classic text, whilst making it relevant and appealing to a new audience? Thankfully, the task fell to Gwen Hall, who although understandably daunted, responded with enthusiasm, dedication and that rare brand of common sense for which she is famed.

Diabetes care is changing. The epidemic that threatens to engulf healthcare systems has led to new therapies, new approaches and inevitably new political initiatives. These are all met head on in this edition, which is bang up to date and intensely relevant.

There is a helpful glossary, an incisive overview and clear sections on management. I personally found the chapter on 'Aspects of Culture' especially informative. The evolving field of therapeutic education is sensitively handled, and the chapter on 'New Insights' carefully guides the reader through the maze of new, and often confusing, research. The whole book is also peppered with useful patient information and is very thoroughly referenced.

All in all, there is something for everyone involved in diabetes care in this book, from the new practice nurse struggling to get to grips with a diabetes clinic, to the seasoned, world-weary GP.

Gwen Hall is to be congratulated in retaining the spirit of the original but imbuing it with her own personality. The best just got better. Treasure it.

Eugene Hughes
Chairman, Primary Care Diabetes Europe

Acknowledgements

In addition to those who assisted with previous editions of this book, I would like to thank the following for helping me in many ways with this update:

Vasso Vydelingum – for wise counsel on culture.
Maggie Cooper – for help with women's health.
Sally Wakelin-Harkett – for dipping her foot in it.
Dr Peter Evans – for relieving the pain of writing on neuropathy.
Sue Curnow and Bridget Turner of Diabetes UK – for support, patience and coffee.
Henri Mulnier – for more research data than I could imagine (and for sharing an offfice).
Dr Eugene Hughes and Dr Roger Gadsby – for general encouragement.
Dr Patricia Cremin for practical suggestions.
Rosie Walker for the final push.
All the staff at Haslemere Health Centre for support, encouragement and putting up with me for 19 years.

. . . and of course Mary MacKinnon, for getting me into all this.

Dear Gwen,

Thank you for taking on the 5th Edition of *Providing Diabetes Care in General Practice*. The first edition was published in 1993 and although there have been many changes in the Health Service and in the world of diabetes over the last thirteen years, the standards for first class diabetes care that you and I believe in, have not changed.

This book is about translating theory into clinical practice for the primary care team with the aim of enabling practice nurses, general practitioners and others to care for and help those who live with diabetes to look after themselves.

Gwen, you have been in my sights to update my book for a very long time! You have many years of experience of providing diabetes care in general practice, you 'practise what you preach' and you preach so well! You write concisely and with eloquence. Most of all, you uphold the philosophy of the person with diabetes and the family to be central to the care you give.

My grateful thanks to you for all the effort you have put in to the 5th Edition. I hope you have enjoyed it!

With every good wish,

Mary

Dear Mary,

How could I not be honoured to be asked to take on your book? You have been my guide, inspiration and mentor these many years. I wonder if you remember, as I do, your telephone call to me when the 1st edition came out.

There I was, oblivious to the demands of having to think up good ideas for diabetes management because someone called Mary MacKinnon had written the definitive book for me. This book not only gave me the background to diabetes, it also provided me with the tools to do the job.

I was then a practice nurse enjoying the challenge of general practice. I knew nothing of the people who were influencing changes to diabetes care such as yourself but I had written some short articles for *Practice Nurse* journal. I thought then, as now, that this Mary MacKinnon must be a very clever person to write so well. I thought I would put pen to paper and tell her so. I had the pen in my hand. That was when you rang. Well, I nearly dropped the phone in my surprise. Probably not as surprised as you when I agreed to do what you asked without waiting to hear what it was! Do you know, I still cannot remember what you wanted but I knew that the author of THAT book would not ask me to become involved in anything unworthy of my time. Little did I know that this gave you carte blanche to involve me in all sorts of things ever since.... And for that, I thank you hugely. Life has been all the more interesting for it.

Thank you Mary, I have enjoyed updating your book. I feel as though I have been entrusted with a precious child – I hope I nurture it in your best traditions. I value your faith in my abilities but, more than that, I truly value your friendship and hope that I have done justice to your work.

If not – you know where I live!

Keep up the good work and keep in touch.

Kindest regards,

[signature]

Introduction

I take on this book with some trepidation. It has been my 'bible' of primary diabetes care since 1993 when I first appreciated Mary MacKinnon's wisdom not only in recognising my plight in providing diabetes care, but also in giving me the tools to do the job. This book has formed the backbone of the care I aspire to give.

But changes are afoot in diabetes care – and with them a change in the author of this book. Readers of previous editions will recognise much of the common sense contained herein: Mary's text that is still relevant today is kept while changes affecting the provision of diabetes care have been incorporated into the original format of the book. The Internet has opened up the availability of information to all, and websites and online references have become a feature of everyday life for primary care teams and patients alike. This book, whilst not attempting to be a reference book, now provides links to online evidence and guidance from a variety of reputable sources, as well as references to major publications.

New chapters on the General Medical Services (GMS) Contract and nurse prescribing reflect the gradual shift of care from specialist services to general practice. Changes are affecting the way in which primary care teams work. More and more emphasis is on 'putting the patient at the centre of care'. The proof is there that this is the way to achieve improvements in health (Department of Health, *Supporting People with Long Term Conditions to Self Care. A Guide to Developing Local Strategies and Good Practice*, London, DoH, 2006). Yet people with diabetes and their carers involved in an online forum set up by the All-Party Parliamentary Group for Diabetes (2005) quite strongly expressed their views that this was happening more in written guidance than in actuality. The purpose of this book is to provide health professionals, and increasingly other carers, with a practical approach to making this happen.

The text is set out in three sections:

Part 1: Diabetes – an overview. This sets the scene and includes the roles and educational needs of the primary care team in providing care that is centred around patients and their carers.

Part 2: Providing diabetes care. This describes how to provide a systematic service for people with diabetes and new ways of working to achieve success.

Part 3: About diabetes. This provides further information about the metabolic syndrome, diabetes and complications of diabetes.

Further helpful information for people with diabetes, carers and members of the primary care team can be found in the Appendices, and an extensive index is available to locate specific topics. The quotations opening the chapters all come from Audit Commisssion (*Testing Times*, London, Audit Commisssion, 2000).

I hope you enjoy reading this book as much as I have enjoyed the challenge of updating it.

Part I

Diabetes: an overview

1   Diabetes mellitus in the United Kingdom

Questions this chapter will help you answer

- What is the prevalence of diabetes in the UK?
- Which ethnic groups are more affected?
- How is diabetes care organised in the UK?
- What role do specialists outside the practice play?
- How does Diabetes UK help?

> *... few professionals in the field doubt that effective prevention, management and early detection of problems is cost-effective in the long run.*
>
> Audit Commission (2000)

Physically active people have a 20–30% reduced risk of premature death and up to a 50% reduced risk of major chronic disease such as coronary heart disease, stroke, diabetes and cancer.

Prevalence and incidence

The prevalence of diabetes in the UK (Figure 1.1) suggested by most authorities is now well over 3%, and undiagnosed diabetes existing in the population may account for a further 2%. The prevalence of diabetes is considerably increased in certain ethnic groups (South Asians, i.e. Asians from the Indian subcontinent, and those of African/Caribbean descent) and is higher in the older age range of all groups. Over the age of 75 years, this figure may increase to as much as 10% of the population. The increase in prevalence of diabetes in the UK population relating to age is shown in Figure 1.2.

Figures available for the prevalence of diabetes in children and young people show that this condition has become more common over the

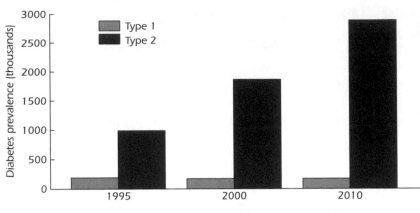

Figure 1.1 Prevalence of diabetes in the UK
(Data from Amos et al, Diabetes Med 1997 14 [Suppl. 5], S1–S85)

past 20 years and that the increase is mainly in social classes I and II. The prevalence of type 1 (previously known as insulin-dependent) diabetes in people under the age of 20 years is 0.14% (1.4 per 1000), which means that there are probably more than 20 000 young people with diabetes in the UK. There is a rising trend in the incidence of diabetes in this age group.

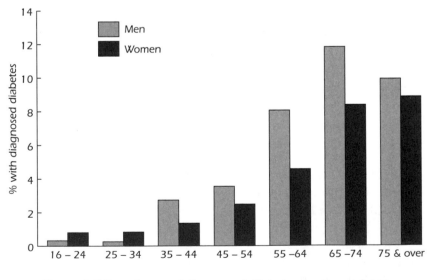

Figure 1.2 Prevalence of diagnosed diabetes by sex and age, England, 2003
(From Joint Health Surveys Unit, 2004, with permission)

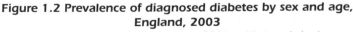

People with type 2 (previously known as non-insulin-dependent) diabetes may remain undiagnosed for months or years. The condition may be recognised only by coincidence, after routine screening (e.g. at a medical examination, a routine outpatient visit or before surgery) or during a hospital admission.

Type 2 diabetes is thought of as a condition of the older person. However, in the age range 15–44 years, almost 100 000 people in the UK have type 2 diabetes. This is due to changes in lifestyle with decreasing activity and increasing waistlines. If a woman has a waistline of over 35 inches (89 cm), she is at risk of type 2 diabetes. For a man, the corresponding figure is 40 inches (102 cm).

Type 2 diabetes is said to be a time bomb in terms of coronary heart disease. People are living longer, becoming less active and eating a diet higher in saturated fat than in previous decades. Men with type 2 diabetes have a 2–4 times greater annual risk of coronary heart disease, whereas women fare even less well, especially after the menopause when they lose their cardioprotection. This gives them a 3–5 times increased risk. Guidelines to assess the 10-year risk have been published in the journal *Heart* (Wood et al, 1998), but this has largely been superseded by the Joint British Societies (2005) guidance on the prevention of cardiovascular disease in clinical practice, which considers that all people with diabetes should be treated as though they have already suffered a coronary event (see Chapter 24).

Type 2 diabetes is only one part of the metabolic syndrome of dyslipidaemia, hypertension and obesity. All of these need tackling if we are to avoid an escalation in mortality through diabetes. By the time they are diagnosed with type 2 diabetes, 50% of people have evidence of complications (Diabetes UK, 2004).

In the UK, there are over 2 million adults with known diabetes; most of these (75–90%) have type 2 diabetes mellitus. It is estimated that there are another million people with undiagnosed diabetes in the UK.

Type 2 diabetes is associated with insulin resistance (see Chapter 7).

Ethnic variations

In contrast to the 3% prevalence of diabetes in the general population, the condition affects about 20% of the South Asian community and 17% of the African/Caribbean community (Table 1.1). As in the general population, the prevalence rises with age, and significant increases are seen in older people of certain ethnic groups. Both these populations are more at risk of cardiovascular disease.

The consequences of diabetes: microvascular complications

These include retinopathy, nephropathy, neuropathy and peripheral vascular disease.

Retinopathy

Damage to the eye is caused when the blood vessels in the retina become blocked or leaky, or grow haphazardly. This may not affect the eyesight

Age	16–34 years (%)	35–54 years (%)	55 years and over (%)	All ages (%)
Table 1.1 Prevalence of diagnosed diabetes by sex and ethnic group in England, 1999				
Men				
Bangladeshi	19.0	2.4	10.6	30.6
Black Caribbean	8.3	1.9	3.2	17.6
Chinese	4.8	–	2.2	16.1
Indian	9.8	0.7	8.0	19.2
Irish	4.5	1.6	0.8	11.8
Pakistani	17.9	0.8	9.6	39.0
General population	3.3	0.5	2.2	6.9
Women				
Bangladeshi	14.6	0.4	12.1	26.0
Black Caribbean	10.5	0.4	3.9	25.7
Chinese	5.3	1.6	0.7	11.8
Indian	7.2	0.6	4.4	15.3
Irish	2.6	–	1.9	5.9
Pakistani	14.0	1.1	7.4	28.3
General population	2.5	1.3	3.4	5.3

Data from the 1999 Health Survey for England (2001)

until it has become advanced, and only early screening will pick up potential problems in time to save the individual's sight.

A key target of the National Service Framework for Diabetes (Department of Health, 2001) is that, by 2006, a minimum of 80% of people with diabetes are to be offered screening for the early detection and treatment of diabetic retinopathy, rising to 100% by the end of 2007. A position statement from Diabetes UK (2005) suggests, however, that this target is unlikely to be met in many areas. Funding has been made available for digital cameras, and a quality assurance scheme has to be in place to ensure an effective service.

- Diabetes is the leading cause of blindness in people of working age in the UK (Kohner et al, 1996).

- People with diabetes are up to 20 times more likely to go blind than people without diabetes (Hamilton et al, 1996).

- Treatment can prevent blindness in 90% of those at risk if applied early and adequately (Department of Health/British Diabetic Association, 1995).

- Twenty years after diagnosis, nearly all people with type 1 diabetes will have some form of retinopathy (Campbell and Lebowitz, 1996). Blindness is more prevalent in people who have type 1 diabetes than in the population at large (Krentz, 2000).

- Twenty years after diagnosis, 60% of those with type 2 diabetes will have some degree of retinopathy (Department of Health/British Diabetic Association, 1995).

Appropriate interventions including lifestyle changes and the control of blood pressure and blood glucose, as well as specific treatment through eye clinics, may prevent 60–70% of individuals with maculopathy and 90% of those with proliferative retinopathy going blind in at least one eye. The cost of introducing effective eye screening is high, but the National Screening Committee accepts that the cost in terms of disability and social care, not to mention individual suffering, outweighs this. Lack of screening may also result in costly compensation claims. Scotland introduced a national eye screening programme in 2002.

Nephropathy

Nephropathy is a major cause of kidney failure and death, yet Diabetes UK found that almost half of local health services do not ensure access to jointly run diabetes and renal clinics. Nephropathy is caused by protracted poor glycaemic and blood pressure control. Good communication between renal and diabetes teams enhances care.

- Diabetic nephropathy (diabetic kidney disease) develops in about one third of people with diabetes (International Diabetes Federation, 2003).

- Diabetes is now the leading cause of end stage renal failure (Harvey, 2003).

- Approximately 20% of people with type 1 diabetes will reach end stage kidney disease (Krentz, 2000).

- The risk of kidney damage increases with the duration of diabetes. Twenty-five years after diagnosis, the risk is 40–50% for both types of diabetes (Hasslacher and Bohm, 2004).

- Approximately 1000 people in the UK go onto dialysis each year because of their diabetes (UK Renal Registry, 2002).

Neuropathy and peripheral vascular disease

Foot ulceration is at least 50 times more common in people with diabetes than in those without. If the ulceration is the result of peripheral vascular disease, amputation is often the outcome. In the UK, diabetes is the second most common cause of lower limb amputation and the most common cause of non-traumatic amputation (Department of Health, 2001).

- The rate of lower limb amputation in people with diabetes is 15 times higher than in people without diabetes (Williams and Pickup, 2004).

- 15% of foot ulcers will lead to amputation (Defronzo et al, 2004).

- 5% of, or around 90 000, people with diabetes may develop a foot ulcer in 1 year (National Institute for Health and Clinical Excellence, 2004).

- Uncontrolled studies have shown that the rate of amputation may be reduced by 40% or more through screening, education and the development of multidisciplinary diabetes foot care teams (Ross and Gadsby, 2004).

Evidence of neuropathy may be found in up to 40% of people with diabetes (30% of those in hospital studies but over 50% of patients with type 2 diabetes), causing problems for about one third of them. One of the most distressing and often hidden problems is that of male impotence: varying degrees of erectile dysfunction can affect one in two men with diabetes.

The consequences of diabetes: macrovascular complications

Heart disease and stroke

Cardiovascular disease includes coronary heart disease and stroke. It is the major contributory factor in the mortality of type 2 diabetes: 80% of people with diabetes will die from cardiovascular complications (Barnett and O'Gara, 2003).

Diabetes, hypertension and heart disease (all part of the metabolic syndrome) are the most frequent cause of stroke. As obesity and physical inactivity increase, so does the incidence of stroke – and it is affecting an increasingly younger age group.

As mentioned above, 50% of people with type 2 diabetes will have complications at diagnosis. Most of these will have evidence of cardiovascular disease as well as other problems. Over 3% of the population are diagnosed with diabetes, yet they account for between 10% and 15% of those admitted to hospital with a heart attack and 20% of those who die from one.

- People with diabetes have up to a fivefold increased risk of developing cardiovascular disease.

- Middle-aged men with diabetes are five times more likely to die of cardiovascular disease than men without diabetes (Laing et al, 1999).

- Women with diabetes are eight times more likely to die of cardiovascular disease than women without diabetes (Laing et al, 1999).

- Cardiovascular disease is rare in people with type 1 diabetes in the 30 years following diagnosis. At 40 years after diagnosis, however, cardiovascular disease accounts for 30% of deaths in this group (British Medical Association, 2004).

- People with diabetes are five times more likely to suffer heart failure (Yudkin et al, 1996).

- People with diabetes have a 2–3 times increased risk of having a stroke compared with those without the condition (Laing et al, 1999).

- African/Caribbean and South Asian men with diabetes have a 40% and 70%, respectively, higher risk of stroke than the general population (Burlace, 2001).

Life expectancy and mortality rates

It is recognised that people with diabetes die earlier than those of a similar age and sex without the condition. Death may be directly caused by diabetes (e.g. diabetic ketoacidosis or renal failure resulting from diabetes). More commonly, however, death is caused by macrovascular complications, particularly myocardial infarctions and strokes.

The National Service Framework (Department of Health, 2001) confirms that life expectancy is reduced by on average more than 20 years in type 1 diabetes and up to 10 years in type 2 diabetes. Early mortality rates are up to five times higher for people with diabetes (Kanters et al, 1999).

Type 2 diabetes is a condition that affects the least affluent of our society, and the incidence is highest in deprived areas with a high ethnic mix. The outcome in these areas is also poorer than that for people in wealthier parts of the UK.

Figures on death rates due to diabetes are not reliable as death certificates often fail to record diabetes as an underlying cause. The same is true of hospital admissions: figures are thought to be much higher than declared as diabetes is regularly left out of the reason for admission.

The World Health Organization Global Burden of Disease Project (Murray and Lopez, 1996) suggests that, in established market economies such as the UK, about five times as many deaths are indirectly attributable to diabetes as directly attributable. This would mean that there are about 35 000 deaths a year in the UK attributable to diabetes – or about 1 in 20 of all deaths.

In the UK, apart from natural causes, diabetes is in the top five leading causes of death (Yuen, 2005):

- coronary heart disease and pulmonary circulation (although it is not known whether Yuen also took diabetes into account here);

- all cancers;

- pneumonia;

- cerebrovascular disease (again, it is likely that diabetes was present in a proportion of these individuals);

- diabetes.

The two most common causes of death for people with diabetes under the age of 50 were heart attacks and kidney failure. In those aged under 20 years, ketoacidosis is the most common cause of death.

The cost of diabetes

The exact costs of diabetes are inestimable. One study (Currie et al, 1997) suggested that diabetes accounts for around 9% of the annual UK National Health Service (NHS) budget. This represents a total of approximately £5.2 billion per year.

Diabetes UK (2001) considers that the exact costs of diabetes are hard to pin down:

- *Costs linked directly to the diagnosis and management of diabetes itself,* for example the cost of inpatient and outpatient care and of insulin, tablets, syringes and blood-testing and urine-testing equipment.

- Costs related to the complications of diabetes – quantifying these is difficult because many conditions people with diabetes are at risk of, such as heart disease and stroke, are common. This makes it hard to ascertain what proportion of costs arise from diabetes alone. In addition, diabetes can complicate other unrelated medical or surgical procedures, adding to the costs of care.

- *Less tangible indirect costs* relating to wider aspects of diabetes, such as the ability to work and the quality of life.

Impact of diabetes on the individual

The cost of diabetes to the government is paralleled by its potentially devastating impact on the health of individuals in the form of complications such as heart disease, stroke, kidney disease, blindness and amputation.

The increase in the number of people with diabetes will undoubtedly increase NHS costs, but health costs to people with diabetes can be ameliorated through effective management of their condition and patient education. New, effective models of diabetes care are emerging that encourage participation and empowerment on the part of those with diabetes. They are by no means universally welcomed with open arms by those who have diabetes, but the onus of responsibility for an individual's health rests firmly with that individual – it is up to health professionals, and others, to provide people with diabetes with the education and support they need to motivate themselves in self-care.

Evidence of good practice is available that could reduce costs, for example:

- *new ways of working*: as the number of people with diabetes increases, we need to find new ways to tackle diabetes care. Examples are given by the NHS Modernisation Agency (2003);

- *a 'whole-systems' approach* involving health and social care, charitable agencies and people with diabetes in service planning;

- *adequate education* facilities for people with diabetes and their families; National Institute for Health and Clinical Excellence, Technology Appraisal No. 60 on *Structured Patient Education in Diabetes* (National Institute for Health and Clinical Excellence, 2003; Diabetes UK/Department of Health 2005) has to be implemented by primary care organisations (see Chapter 16);

- *resources and support for general practitioners* (GPs) and their teams, including new initiatives involving modern matrons and intermediate care nurses to help prevent unplanned hospital admissions (National Diabetes Support Team, 2005).

Reducing the costs of diabetes may be achieved through:

- primary prevention – targeting at-risk groups;

- the prevention of complications;

- the implementation of agreed standards of care;

- a reduction in the number of inappropriate admissions to hospital;

- an examination of the costs and benefits of the management, screening and treatment options available;

- engaging people with diabetes in self-care plans.

Effectiveness of treatment for people with diabetes

The maintenance of a near-physiological blood glucose, blood pressure and lipid levels, combined with a healthy lifestyle, reduces the risk of development of long-term complications of diabetes. The early detection and treatment of established complications can reduce morbidity and costs. For example, in retinopathy, the detection of early changes, followed by laser treatment, can prevent blindness.

Planned follow-up with screening for complications is essential. Living with diabetes involves lifestyle modification to achieve optimal control of the condition. Time spent in listening, responding to questions and providing information and support is as essential to treatment as the prescription of diet, activity and medication.

The Diabetes Control and Complications Trial showed that greater efforts to control blood glucose levels led to a reduction in risk of all the complications of diabetes (Diabetes Control and Complications Trial Research Group, 1993). The study included only those with type 1 diabetes, so these findings cannot be extrapolated to type 2 diabetes.

A further study in the UK was carried out on those with type 2 diabetes – the UK Prospective Diabetes Study (UK Prospective Diabetes Study Group,1998a, 1998b). The findings showed that a strict control of blood pressure was significant in preventing macrovascular complications, mainly coronary heart disease; glucose control was similarly effective for microvascular complications (Box 1.1).

The aims of diabetes care

The overall aims of any system of diabetes care are to facilitate diabetic self-management and control, enabling people with diabetes to make the necessary adjustments to retain a good quality of life, to reduce mortality, morbidity and hospitalisation, and to improve the early detection of complications by effective surveillance.

Box 1.1 United Kingdom Prospective Diabetes Study (UKPDS) outcomes

An intensive glucose control policy of HbA_{1c} 7.0% versus 7.9% reduces the risk of:

■ any diabetes-related end points   12%   *P*=0.030

■ microvascular end points   25%   *P*=0.010

■ myocardial infarction   16%   *P*=0.052

A tight blood pressure control policy of 144/82 mmHg versus 154/87 mmHg reduces the risk of:

■ any diabetes-related end point   24%   *P*=0.005

■ microvascular end points   37%   *P*=0.009

■ stroke   44%   *P*=0.013

HbA_{1c}, glycated haemoglobin.

How is diabetes care organised in the UK?

In 2000, the Audit Commission identified that there was considerable variation in the standard of care provided for people with diabetes. Most districts have specialist diabetes clinics, although these vary in quality. In some districts, people with diabetes are followed up in general medical clinics, but hospital and GP specialist clinics are increasingly being set up collaboratively for special problems. There may be joint clinics with obstetricians, joint renal clinics and foot clinics, including the expertise of vascular surgeons, chiropodists/podiatrists and orthotists (fitters of shoes and other appliances).

In many districts, clinics for children with diabetes are organised and run by a paediatrician with a special interest in diabetes. Out-of-hours peripheral clinics are available in some areas, providing a service for the adolescent and working populations.

Many people with diabetes regularly attend a hospital clinic with the specialist facilities that this provides. Those attending the hospital are mainly the younger population (treated with diet and insulin) and those with established complications requiring particular surveillance and treatment. Shared care, with excellent communication between primary and secondary care, is good.

Many people either may be cared for by their GP and team or receive no structured care at all. The General Medical Services contract of 2004 provided the stimulus to organise diabetes care within general practice. This system rewards practices for achieving targets and organising care rather than providing a *per capita* sum to GPs for everyone on their register (see Chapter 3).

On the whole, interested GPs and their teams are looking after people with type 2 diabetes and those with few complications. This type of diabetes has often been regarded as 'mild', but there is no such thing as mild diabetes. Over 75% of people diagnosed with diabetes will have type 2, and as many as half of these will have complications at diagnosis. In addition, for every person diagnosed there will be many more who do not know that they have it. It is vitally important to screen people with hypertension, dyslipidaemia, obesity or a strong family history of diabetes, especially in ethnic groups, for type 2 diabetes.

The organisation of diabetes care is complex and ever-changing in the life of a person with diabetes, not only from the person's own perspective, but also in terms of the multitude of relatives and professionals who may be involved in his or her care, individually or collectively.

Support, education, good communication and an understanding of the availability of appropriate care by the person with diabetes, the relatives and healthcare professionals are as important as the treatment of the condition.

The role of the specialist team

The specialist team in diabetes care has evolved over a number of years. The team includes the:

- specialist physician/paediatrician;
- diabetes specialist nurse (DSN); DSNs may be hospital or community based, or both;
- specialist dietitian;
- specialist chiropodist/podiatrist.

Good communications and liaison with other specialist teams is paramount owing to the nature of diabetes and the organs it affects. The team may be extended to include an:

- obstetrician;

- vascular surgeon;

- ophthalmologist;

- renal physician;

- psychologist;

- cardiologist;

- diabetes facilitator.

In primary care, links to community pharmacists and optometrists may be appropriate.

The team should provide the expertise (based on training and experience) for the management of care of diabetes in the hospital setting and be available as a resource for care in the community.

The specialist physician (diabetologist)

The specialist physician:

- has a specialist interest, training and experience in the management of diabetes;

- may have research interests;

- should be involved in the leadership of diabetes care in a district;

- should be a resource for medical practitioners and healthcare professionals;

- is dedicated to raising awareness of diabetes.

It is important that GPs and their teams providing diabetes care are aware of those district physicians and GPs with a specialist interest. Should problems arise, they will be quickly resolved where links have been established and communication is easy. Effective shared care aids both the medical management of diabetes and access to care by people with diabetes.

Most centres also have a paediatrician with a particular interest and training in the care of children and young people with diabetes. The paediatrician's team will consist of a nurse specialist (preferably trained to work with children) and a dietitian specialising in the needs of children. Ideally, as children move towards adulthood, a collaborative service should be available in which the paediatrician and physician caring for adults work together with appropriate teams to ensure that the transition from childhood care to adult care is as smooth as possible.

The role of community diabetologist is becoming more common, and new ways of providing specialist care are emerging.

GPs with a special interest

The number of GPs with special interests (GPwSI; generally pronounced 'gypsy') has been growing since 2003. These GPs may have specialist knowledge and skills in a variety of settings, including diabetes. Working with a specialist team, undertaking additional training and experience in the field may all contribute to the role. GPwSI services will reflect local need but might include:

- influencing and leading on the organisation and commissioning of services at a strategic level, be it primary care organisation or trust;

- assisting with the provision of training/mentoring for other health professionals locally;

- acting as a resource to other GPs to ensure appropriate referral to specialists;

- providing a specialist clinic in primary care to assess the needs of individuals with more complicated cases who may not warrant hospital referral.

The DSN

The DSN is a trained nurse with extended knowledge and skills in diabetes management as an educator, manager, researcher, communicator and innovator held responsible for his or her actions.

DSNs generally work wholly in diabetes care, either full or part time, usually as part of the specialist team but increasingly in the community through primary care organisations. Historically, their role was set up to provide help and support for people being treated with insulin, but this is now broadening to encompass more holistic care and complication management.

The DSN may be based in a hospital or community but may visit individuals in either depending on need. The nurse works with either adults or children with diabetes and their families, or with both. He or she is a resource and adviser in diabetes for other health professionals. The specialist nurse acts to educate colleagues in nursing and other disciplines in the hospital and community and, working within the diabetes care team, will provide some, if not all, of the following services:

- Working with people newly diagnosed with diabetes, particularly those with type 1 receiving insulin; this involves working with family and carers to help them understand and come to terms with the condition.

- Education for new and ongoing care for people with diabetes.

- Continuing support for and stabilisation of those new to insulin.

- Training and education on blood glucose monitoring systems and interpreting the results.

- Education and training on the recognition, prevention and treatment of hypoglycaemia.

- Advice on the recognition, prevention and treatment of hyperglycaemia (e.g. during illness), ketoacidosis and hyperosmolar non-ketotic coma.

- Changing and advising on insulin regimens or insulin injection systems.

- Training in and management of diabetic complications, including advice on screening, interpreting results, therapies and ongoing management.

- The management of special cases, for example where there is an eating disorder, dialysis or percutaneous endoscopic gastrostomy feeding.

- The prevention of foot problems (in liaison with podiatrists).

- Education on all aspects of diabetes, individually or in groups for people with diabetes and for the DSN's colleagues.

- Crisis management, in particular where there are psychological, social or family problems.

- Facilitating all aspects of diabetes care with appropriate healthcare professionals and others (e.g. teachers and employers).

- Providing the necessary expertise and materials or resources where requested or required.

- Travel advice for coping with long-haul travel, extra activity and care of equipment.

- In association with other team members, developing protocols, undertaking audit and setting standards.

DSNs have incorporated into their job description the necessary authorisation to alter insulin and medication in the treatment of diabetes. In addition, an increasing number of DSNs are trained to prescribe.

Many specialist nurses provide an out-of-hours, weekend advisory service. It is well recognised that this is valued by people with diabetes, particularly by adults and children who have recently been diagnosed, and their families and carers. A telephone call for advice may prevent an emergency situation arising.

The specialist dietitian

The particular responsibilities of the dietitian in diabetes care include:

- assessment of eating habits (for individuals and their families);
- advice on buying and cooking food;
- ensuring adequate nutrition (especially with young and elderly people);
- promoting healthy eating;
- helping people to reduce weight;
- helping people to stabilise their weight;
- meal-planning (especially regular meals);
- advice and planning for special dietary needs (e.g. for people with renal failure or who are terminally ill).

Interested dietitians are often involved in all aspects of diabetes support and education, for either individuals or groups. They may also, however, be involved in the provision of other dietetic services. In general, dietitians are hospital based, working with their colleagues and linking in with the diabetologist and nurse specialist, although they may increasingly be working with primary care organisations to provide care and education in the community. If nurses and other health professionals in primary care are providing first-line advice for people with diabetes, there should be an ongoing system of education in place for them.

The dietitian should be an important resource in the provision of training and continuing education for all those providing diabetes care in the community. More community dietitians are required to meet this need.

The specialist chiropodist/podiatrist

Within the UK NHS, each district provides a chiropody/podiatry service in community clinics and hospitals and at home for house-bound patients. Some hospitals and general practices provide chiropody within their diabetic clinics. The NHS employs only state-registered chiropodists who have trained for 3 years at one of the recognised schools. State-registered chiropodists also practise privately. Since 2003, only those who have completed the relevant training are allowed to use the title 'chiropodist' or 'podiatrist', and they must be registered with the Health Professional Council.

Chiropody/podiatry services are highly relevant for people with diabetes. Both neuropathic and ischaemic ulcers are common in people with diabetes. The chiropodist has an important role in teaching about all aspects of foot care, including advice about nail-cutting and shoes to avoid the development of foot ulcers, and about the management of existing ulcers. A specialised multidisciplinary foot clinic can halve the number of amputations carried out on patients with diabetes as long as referral to these clinics is appropriate and occurs in good time.

Most health authorities expect chiropodists/podiatrists to provide services for patients in four official priority groups:

- senior citizens;

- children attending school;

- people with a mental or physical handicap;

- pregnant women.

Surprisingly, people with diabetes are not officially recognised as a priority group, but many chiropody/podiatry services do accept the referral of people with diabetes and other high-risk groups. At present, most district health authorities do not purchase chiropody for otherwise well people between the ages of 16 and 65 years. Ideally, a range of foot problems should be officially recognised by the NHS. A more coherent policy is required, based on unmet need and its associated morbidity.

Chiropodists/podiatrists with an up-to-date knowledge of diabetes care have an important role in preventing disability in their management of diabetic foot problems. Their expertise includes:

- the assessment of foot structure and function;

- the manufacture of orthotics (insoles, padding, special shoes);

- advice on shoes and shoe-fitting;

- ongoing surveillance;
- treatment (e.g. reducing callus, nail care, debriding ulcers).

A list of state-registered chiropodists/podiatrists employed by the health authority is available in every district, in primary care organisations' headquarters or community units. Lists of private state-registered chiropodists are available in the *Yellow Pages* or online (see Appendix 4). Fees for private chiropody services vary; home visits are more costly than visits to a surgery.

Diabetes centres

The diabetes centre is a base for the specialist team and a focus for care provision and resources within the district. Its functions ideally include provision of the following:

- A register of all patients in the district. Registers are commonly practice based, and it is important that a system is in place to ensure that everyone on the register, wherever it is held, is offered an ongoing, regular, review of their diabetes.

- The appropriate organisation and a pleasant environment for effective patient education (individually or in groups) that ensures the development and achievement of agreed objectives with:
  - primary education programmes for people newly diagnosed with diabetes (and their families and carers);
  - secondary education: counselling to achieve long-term diabetes control, and the maintenance and reinforcement of any changes in behaviour;
  - support for patients in hospital.

- A communication centre to:
  - provide a reference point for patient enquiries;
  - ensure coordination between members of the diabetes team, thus enabling the formulation and implementation of agreed objectives;
  - provide integration with other hospital departments and staff in order to achieve common treatment policies;
  - help GP cooperative care schemes to achieve common goals;
  - act as a focal point for training medical and non-medical staff;
  - streamline organisation and improve cost-effectiveness.

- A comprehensive system of clinical care and evaluation that should ensure:
  - outpatient care for all new and follow-up patients;
  - effective screening and surveillance procedures for complications;
  - the availability of facilities to treat diabetic complications, and referral for non-diabetic medical problems;
  - the development, maintenance and support of GP cooperative care schemes.

Diabetes UK

Diabetes UK (formerly known as the British Diabetic Association; see Appendix 4 for contact details) is a unique patient/professional organisation and the leading charity for people with diabetes. One of the greatest strengths of the organisation lies in the partnership between professionals and those with diabetes, which is reflected in its membership. Its mission is to improve the lives of people with diabetes and work towards a future without diabetes by supporting those who live with the condition and those who work in diabetes care and research.

Since it was set up in 1934 by an individual with diabetes and a physician, Diabetes UK has always advocated integrated, patient-centred care. It provides a two-way information and support network for those working in research and clinical care, and those involved with the education of both professionals and people with diabetes.

Diabetes UK is the largest patient organisation in Europe and also has over 6000 professional members from all areas of care and research. There are numerous benefits associated with professional membership of Diabetes UK (see Appendixes 3 and 4).

Diabetes UK has four national offices and eight regional offices throughout England. There are also around 430 local Diabetes UK groups across the UK, all run voluntarily by people living with diabetes. There are also some specialist groups – for parents and young people with diabetes, self-help groups, Asian support groups and a group for the visually impaired, based in Edinburgh.

Science Information Team

The Science Information Team handles research-based queries from healthcare professionals, students and the general public.

Diabetes UK Careline

This was established in 1994 to provide information and support to people with diabetes, their families and carers, healthcare professionals and the general public. It is considered a lifeline by many of the thousands of people who call it each year. This is especially true for those who have recently been diagnosed, as they often need to share their anxieties, and benefit from receiving reassurance and assistance from dedicated professionals. (See Appendix 4 for contact details.)

Research

Diabetes UK is one of the largest funders of diabetes research in the UK, with an annual research budget of £4.5 million at the time of going to press. Diabetes UK currently funds around 150 projects throughout the UK, focusing on three areas of equal importance: care and treatment, cause and prevention, and cure. *Research Matters*, published shortly after each grant round, provides updates on research funded by the organisation. (See Appendix 4 for contact details.)

The Diabetes UK website

The Diabetes UK website (see Appendix 4) is an excellent source of information and support for both those with diabetes and healthcare professionals, the latter having a specific section dedicated on the site. This includes information on clinical audit and the various national service frameworks for diabetes, care recommendations and information on and examples of good practice in diabetes care. The examples of good practice look at a wide variety of areas including early identification, innovative care, education for those with diabetes, patient-held records, physical activity, retinal screening, user involvement and weight management.

Events for people with diabetes

Every year, Diabetes UK organises a range of events around the UK for people with diabetes, their carers and healthcare professionals. Events such as 'Living with Diabetes' and 'Diabetes for Life' days give people with diabetes and their families and carers an opportunity to find out more about their condition and learn from each other and from healthcare professionals. Care support and family events also provide a unique opportunity for people with diabetes to share and learn from each other.

The Professional Advisory Council of Diabetes UK

The organisation is advised by the UK Advisory Council (UKAC), which comprises elected representatives of the lay and professional membership. The Professional Advisory Council (PAC; see Appendix 4) is an integral part of the UKAC and contributes enormously to the operational aspects of the organisation, providing direct professional expertise and experience from those working in care and research. The members of the PAC meet regularly and also form part of the Conference Organizing Committee, responsible for the Annual Professional Conference Programme, one of the largest events for diabetes professionals in the UK.

Each member sits on one of three multidisciplinary/multisector Working Groups dedicated to Healthcare Delivery, Professional Support and Development, or Science and Research. The members of the PAC liaise and work with other professional bodies (including the Department of Health and many of the Royal Colleges) on behalf of the Diabetes UK to raise standards of knowledge, awareness and support for those working in diabetes, and to improve standards of care. The PAC Executive guides and coordinates the work of the PAC and is responsible for promoting the interests and concerns of the professional membership. Elections to the PAC take place every year.

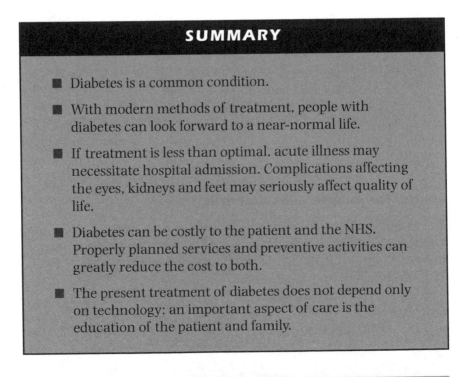

SUMMARY

- Diabetes is a common condition.

- With modern methods of treatment, people with diabetes can look forward to a near-normal life.

- If treatment is less than optimal, acute illness may necessitate hospital admission. Complications affecting the eyes, kidneys and feet may seriously affect quality of life.

- Diabetes can be costly to the patient and the NHS. Properly planned services and preventive activities can greatly reduce the cost to both.

- The present treatment of diabetes does not depend only on technology: an important aspect of care is the education of the patient and family.

References

Audit Commission (2000). *Testing Times: A Review of Diabetes Services in England and Wales*. London: Audit Commission

Barnett A (ed.) (1998). *The Insulin Treatment of Diabetes: A Practical Guide*. London: EMAP Healthcare.

Barnett AH, O'Gara MG (2003). *Diabetes and the Heart*. Oxford: Churchill Livingstone.

British Medical Association Board of Science and Education (2004). Diabetes Mellitus: An Update for Healthcare Professionals. www.bma.org.uk.

Burlace S (2001). Reducing stroke risk in ethnic minorities. *Best Practice* 18 July: 14–15.

Campbell N, Lebovitz H (1996). *Diabetes Mellitus Fast Facts*. Oxford: Health Press.

Currie CJ, Draus D, Morgan CL et al (1997). NHS acute sector expenditure for diabetes: the present, future, and excess in-patient cost of care. *Diabetic Medicine* **14**: 686–692.

Defronzo RA, Ferrannini E, Keen H, Zimmet P (eds) (2004). *International Textbook of diabetes*, 3rd edn. Chichester: John Wiley & Sons.

Department of Health (2001). *National Service Framework for Diabetes: Standards*. London: DoH.

Department of Health/British Diabetic Association (1995). *St Vincent Joint Task Force for Diabetes (Visual Impairment Subgroup)*. London: British Diabetic Association (now Diabetes UK).

Diabetes Control and Complications Trial (DCCT) Research Group (1993). The effect of intensive treatment of diabetes on the development and progression of long-term complications in insulin-dependent diabetes mellitus. *New England Journal of Medicine* **329**: 977–986.

Diabetes UK (2001). Diabetes: Cost and Implications. Factsheet No. 3. London: Diabetes UK.

Diabetes UK (2004). *Diabetes in the UK 2004. A Report from Diabetes UK*. London: Diabetes UK.

Diabetes UK (2005) *Position Statement on Eye Screening*. London: Diabetes UK.

Diabetes UK/Department of Health (2005). *Structured Patient Education in Diabetes. Report from the Patient Education Working Group*. London: Diabetes UK.

Hamilton AMP, Polkinghorne P, Ulbig M (1996). *Management of Diabetic Retinopathy*. London: BMJ Books.

Harvey JN (2003). Trends in the prevalence of diabetic nephropathy in type 1 and type 2 diabetes. *Nephrology and Hypertension* **12**: 317–322.

Hasslacher C, Bohm S (2004). *Diabetes and the Kidney*. Chichester: John Wiley & Sons.

International Diabetes Federation (2003). Diabetes and Kidney Disease: Time To Act. www.idf.org.

Joint British Societies (2005). Guidelines on prevention of cardiovascular disease in clinical practice. *Heart* **91**: 1–52.

Joint Health Surveys Unit (2004). *Health Survey for England 2003*. London: Stationery Office.

Kanters SD, Banga JD, Stolk RP, Algra A (1999). Incidence and determinants of mortality and cardiovascular events in diabetes mellitus: a meta analysis. *Vascular Medicine* **4**: 67–75.

Kohner E, Allwinkle J, Andrews J et al (1996). Report of the Visual Handicap Group. *Diabetic Medicine* **13** (Suppl. 4): S13–S26.

Krentz AJ (2000). *Churchill's Pocketbook of Diabetes*. Oxford: Churchill Livingstone.

Laing SP, Swerdlow AJ, Slater SD et al (1999). The British Diabetic Cohort Study. II. Cause-specific mortality in patients with insulin treated diabetes mellitus. *Diabetic Medicine* **16**: 466–471.

Murray CJL, Lopez A (1996). *The Global Burden of Disease*. Geneva: World Health Organization.

National Diabetes Support Team (2005). *Working Together To Reduce Length of Stay for People with Diabetes*. Factsheet No. 10. London: NDST.

National Institute for Health and Clinical Excellence (2003). *Guidance on the Use of Patient-education Models for Diabetes*. Technology Appraisal No. 60. London: DoH.

National Institute for Health and Clinical Excellence (2004). *NICE Guideline: Type 2 diabetes: Prevention and Management of Foot Problems*. London: NICE.

NHS Modernisation Agency (2003). *Workforce Matters: A Guide to Role Redesign in Diabetes Care*. London: Department of Health.

Ross S, Gadsby R (2004). *Diabetes and Related Disorders*. London: Elsevier.

UK Prospective Diabetes Study Group (1998a). Tight blood pressure control and risk of macrovascular and microvascular complications in type 2 diabetes (UKPDS 38). *British Medical Journal* **317**: 703–713.

UK Prospective Diabetes Study Group (1998b). Intensive blood-glucose control with sulphonylureas or insulin compared with conventional treatment and risk of complications in patients with type 2 diabetes (UKPDS 33). *Lancet* **352**: 837–853.

UK Renal Registry (2002). UK Renal Registry Report. www.renalreg.com.

Williams B, Poulter NR, Brown MJ et al (2004) Guidelines for management of hypertension: report of the fourth working party of the British Hypertension Society. 2004 – BHS IV. *Journal of Human Hypertension* **18**: 139–185.

Williams G, Pickup JC (2004). *Handbook of Diabetes*, 3rd edn. Oxford: Blackwell Publishing.

Wood D, Durrington P, Poulter N et al (1998). Joint British Recommendations on Prevention of Coronary Heart Disease in Clinical Practice. *Heart* **80** (Suppl. II): S1–S29.

World Health Organization (1985). *Diabetes Mellitus: Report of a WHO Study Group*. WHO Technical Report Series No. 727. Geneva: WHO.

Yudkin JS, Blauth C, Drury P et al (1996). Prevention and management of cardiovascular disease in patients with diabetes mellitus: an evidence base. *Diabetic Medicine* **13** (Suppl. 4): S101–S121.

Yuen P (2005). *The Compendium of Health Statistics*, 16th edn, 2004–2005. London: Office of Health and Economics.

Further reading

Department of Health (2001). *National Service Framework (NSF) for Older People*. London: DoH.

Department of Health/Royal College of General Practitioners (2003) *Guidelines for the Appointment of General Practitioners with Special Interests in the Delivery of Clinical Services. Diabetes*. London: Department of Health.

Diabetes UK (1998). *Diabetes Centres in the UK. Report*. London: Diabetes UK.

Diabetes UK (2001). *Diabetes UK Report: Missing Millions*. London: Diabetes UK.

Kings Fund (1996). *Counting the Cost: The Real Impact of Non-insulin-dependent Diabetes*. London: King's Fund/British Diabetic Association.

National Institute for Health and Clinical Excellence publications; available at www.nice.org.uk.

- Management of Type 2 Diabetes. *Management of Blood Pressure and Blood Lipids*. Inherited Guideline H. London: NICE; 2002.

- *Management of Type 2 Diabetes. Management of Blood Glucose*. Inherited Guideline G. London: NICE; 2002.

- *Management of Type 2 Diabetes. Renal Disease – Prevention and Early Management*. Inherited Guideline F. London: NICE; 2002.

- *Management of Type 2 Diabetes. Retinopathy – Screening and Early Management*. Inherited Guideline E. London: DoH; 2002.

United Kingdom Prospective Diabetes Study publications:

- Risk factors for coronary artery disease in non-insulin dependent diabetes mellitus (UKPDS 23). *British Medical Journal* 1998; **41**: 823–828.

- Effect of intensive blood-glucose control with metformin on complications in overweight patients with type 2 diabetes (UKPDS 34). UK Prospective Diabetes Study (UKPDS) Group. *British Medical Journal* 2000; **321**: 405–412.

- Association of systolic blood pressure with macrovascular and microvascular complications of type 2 diabetes: prospective observational study (UKPDS 39). *British Medical Journal* 1998; **317**: 713–720.

2 Responsibilities of those involved in the provision of diabetes care

Questions this chapter will help you answer

- Who are the key members of my primary care diabetes team and how do I interact with them?

- Is my diabetes service accessible to all? Are systems in place to ensure that disadvantaged groups receive as good a service as others?

- Are people with diabetes fully engaged in planning the service and in structured education? Are patients learning rather than being told?

- Do I provide a local contact number for people with diabetes if they want advice that does not warrant a clinic visit?

- Do I make effective use of non-clinical staff (receptionists, clerical staff, healthcare assistants) in organising the best possible care for my patients?

> *... diabetes is an area of significant and growing spend for the NHS.*
>
> Audit Commission (2000)

The general practitioner

The general practitioner (GP) takes overall clinical responsibility for the provision of care. In addition, the GP, as an employer, is bound by the code of conduct of the General Medical Council. In employing practice nurses, doctors 'must be satisfied that the person to whom they delegate duties is competent to carry out such treatments and procedures'.

The GP's role will depend largely on the training and development of other members of the practice diabetes care team. At best, the GP will be the leader of a team improving their service to people with diabetes through integrated care in which no one slips through the net. The General Medical Services (GMS) contract (Department of Health, 2003a), has encouraged this role through its Quality and Outcomes Framework, which rewards practices for achieving clinical standards. In this case, points literally do mean prizes. Funding is based on achieving set targets. Many of the diabetes standards can be attained by other members of the team. Proposed benefits are shown in Box 2.1.

Box 2.1 Proposed benefits of the quality framework (NHS Employers)

GPs and their practice staff will be resourced to improve the quality of care they provide, and fully rewarded for providing better services to patients.

The patient experience will be put at the heart of primary care with practices rewarded for responding to patient feedback, creating real incentives for improvement.

PCOs will have clear national standards enabling them to work alongside practices in improving the quality of primary care services.

The framework will ensure that excellent management of a wide range of chronic diseases becomes the norm in primary care.

PCO, primary care organisation.

In this new contract, adopted throughout the UK in April 2004 (available via the British Medical Association website; see Appendix 4), funding is provided on the basis of the costs of delivering essential and additional services. Practices have the discretion to decide the staffing complement needed to deliver these services within the amount of money that they have been allocated. Although the GP remains the key member of the team, others may provide the routine, day-to-day, care (see Chapter 3).

The GP's role and responsibilities in diabetes care include:

- providing appropriate medical services;

- ensuring that a full medical review and laboratory/other tests are carried out after diagnosis for all people with diabetes on the practice register;

- instituting an initial programme of treatment, support,

education and surveillance after diagnosis, and at annual review, with the practice and community nurse and others, as appropriate for all people with diabetes on the practice register;

- abiding by locally agreed criteria for referral, ensuring that referrals to specialist teams or other agencies are timely and appropriate;

- in association with other members of the primary care team, ensuring that good communication exists between all parties involved, both verbally and in writing;

- ensuring that other medical problems are taken into account in relation to diabetes management, including addressing those at risk, for example those who are obese or smoke;

- together with the practice nurse, community nurse and members of the team, enabling people with diabetes (and their families and carers) to be informed and supported sufficiently to empower them to control their own diabetes health and to lead as healthy a life as possible.

The practice nurse and community (district) nurse

Practice nurses and community nurses should combine their skills to provide care to all people with diabetes whether or not they are able to attend the practice. The practice and community nurses are the key to good diabetes care, and are often the main point of communication for the practice diabetes team. They are professionally accountable for any nursing service provided, as laid down by the Nursing and Midwifery Council. With a specialist subject, such as diabetes, where particular knowledge (further to that gained in preregistration training and/or acquired only in hospital care or outside a general practice setting) is necessary, it is important that the Nursing and Midwifery Council Code of Professional Conduct (2004) is given particular consideration (Box 2.2).

The role of the *practice nurse* (Figure 2.1) has undoubtedly changed over the years in response to changes in healthcare brought about by the increase in funding after the 1990 GP contract, fundholding and the latest GMS contract. Practice-based commissioning is likely to have an effect, but it is too soon to tell what this will be. Many practice nurses have a coordinating role on top of their traditional clinical element. The word 'linchpin' is often used to describe the role nowadays in general practice.

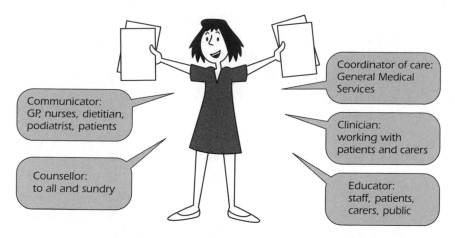

Figure 2.1 The role of the practice nurse

Coordinator of care:
General Medical
Services

Communicator:
GP, nurses, dietitian,
podiatrist, patients

Clinician:
working with
patients and carers

Counsellor:
to all and sundry

Educator:
staff, patients,
carers, public

The *community (district) nurse* may have a role similar to that of the practice nurse, albeit providing diabetes care in settings outside the practice. Community nurses were traditionally employed by primary care organisations but may now be employed in new ways through practice-based commissioning or other organisations. Close links with community diabetes specialist nurses and/or facilitators (or with specialist hospital teams if no community diabetes specialist nurse is available) will be invaluable here to provide care to those with multiple long-term conditions or requiring assistance with medication, including insulin delivery and monitoring.

Working with patients and carers

In the past, patients were recipients of care. Nowadays they are encouraged to be active participants in their own care. This is fostered through the NHS Plan, putting the patient at the centre of care, the National Service Frameworks (NSF) (Department of Health, 2003b) encouraging 'empowerment', patient structured education programmes such as DAFNE (Dose Adjustment for Normal Eating, for type 1 diabetes) and DESMOND (Diabetes Education and Self Management for Ongoing and Newly Diagnosed, for type 2 diabetes; see Chapter 16) and the participation of people with diabetes in planning systems of care at the level of the primary care organisation.

Not all people with diabetes welcome this need to become involved. Nurses are used to treating people as individuals and tailoring care to their needs. This is the true part of the caring role of the nurse and must not be forgotten in the rush to achieve targets and complete records, which the person with diabetes may not see as a priority.

Box 2.2 Extracts from the Nursing and Midwifery Council Code of Professional Conduct: standards for conduct, performance and ethics

As a registered nurse, midwife or specialist community public health nurse, you are personally accountable for your practice. In caring for patients and clients, you must:

- respect the patient or client as an individual
- obtain consent before you give any treatment or care
- protect confidential information
- co-operate with others in the team
- maintain your professional knowledge and competence
- be trustworthy
- act to identify and minimise risk to patients and clients.

You are personally accountable for your practice. This means that you are answerable for your actions and omissions, regardless of advice or directions from another professional.

You may be expected to delegate care delivery to others who are not registered nurses or midwives. Such delegation must not compromise existing care but must be directed to meeting the needs and serving the interests of patients and clients. You remain accountable for the appropriateness of the delegation, for ensuring that the person who does the work is able to do it and that adequate supervision or support is provided.

You must keep your knowledge and skills up-to-date throughout your working life. In particular, you should take part regularly in learning activities that develop your competence and performance.

There is, however, also a need to keep the individual informed through easy-to-read literature and patient-held records, which were advocated in the NSF of 2003. Nurses must thus hone their skills in listening, supporting, advising and teaching/explaining. They must also develop systems for communicating with patients outside normal clinic hours. The NSF outlined the need for a 'local contact'. This need not be out of hours, but if individuals with diabetes have a query, they should know whom to contact and believe that someone will respond within a reasonable length of time. Do you have these systems in place?

Coordinator of care/communicator

You have only to look at the GMS Quality and Outcomes Framework (see Chapter 3) to understand that the clinical indicators are well within the province of nurses involved in providing and coordinating diabetes care – but there is a need for practice nurses, community nurses and others to work together and communicate effectively to put this into practice in order to improve care rather than purely meet targets. Equality of care for all people with diabetes means that the housebound, the elderly, those with learning difficulties and those who speak a different language should not be missed out. Nurses, regardless of their title, can work together to ensure that best practice reaches all – and isn't that what nursing is all about?

Educator/counsellor

If people with diabetes and their carers are to take an increasing role in looking after their own health, by being empowered, they need the tools to do the job. Education has traditionally been provided to patients during the practice clinic or one-to-one nurse consultation. As the number of people with diabetes increases, new ways of providing education are also emerging. Group sessions, such as DAFNE, DESMOND and X-PERT (see Chapter 16), are becoming more common, and self-support groups, for instance Diabetes UK and the Expert Patient Programme (see Appendix 4 for the website address), are being promoted. The National Institute for Health and Clinical Excellence has published guidance for England and Wales, which can be applied elsewhere (Box 2.3).

The NSFs put great stress on the need for psychological support for people with diabetes. In a survey of patients' views, the Audit Commission (2000) found that people with diabetes welcomed continuity of staff in primary care. Nurses build on this and foster trusting relationships with patients that are valued. Psychological support may be required at a level that cannot be provided by the GP or primary care nurses. It is important that the need for psychological healthcare is recognised and that referrals are sensitively handled.

Nurse prescribing

Nurses who have successfully completed a course can now prescribe from the *British National Formulary* within their sphere of competency. In reality, this means that a skilled nurse can prescribe oral hypoglycaemic agents, antihypertensive therapy, statins and insulin if, having considered the Professional Code of Conduct (above; Nursing and

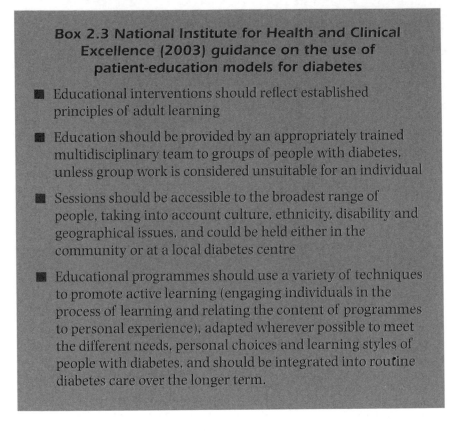

Box 2.3 National Institute for Health and Clinical Excellence (2003) guidance on the use of patient-education models for diabetes

- Educational interventions should reflect established principles of adult learning

- Education should be provided by an appropriately trained multidisciplinary team to groups of people with diabetes, unless group work is considered unsuitable for an individual

- Sessions should be accessible to the broadest range of people, taking into account culture, ethnicity, disability and geographical issues, and could be held either in the community or at a local diabetes centre

- Educational programmes should use a variety of techniques to promote active learning (engaging individuals in the process of learning and relating the content of programmes to personal experience), adapted wherever possible to meet the different needs, personal choices and learning styles of people with diabetes, and should be integrated into routine diabetes care over the longer term.

Midwifery Council, 2004), he or she feels competent to do so. This will reduce the need for the patient to make extra visits to the doctor in order to get a prescription, and will enable nurses to take on a greater role in the provision and monitoring of diabetes care (see Chapter 9 for further information).

The team approach to integrated diabetes care

Diabetes is a condition requiring care from a mix of different people; the GP, nurses, educators, dietitians, podiatrists and others may all play their part. The importance of working as a team and putting into place effective communication systems cannot be stressed enough. The Audit Commission survey (2000) showed that people with diabetes appreciated a consistent message from those who provided their care – that and seeing the same health professional at each visit. The latter is generally easy to arrange in primary care, but health professionals who work together, train together and communicate well will prevent a duplication of visits for patients and a neglect of those who slip through the net. Protecting traditional roles is not an option we can afford, and teams need to decide who are the best people to carry out different roles and support them in their work.

New ways of working in primary care diabetes

New ways of working are appearing that are altering the traditional role of nurses in primary care. Technicians and care assistants are increasing in number and becoming integral members of the diabetes team. This is sometimes seen as threatening to nurses, but the number of people with diabetes is increasing rapidly, and new ways of providing care must be considered and adapted to suit local need. The NHS Modernisation Agency (2002) has produced a useful document on redesigning roles.

Healthcare assistants and technicians

There is a place for skill mix in diabetes care. The increasing number of people with diabetes, particularly type 2 diabetes, is placing a heavy burden on front-line staff. New ways of working allow healthcare assistants to take over many of the routine tasks of diabetes care: weight measurement, urine testing, stock-taking and ordering, for example. They may assist with call and recall systems to ensure that everyone with diabetes is offered the same level of care. Technicians may take responsibility for quality assurance of blood glucose meters throughout the practice. How healthcare assistants fit into the diabetes primary care team is a local decision, and areas of good practice are emerging as roles increase.

The community pharmacist

The community pharmacy contract (2004) for England and Wales (Pharmaceutical Services Negotiating Committee, 2004), encourages a greater involvement of community pharmacists in health promotion and the management of long-term conditions. This makes admirable sense as many patients with type 2 diabetes have co-morbidities and are taking multiple medicines.

■ Pharmacists can provide expert advice to the primary care team on the management of medicines.

- Community pharmacists will be able to undertake a review of patients' medication (a medicines use review) and intervene if appropriate (prescription intervention), in agreement with local service providers.

- Community pharmacists are already working on repeat prescribing, allowing patients easy access to repeat medication without the need to visit their GP.

- Through the ability to prescribe, community pharmacists who have successfully completed the training course will be able to prescribe directly.

Funding issues are being addressed, but this demonstrates another new way of working involving healthcare professionals who have not historically been included in the primary care team and who are ideally placed to advise on medicine use.

The new contract is made up of three different service levels:

- *essential services*: provided by all contractors;

- *advanced services*: which can be provided by all contractors once accreditation requirements have been met;

- *enhanced services*: commissioned locally by primary care organisations in response to the needs of the local population.

Community pharmacists may supply a variety of services for people with diabetes. They may:

- offer advice after consultation;

- dispense prescriptions;

- provide supplies (blood glucose meters, hypoglycaemia treatments and foot care products) for sale;

- operate a service for the disposal of 'sharps';

- provide facilities for customers to weigh themselves;

- liaise with other community pharmacists, the primary care team and secondary care services;

- deliver prescriptions to the home;

- provide out-of-hours/emergency pharmacy services;

- advise on drugs, including doses, timing, routes of administration, side effects, interactions and disposal.

The community link worker

Healthcare for specific ethnic populations, who may have language, cultural and other personal barriers to overcome, will be improved where suitably trained link workers are included in the team and are available when needed. Language Line is a translation service that can cope with telephone or written queries. Some organisations subscribe to Language Line, the cost depending on frequency of use. More information can be found on their website (see Appendix 4). Diabetes UK Careline also offers a translation service.

Receptionists, clerical staff and practice managers

Administrative staff in a practice have increasing responsibilities. Most important are those in contact every day with patients, relatives and visitors to the practice, either in person or by telephone. Administrative staff are in a unique position in the identification of the diabetic population with their knowledge of those attending the practice, as receivers of information and in the organisation of prescriptions. An accurate input of information on demography, care provision, treatment changes and other data to computer systems is vital in the audit of diabetes care and in the assessment of needs for the future.

Receptionists are definitely in the 'front line'. Their attitude, knowledge and understanding of the problems of people telephoning or attending the practice may have a bearing on whether help is sought when needed.

Clerical staff also have an important part to play in the secretarial and administrative aspects of healthcare – particularly where the computerisation of prescriptions, information, registers and recall systems has been implemented.

In small practices, the staff may know the patients well and readily identify those already diagnosed with diabetes and whether they are due for recall. In a large practice or a practice with several branch surgeries, there may be many part-time staff working in shifts, communications being passed from one to the other in writing. It is unlikely in this situation that the 'front line' will have as much knowledge of their diabetic population. Electronic mail and instant on-screen messages aid rapid communication and are rapidly becoming more acceptable in computerised practices.

Larger practices have for many years required the employment of a practice manager to run the business side of the practice. The practice manager has an increasing responsibility in developments related to the GMS contract or Personal Medical Services.

An understanding of the roles and responsibilities of administrative staff is important in diabetes care in general practice. Educating the practice manager, receptionists and clerical staff about diabetes, its treatment and acute problems requiring immediate access to the doctor or nurse enables them to understand the problems encountered by people with diabetes and dispels some of the fear, ignorance, mystery and 'old wives' tales' surrounding this condition.

Other members of staff

The roles of the dietitian, chiropodist (podiatrist) and optician (optometrist) are discussed in Chapters 10, 13 and 14.

Note: Not all members of the primary care team who might be involved in providing care are necessarily included here. It is also important to recognise that members of the diabetes team may be involved in primary diabetes care, bridging the gap between primary and specialist services. These may include, for example, community diabetologists, diabetes specialist nurses, facilitators, 'specialist' dietitians and chiropodists (podiatrists).

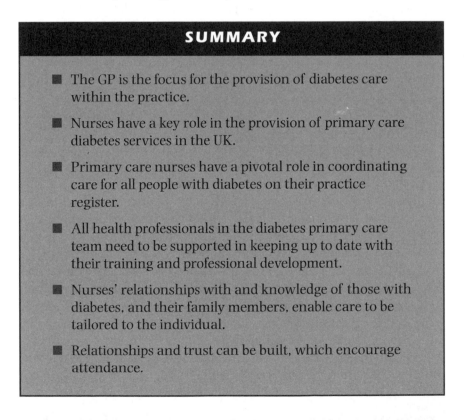

SUMMARY

■ The GP is the focus for the provision of diabetes care within the practice.

■ Nurses have a key role in the provision of primary care diabetes services in the UK.

■ Primary care nurses have a pivotal role in coordinating care for all people with diabetes on their practice register.

■ All health professionals in the diabetes primary care team need to be supported in keeping up to date with their training and professional development.

■ Nurses' relationships with and knowledge of those with diabetes, and their family members, enable care to be tailored to the individual.

■ Relationships and trust can be built, which encourage attendance.

- The practice nurse is in an ideal position to organise and coordinate a protected but flexible service in the practice setting.

- New ways of working are emerging to cope with rising demand, and nurses are in an ideal position to lead this change.

- Prescribing by nurses will prevent the duplication of visits for patients and healthcare staff alike.

- Healthcare assistants, technicians and link workers all have their place in the evolving team.

- Community pharmacists are ideally placed to become active members of the diabetes primary care team.

- Administrative and clerical staff are invaluable allies in managing data and queries on diabetes.

References

Audit Commission (2000). *Testing Times: A Review of Diabetes Services in England and Wales.* London: Audit Commission.

Department of Health (2003a). *The New General Medical Services Contract.* London: British Medical Association.

Department of Health (2003b). *National Service Framework for Diabetes: Delivery Strategy.* London: DoH.

National Institute for Health and Clinical Excellence (2003). *Guidance on the Use of Patient Education Models for Diabetes.* Technology Appraisal No. 60. London: Department of Health.

NHS Modernisation Agency (2002). *Workforce Matters. A Guide to Role Redesign in Diabetes Care.* London: Department of Health.

Nursing and Midwifery Council (2004). *Code of Professional Conduct: Standards for Conduct, Performance and Ethics.* London: Nursing and Midwifery Council.

Pharmaceutical Services Negotiating Committee (2004) New Community Pharmacy Contract. www.psnc.org.uk.

Further reading

Department of Health (2001). *National Service Framework for Diabetes: Standards.* London: DoH.

National Primary and Care Trust Development Programme (2003). *The Role of Nurses under the New GMS Contract.* London: Department of Health.

Pierce M, Agarwal G, Ridout D (2000). A survey of diabetes care in general practice in England and Wales. *British Journal of General Practice* **50**: 542–545.

3 The General Medical Services contract and practice-based commissioning

Questions this chapter will help you answer

- Does my diabetes register accurately reflect the prevalence of diabetes in my locality?

- Does my practice have an effective call and recall system that includes those not able to attend the practice?

- Data must be recorded in a unified manner with all members of the team using pre-set Read codes. Are we all recording information in the same way?

- The targets in the GMS are funding targets – not evidence-based metabolic targets. Am I using the correct targets to prevent complications?

> *There is (good) evidence in the field of diabetes about what works and a growing recognition of the serious nature of the disease.*
>
> Audit Commission (2000)

The General Medical Services (GMS) contract came into effect on 1st April 2004 and was updated in February 2006 (British Medical Association, 2006) for implementation from April that year. The contract's key principles are:

- *A practice-based contract.* The new contract is between the primary care organisation (PCO) and the general practice, as opposed to the previous contract, which was with each general practitioner (GP). This is intended to allow greater freedom to adapt care to local circumstances in conjunction with practice-based commissioning (PBC; see below).

- *Workload control.* The contract includes new proposals to help GPs manage their workload by enabling practices to transfer responsibility for providing some services – including out-of-hours care – to their PCO.

- *A focus on quality and outcomes.* The Quality and Outcomes Framework (QOF) rewards practices for meeting targets, many of which are clinical (see below). Practices can set the targets they aspire to.

- *Fairer funding.* The new contract structure removes inequalities in funding associated with the previous payment for the numbers of people on lists rather than how they were cared for.

- *A wider range of services.* 'Enhanced services' will encourage the management of long-term conditions such as diabetes in primary care, continuing the shift of care from secondary care and hospital services to general practice and PCOs.

- *Maximising the contribution of practice staff.* Nurses, pharmacists, practice managers and other allied health professionals will be able to sign up as equal parties to the contract as long as they have the knowledge and skills to do so.

The original contract contained three categories of service: essential, additional and enhanced. The updated version, based on evidence from how the implementation of the original contract had worked in practice, contained some revisions:

- A review of the QOF, with several new or revised areas.

- In England, new directed enhanced services for PBC, access, information management and technology and patient choice and booking.

- In England, the introduction of a new patient experience survey.

- In Scotland, new directed enhanced services for cardiovascular disease risk database, learning disabilities, carers and cancer referral and re-badging of the 50 QOF points for access into a new directed enhanced service.

- In Wales, new directed enhanced services for access, information technology, learning disabilities and severe mental health.

- In Northern Ireland, new directed enhanced services for access and long-term chronic disease.

- In England and Wales, a new system for paying dispensing doctors and more transparent arrangements for reimbursing VAT.

The QOF framework

The QOF rewards four areas of care called domains:

1 *Clinical* – 18 long-term conditions listed in Table 3.1. (Heart failure, palliative care, dementia, depression, chronic kidney disease, atrial fibrillation, obesity and learning disabilities were added in April 2006.)

2 *Organisational* standards relating to records and information, communicating with patients, education and training, medicines management, and clinical and practice management.

3 *Additional services*, which covers cervical screening, child health surveillance, maternity services and contraceptive services.

4 *Patient experience*, based on patient surveys and the length of consultations.

Quality is assessed through an annual audit of specific indicators and points rewarded with funding if they are achieved. The clinical domain covers many of the areas traditionally managed by practice nurses.

How to gain points and improve diabetes care

Practice nurses will be key players in achieving the clinical quality indicator points that attract additional funding. But it is not all about gaining financial points – in this case points do mean prizes in terms of enhanced patient care and well-being.

The management of long-term conditions, including diabetes, is an essential service. It must be provided by all participating practices, although they can decide to provide a higher-quality service for diabetes through the QOF. This will attract additional funding.

Table 3.1 Clinical standards in the General Medical Services contract 2006/07 (data from www.bma.org.uk, accessed 2 March 2006)

Long-term condition	Number of points	Comments relating to diabetes
Asthma	45	
Atrial fibrillation	30	
Cancer	11	
Chronic kidney disease	27	Diabetes is the largest cause of chronic kidney disease
Chronic obstructive pulmonary disease (COPD)	33	
Dementia	20	
Depression	33	Up to 50% of people with diabetes may have some form of depression
Diabetes mellitus	93	
Epilepsy	15	
Heart failure	20	
Hypertension	83	Up to 70% of people with diabetes will suffer from hypertension
Hypothyroidism	7	
Learning disabilities	4	
Mental health	39	
Obesity	8	Obesity and type 2 diabetes are strongly linked and numbers are rising to epidemic proportions
Palliative care	6	
Secondary prevention of coronary heart disease	89	Around 80% of people with type 2 diabetes have coronary heart disease
Smoking indicators	68	
Stroke and transient ischaemic attack	24	Type 2 diabetes doubles or triples the risk here

The specific indicators and points available for diabetes are listed in Table 3.2. The minimum target that can be set was originally 25%, and increased to 40% from April 2006, but the majority of practices have opted for higher levels.

Table 3.2 Quality indicators for diabetes (updated 2006)

Diabetes mellitus (diabetes)		All minimum thresholds are 40%
Indicator	Points	Maximum threshold
Records		
DM 19. The practice can produce a register of all patients aged 17 years and over with diabetes mellitus, which specifies whether the patient has type 1 or type 2 diabetes	6	
Ongoing management		
DM 2. The percentage of patients with diabetes whose notes record body mass index in the previous 15 months	3	40–90%
DM 5. The percentage of diabetic patients who have a record of HbA$_{1c}$ or equivalent in the previous 15 months	3	40–90%
DM 20. The percentage of patients with diabetes in whom the last HbA$_{1c}$ is 7.5% or less (or the equivalent test/ reference range depending on the local laboratory) in the past 15 months	17	40–50%
DM 7. The percentage of patients with diabetes in whom the last HbA$_{1c}$ reading is 10% or less (or the equivalent test/reference range depending on the local laboratory) in last 15 months	11	40–90%
DM 21. The percentage of patients with diabetes who have a record of retinal screening in the previous 15 months	5	40–90%
DM 9. The percentage of patients with diabetes with a record of the presence or absence of peripheral pulses in the previous 15 months	3	40–90%
DM 10. The percentage of patients with diabetes with a record of neuropathy testing in the previous 15 months	3	40–90%
DM 11. The percentage of patients with diabetes who have a record of their blood pressure in the past 15 months	3	40–90%
DM 12. The percentage of patients with diabetes in whom the last blood pressure is 145/85 mmHg or less	18	40–60%
DM 13. The percentage of patients with diabetes who have a record of microalbuminuria testing in the previous 15 months (exception reporting for patients with proteinuria)	3	40–90%
DM 22. The percentage of patients with diabetes who have a record of estimated glomerular filtration rate (eGFR) or serum creatinine testing in the previous 15 months	3	40–90%

Table 3.2 Quality indicators for diabetes (updated 2006) cont'd

Indicator	Points	Maximum threshold
DM 15. The percentage of patients with diabetes with proteinuria or microalbuminuria who are treated with ACE inhibitors (or A2 antagonists)	3	40–80%
DM 16.The percentage of patients with diabetes who have a record of total cholesterol in the previous 15 months	3	40–90%
DM 17.The percentage of patients with diabetes whose last measured total cholesterol within previous 15 months is 5 mmol/l or less	6	40–70%
DM 18.The percentage of patients with diabetes who have had influenza immunisation in the preceding 1 September to 31 March	3	40–85%

ACE, angiotensin-converting enzyme; HbA_{1c}, glycated haemoglobin

QOF points explained

DM19 (updated from the original DM1): The practice can produce a register of all patients aged 17 years and over with diabetes mellitus, which specifies whether the patient has type 1 or type 2 diabetes

The national prevalence of diabetes is around 3.6% and rising. Areas of high ethnicity, especially in terms of those of South Asian and African/Caribbean origin, will have figures higher than this.

- Everyone on this register should be the subject of regular review through call and recall, and the practice needs to agree codes to be used to record information on computer systems.

- A flexible approach to review is important and should be tailored to the needs of the patient: it is not necessary to check all the quality indicator boxes at one visit.

- It is important to record those who are under specialist review to prevent them slipping through the net, and to consider how to involve the wider team to ensure that those unable to attend are not missed.

DM 2. The percentage of patients with diabetes whose notes record a body mass index during the previous 15 months

There is evidence linking obesity and diabetes with heart disease (Abate, 2002). Little emphasis is put on the prevention of diabetes so primary care teams should develop systems to engage patients in weight loss, for example exercise referral or Weight Watchers programmes. Extra QOF Clinical Indicator points are available for having an obesity register.

DM 3 and 4. These have been withdrawn from the diabetes section and updated in the Smoking Indicators from April 2006

DM 5. The percentage of diabetic patients who have a record of HbA_{1c} or equivalent in the previous 15 months

DM 20 (Updated April 2006 from DM6). The percentage of patients with diabetes in whom the last HbA_{1c} is 7.5% or less (or equivalent test/reference range depending on local laboratory) in the previous 15 months

DM 7. The percentage of patients with diabetes in whom the last HbA_{1c} is 10% or less (or equivalent test/reference range depending on local laboratory) in the previous 15 months

Trials (Diabetes Control and Complications Trial Research Group, 1993; Gray et al, 2002) have demonstrated that improved glycaemic control reduces the risk of the complications of diabetes or can halt their progression. Regular HbA_{1c} (glycated haemoglobin) tests are recommended, but this target does not take into account evidence advising an HbA_{1c} value of as near 6.5% as possible (Diabetes UK, 2005, Joint British Societies, 2005). The rewards do not match the possible health gains from lowering higher levels of HbA_{1c}. Home blood glucose monitoring may help here if patients know what action to take if their levels are not as expected and whom to contact.

DM 21 (Updated from April 2006 from DM8). The percentage of patients with diabetes who have a record of retinal screening in the previous 15 months

This is a key element of the National Service Framework for diabetes; 80% of patients were to be offered screening by 2006 and 100% by the following year. This will be achieved by digital camera screening using call-and-recall schemes, but it is the responsibility of those providing diabetes care to ensure that people with diabetes are offered screening now and that it is recorded. This may be by an organised scheme, through opticians/optometrists or by hospital clinics or some other local initiative. If no system exists locally, the practice should liaise with its local PCO on future developments, but they should agree how to tackle any gaps in the current service. (See Chapter 13 for further information.)

DM 9. The percentage of patients with diabetes with a record of the presence or absence of peripheral pulses in the previous 15 months

DM 10. The percentage of patients with diabetes with a record of neuropathy testing in the previous 15 months

Diabetes is a major cause of lower limb amputations, yet much could be achieved by regular foot checks (see Chapter 14 for further information). Agree referral policies with your local podiatrists and specialist team. Make sure results are recorded in an agreed format.

DM 11. The percentage of patients with diabetes who have a record of their blood pressure within the past 15 months

DM 12. The percentage of patients with diabetes in whom the last blood pressure reading is 145/85 mmHg or less

Good blood pressure control is essential for preventing coronary heart disease. Eighty per cent of people with diabetes will die from heart disease, much of which could be prevented by lifestyle changes, particularly in terms of diet, increased activity and smoking cessation, but blood pressure control plays a major role (National Institute for Health and Clinical Excellence, 2002). Current evidence suggests a target of 135/75 mmHg if control is to be beneficial in preventing complications. Many practices already provide hyper-tension clinics, and the same level of support should be given to people with diabetes.

DM 13. The percentage of patients with diabetes who have a record of microalbuminuria testing in the previous 15 months (the exception being reporting for patients with proteinuria)

DM 22 (Updated DM 14 from April 2006). The percentage of patients with diabetes who have a record of estimated glomerular filtration rate (eGFR) or serum creatinine testing in the previous 15 months

DM 15. The percentage of patients with diabetes with a diagnosis of proteinuria or microalbuminuria who are treated with ACE inhibitors (or A2 antagonists)

The early detection of small amounts of protein in the urine (microalbuminuria) and creatinine testing can lead to treatments that limit the progression of renal disease. Various systems are in place to detect microalbuminuria, and new ones are being developed. Any patient albumin-positive on urine testing can be excluded from DM 13 as microalbumin testing is not indicated. The results need to be recorded and any abnormalities acted upon. A local protocol for testing for microalbuminuria should be agreed as diagnosis is usually confirmed from three samples and ACE (angiotensin-converting enzyme) inhibitors or A2 antagonists initiated where indicated.

DM 16. The percentage of patients with diabetes who have a record of their total cholesterol level within the previous 15 months

DM 17. The percentage of patients with diabetes whose last measured total cholesterol level within previous 15 months is 5 mmol/l or less

The National Institute for Health and Clinical Excellence recognises that many people with type 2 diabetes have an increased coronary event risk and that early treatment will lessen that risk (National Institute for Health and Clinical Excellence, 2002). It also recommends recording fasting lipid levels 'if feasible'. Primary care teams should adhere to local protocols for lipid testing or agree plans with specialists, especially with regard to fasting if people are on insulin or sulphonylureas (such as gliclazide or glibenclamide), which can cause hypoglycaemic episodes ('hypos'). The National Institute for Health and Clinical Excellence suggests that fasting lipids should be recorded, again if feasible, at diagnosis and annually thereafter if levels are normal, but more frequently if any abnormalities are found.

DM 18. The percentage of patients with diabetes who have had influenza immunisation in the preceding 1st September to 31st March

People with diabetes are more prone to infections and, unless contraindicated, should be encouraged to have influenza and pneumonia vaccination.

QOF results

The percentages of points achieved in the QOF are shown in Figure 3.1.

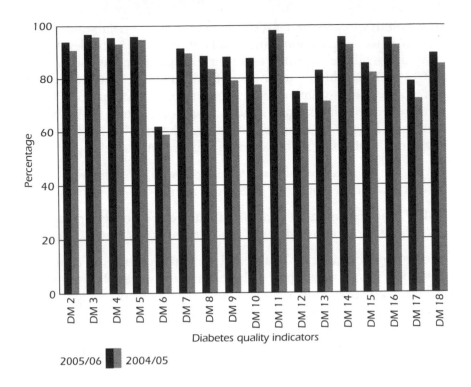

2005/06 ▓ 2004/05

Figure 3.1 The percentages of points achieved in the QOF

Nurses in the GMS contract

(National Primary and Care Trust Development Programme, 2003)

- Front-line nurses can extend their interests from clinical to business aspects of a practice.

- They can take on a more strategic role within primary care.

- They can become partners in the practice.

- Forward-thinking nurses can form a limited company (provided at least one GP is a signatory on the contract).

- New ways of working are emerging (NHS Modernisation Agency, 2002).

Practice-based commissioning

PBC is a method for GPs in England to develop services through commissioning them from local sources. It is likely to have an impact on other areas of the UK too. PBC is most likely through clusters of local practices working together while monitoring referrals at practice level. It has two aims:

1 To involve GPs and practices more directly in the process of commissioning (buying in services), as well as giving them a central role in planning *what* services their patients need and deciding *how* these services will be provided.

2 To encourage and support GPs in managing referrals more effectively so that money that previously went into secondary referrals can be reinvested in primary care. The scheme will be available to all practices, both GMS and Personal Medical Services. It is not compulsory.

The intention is for practices to examine their localities and band together to provide services. Concerns have been expressed about who will provide services such as community staff:

■ Alternative Provider Medical Services are a significant threat to general practice. Patients are being diverted to a multiplicity of private sector primary care providers.

■ PBC has the ability to develop NHS general practice and move resources into primary care if sufficient funding is identified.

■ If GPs decide not to hold budgets, others, such as community matrons and/or district nurses or private providers, may be willing to do so.

■ Detail is lacking, and local medical committees and practices will need to attempt to fill in the gaps through local negotiations with primary care organisations.

References

Abate N (2002). Obesity and cardiovascular disease. Pathogenic role of the metabolic syndrome and therapeutic implications. *Journal of Diabetes and its Complications* 14: 154–174.

Audit Commission (2000). *Testing Times: A Review of Diabetes Services in England and Wales*. London: Audit Commission.

British Medical Association (2006). *Revisions to the GMS Contract 2006/7 Delivering Investment in General Practice*. London: BMA.

Diabetes Control and Complications Trial Research Group (1993). The effect of intensive treatment of diabetes on the development and progression of long-term complications in insulin-dependent diabetes mellitus. *New England Journal of Medicine* **329**: 977–986.

Diabetes UK (2005). *Recommendations for the Provision of Services in Primary Care for People with Diabetes*. London: Diabetes UK.

Gray A, Clarke P, Farmer A, Holman R (UKPDS Group) (2002). Implementing intensive control of blood glucose concentration and blood pressure in type 2 diabetes in England: cost analysis (UKPDS 63). *British Medical Journal* **325**: 860–863.

Joint British Societies (2005). Guidelines on prevention of cardiovascular disease in clinical practice. *Heart* **91**: 1–52.

National Institute for Health and Clinical Excellence (2002). *Management of Type 2 Diabetes. Management of Blood Pressure and Blood Lipids*. Inherited Clinical Guideline H. London: NICE.

National Primary and Care Trust Development Programme (2003). *Briefing. The Role of Nurses under the New GMS Contract*. London: NatPaCT.

NHS Modernisation Agency (2002). *Workforce Matters. A Guide to Role Redesign in Diabetes Care*. London: DoH.

Further reading

Department of Health (2005). *Practice Based Commissioning. Promoting Clinical Engagement*. London: DoH.

Gadsby R (2005). *Delivering Quality Diabetes Care in General Practice*. London: Royal College of General Practitioners.

The educational needs of the team

Questions this chapter will help you answer

- Can I assess gaps in my learning and professional development plan?

- Am I trained to assess learning in patients rather than provide advice?

- Are people with diabetes offered structured education?

- What practical educational resources are available locally for healthcare professionals?

> *... the incidence of Type 2 diabetes could be reduced by lifestyle changes in the broader community.*
>
> Audit Commission (2000)

With a complex subject such as diabetes, up-to-date knowledge applied appropriately is a prerequisite for the effective clinical management and education of people with diabetes. But if you are working with diabetes on a daily basis, it can be quite a challenge to assess what you actually need at any particular time to enable you to remain as well informed as possible when providing education and support to people living with diabetes.

There are particular difficulties with knowing what 'you don't know', so one way of finding out what each team member needs to know is for all team members (mainly doctors and nurses) to begin by identifying their own learning needs using a 'diabetes topic' list (Box 4.1). This list does not include every topic, but it encompasses many subjects relating to clinical management, information and explanation on which individuals with diabetes, either newly diagnosed or during their life with diabetes, expect the doctor or nurse to have a certain level of knowledge. It is therefore intended to stimulate enquiry.

Box 4.1 Diabetes knowledge – needs assessment

Please fill in the appropriate box using the following key:

0 = No knowledge of topic
1 = Some knowledge of topic – insufficient
2 = Good knowledge of topic – sufficient

Types of diabetes	☐	Hypos	☐
Causes of diabetes	☐	Practical aspects	☐
Inheritance	☐	Unproven methods of treatment	☐
Physiology	☐	Alternative therapy	☐
Symptoms	☐	Control	☐
Related conditions	☐	Monitoring	☐
Diet	☐	Blood glucose	☐
Overweight	☐	Urine glucose	☐
Tablets	☐	Glycated haemoglobin (HbA$_{1c}$)/fructosamine	☐
Insulin	☐	Thrush	☐
Management (of diabetes care)	☐	Hormone replacement therapy (HRT)	☐
Brittle diabetes	☐	Termination of pregnancy	☐
Sport	☐	Infertility	☐
Eating out	☐	Genetics	☐
Holidays	☐	Pre-pregnancy	☐
Travel	☐	Pregnancy	☐
Work	☐	Gestational diabetes	☐
Other illness	☐	Baby with diabetes	☐
Sick day rules	☐	Child with diabetes	☐
Surgical operations	☐	Diabetes in adolescence	☐
Investigations	☐	A cure?	☐
Driving	☐	Complications	☐

Alcohol	☐	Feet, footwear	☐
Drugs	☐	Chiropody/podiatry	☐
Smoking	☐	Retinopathy	☐
Impotence	☐	Vision	☐
Contraception	☐	Transplantation	☐
Hypertension	☐	Insulin pumps	☐
Cardiovascular problems	☐	Artificial pancreas	☐
Psychological aspects	☐	New insulins	☐
Diabetes UK	☐	Oral insulins	☐
Emergency treatment of hyperglycaemia	☐	Emergency treatment of hypoglycaemia	☐
Life insurance	☐	Medical insurance	☐

Members of the team may find it helpful to score themselves and note further topics of identified educational need from this book.

Topic	Score	Page number

Diabetes education for the primary care team – what is available?

Philosophy of practice

Changes are taking place in education for both health professionals and people with diabetes themselves. Both are having to get to grips with changes that place the patient at the centre of education and how it is provided.

Diabetes UK and the Department of Health (2005) recognise two principal models of education:

1   *The traditional medical-centred model.* This focuses on 'the problem' and advice to rectify it, which the person with diabetes may or may not like.

2   *The patient-centred approach.* This engages those with diabetes in their own care, allowing them to identify areas of concern and supporting them in their decision to become experts in their care.

Training and education for health professionals

These changes in the way health professionals provide education are influencing course and study day programmes.

Clinical information is important, but health professionals seeking training should ensure that other areas are covered:

- psychological effects;

- methods of promoting independence;

- motivating change.

Working with a variety of health professionals and putting the patient at the centre of care is the order of the day. Any education undertaken should fit into the individual's personal development plan and that of their organisation. A toolkit is available on the Internet to assist with evaluating the provision of structured education (Diabetes UK/National Diabetes Support Team, 2006).

In 2005, Diabetes UK suggested that the integration of theory and practice should be central to the syllabus, and that the delivery of the programme should support autonomous and reflective thinking, as well as evidence-based practice.

Programmes need to be developed with patient, academic, educational and clinical expert input. See Box 4.2 for sources of further information.

Internationally, the International Diabetes Federation and American Diabetes Association have put their energies into standards for 'educators' in diabetes. This tends to separate educationalists from clinicians, a route not usually followed by the National Health Service. One of the strengths of training and education in the UK is its adherence to the team approach involving multidisciplinary health professionals, trainers and academics. In delivering patient education, those behind the DAFNE (Dose Adjustment for Normal Eating), DESMOND (Diabetes

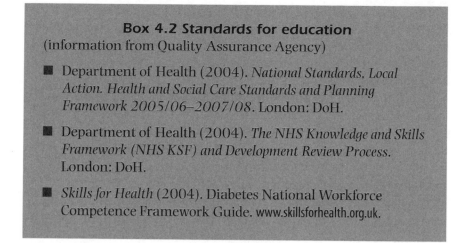

Box 4.2 Standards for education
(information from Quality Assurance Agency)

- Department of Health (2004). *National Standards, Local Action. Health and Social Care Standards and Planning Framework 2005/06–2007/08*. London: DoH.

- Department of Health (2004). *The NHS Knowledge and Skills Framework (NHS KSF) and Development Review Process*. London: DoH.

- *Skills for Health* (2004). Diabetes National Workforce Competence Framework Guide. www.skillsforhealth.org.uk.

Education and Self Management for Ongoing and Newly Diagnosed) and X-PERT programmes (see below) have identified specific learning objectives for 'Train the Trainers' courses that match to these.

'Train the Trainers' programmes

The Department of Health has announced that all primary care organisations in England and Wales will need to implement guidance from the National Institute for Health and Clinical Excellence (2005), providing all people with diabetes with high-quality, structured education. Scotland and Northern Ireland have similar guidance in development.

There are excellent, researched programmes in existence, and much can be learned from these (see also Chapter 16):

- DAFNE for type 1 diabetes;

- DESMOND for type 2 diabetes;

- the Diabetes X-PERT Programme, produced by Burnley, Pendle & Rossendale primary care trust – an award-winning education programme for people with diabetes.

Websites are listed in Appendix 4.

Courses

In order to deliver this educational initiative to patients effectively, health professionals must complete a 'Train the Trainers' course. It is recognised that there are problems associated with healthcare professionals taking time away from their clinical service, particularly those working in the primary healthcare setting. Training budgets are tight, but it is incumbent upon all nurses to keep up to date, and access to education may be through various portals. Distance learning may provide this route by fitting into the health professional's personal development plan and home life.

Courses and other educational initiatives are now too numerous to include in this book. Diabetes UK has a list of currently available courses on its website (see Appendix 4), but primary care organisations and local academic institutions may be able to provide more local information. Many local initiatives are run through the diabetes specialist team, and again they will be a useful contact. The University of Warwick (see Appendix 4) has become renowned for its variety of courses at various levels, but it is by no means alone so it is worth checking locally.

- Many organisations are developing diploma, degree and higher degree courses in which diabetes may be a part or a module.

- Credits or Credit Accumulation and Transfer points should be available on all validated courses where assessment is integral to the course.

- Multidisciplinary education is becoming widely available and encourages the team approach.

- District diabetes care should include, in any strategy, a recognition of the need for local training and continuing education for primary care teams.

- Local and district schemes should be planned by specialist teams in conjunction with academic/continuing education institutions.

Practical 'self-help' and continuing personal development

- Reflect on learning from study days and conferences, and build future actions into your personal development plan.

- Visit another practice that is considered to be providing a good service.

- Contact your local GP tutor, primary care organisation and academic institution for relevant further education.

- Diabetes UK and local specialist teams will have reliable literature for people with diabetes and healthcare professionals.

- Individuals or practices should join Diabetes UK to keep up to date with diabetes care and educational events nationally.

- Remember that diabetes is a team event. Involve colleagues and people with diabetes in developing your service.

- Many companies are willing to work with health professionals/practices to organise training 'in house' or across a primary care organisation (if permitted).

Diabetes education for the primary healthcare team – what is needed?

- There should be a clear aim of the study day/course.

- Objectives should be relevant to the participants' areas of work.

- Evaluation of the event should be an integral part of the education.

- Any Credit Accumulation and Transfer points, what level these are and the eventual qualification should be noted.

- Before embarking on the course, what level of work is expected from the participant and whether it is assessed should be understood.

- The content of the event will depend on the timescale and level of education. Potential delegates should be able to see the full programme before registering for the event.

The suggested core content includes:

- the physiology, aetiology and clinical picture of diabetes;

- screening for diabetes and its complications;

- diagnostic criteria including impaired fasting glycaemia and impaired glucose tolerance;

- lifestyle measures: healthy eating, activity levels and management of risk factors;

- the control of glucose, blood pressure and lipids levels;

- care plans for newly diagnosed individuals, as well as ongoing and annual review;

- involving the person with diabetes: empowerment and involvement;

- interviewing techniques, motivational interviewing, psychological issues and the recognition of depression;

- the management of emergencies;

- the management of complications for type 1 and type 2 diabetes;

- current research and its implications in the delivery of future diabetes care;

- providing the service, in practice and within the primary care organisation.

References

Diabetes UK/Department of Health (2005). *Structured Patient Education in Diabetes. Report from the Patient Education Working Group.* London: DoH.

Diabetes UK/National Diabetes Support Team (2006) *How to Assess Structured Diabetes Education. An Improvement Toolkit for Commissioners and Local Diabetes Communities.* London: Department of Health/Diabetes UK.

National Institute for Health and Clinical Excellence (2005). *Diabetes (Types 1 and 2) – Patient Education Models.* Technology Appraisal No. 60. London: NICE.

Further reading

Diabetes UK (2005). *Recommendations for the Provision of Services in Primary Care for People with Diabetes.* London: Diabetes UK.

Part II

Providing
diabetes care

5 The diabetes service in general practice

Questions this chapter will help you answer

- What factors should be considered when planning diabetes care?
- Which diabetes patients will we care for in the practice?
- What resources are available?
- Have I considered new ways of working to cope with increasing demand?

> *I have nobody to contact after hours and sometimes feel very alone with this.*
>
> Audit Commission (2000)

How to set up a system of care

Aims

- To *identify, know and register* the diabetes population covered by the practice.
- To *provide treatment, support, education and surveillance* for people with diabetes not receiving hospital care or where care is 'shared' or 'integrated'. (For a definition of shared/integrated care for people with diabetes, see 'Shared (integrated) care' later in the chapter.)
- To *know and use all available specialist and support services* – referring to these in good time and appropriately.
- To identify a named local contact for advice for peple with diabetes and their carers.

Objectives

1 To enable the organisation of a practice register to support the systematic management and review of people confirmed to have diabetes.

2 To involve people with diabetes in a planned programme of care including:

   a the initial support, assessment and treatment of those newly diagnosed with diabetes, including immediate referral for specialist services where appropriate;

   b initial and staged continuing education that is correct, consistent and up to date;

   c planned appropriate treatment (taking into account age, lifestyle, knowledge and understanding);

   d the agreement of a care plan with the individual, tailoring care to the individual's needs and providing a record appropriate to the person with diabetes;

   e the management of acute complications (such as hyperglycaemia, ketosis and hypoglycaemia);

   f the identification of risk factors for long-term effects of diabetes, such as:

      i obesity;

      ii smoking;

      iii physical inactivity;

      iv hypertension;

      v hyperlipidaemia;

   g early identification, surveillance, treatment (and referral, if appropriate) for long-term complications of diabetes in order to reduce the incidence of:

      i coronary heart disease and stroke;

      ii blindness and visual impairment;

      iii foot ulceration, limb amputation disability;

      iv end stage renal failure.

3 To engage in structured education for patients, carers and staff.

4 To participate in effective communication with others to ensure that appropriate services, for example social services and voluntary groups, are available for people with diabetes.

The General Medical Services contract

In 2004, a new contract was agreed with general practitioners (GPs) that changed the way in which funding was provided to practices (see Chapter 3). This has changed the face of diabetes management and focused practices on providing a service to all those with diabetes on their registers, and on finding new ways of extending that service to those who find it difficult to attend a practice clinic, whether because of working hours, mobility difficulties, communication problems or lack of understanding. Call and recall for all should now be the norm.

There is an argument that achieving set standards gains financial reward without taking account of people's quality of life. Thus, a person who is prone to hypoglycaemic attacks and prefers to run his glucose levels slightly higher than the recommended glycated haemoglobin (HbA_{1c}) level of 7.5% (which is not an evidence-based target but a funding level) will not gain the practice points but may feel safer. Likewise, the older person living alone may suffer an increased risk of a fall during a hypoglycaemic attack owing to attempts to reach this target. Little credit is awarded too for the motivated individuals who have successfully reduced their weight, increased their activity and reduced their HbA_{1c} level from 10% to 8.5%. There is also no incentive to prevent diabetes in the first place.

Despite these limitations, the General Medical Services (GMS) contract has encouraged systematic review, which is a good thing (see Chapter 3).

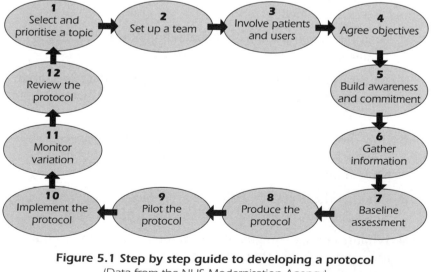

Figure 5.1 Step by step guide to developing a protocol
(Data from the NHS Modernisation Agency)

Prior to planning the service, it is good practice to agree a protocol so that each participant understands his or her role. The NHS Modernisation Agency has published useful information with practical examples and step-by-step guidance to assist in forming effective protocols (Figure 5.1), as well as some examples of protocol-based care (NHS Modernisation Agency, 2004).

Planning the service

To plan for the future of diabetes care, the primary care diabetes team should assess the following:

■ Their total population with diabetes and how much time is available to provide adequate care (Box 5.1).

■ Who is providing that care: is it primary, secondary or shared? Is there a protocol for shared care? A referral pathway? A home service?

■ How the care will be organised and how to reach special groups, for example those in care, refugees and mobile populations.

■ Whether the necessary skills are available; training and education may be needed for all members of the team.

■ What necessary equipment, education material and resources are required (other than those currently available in the practice).

- The methods of record-keeping to be employed, which may demand computer training and an agreement of the accepted codes to be used.

- Whether the current system is working effectively; audit should form an integral part of the service and could include patient satisfaction. (See Chapter 19.)

Involvement and discussion on the part of members of the team will identify possible organisational problems and resource implications early on. It may be helpful for a member of the local hospital specialist team, primary care organisation or specialist facilitator to be invited to the practice when any new services or changes to existing systems are being planned. This would have the advantages of:

- establishing a relationship and communication between the practice and the hospital diabetes team;

- signifying the practice's intentions and plans for its service so that the specialist team and diabetes lead for the primary care organisation are aware of them;

- providing awareness of the diabetes specialist and support facilities available locally and nationally;

- setting up the necessary links for sharing care;

- discussing diabetes management and local protocols for care, criteria for referral and mechanisms for urgent referral (such as those for a child newly diagnosed with diabetes or an adult with foot ulceration);

- training or updating requirements by the team to be involved in the practice diabetes service.

Various health professionals could be involved in planning – or redesigning – the service:

- *Dietitians*: where and how to access them, waiting time and the availability of structured education for patients and staff alike.

- *Podiatrists*: where and how to access them. In many areas, there are not enough chiropodists/podiatrists to see every patient with diabetes. There should be an agreed referral pathway for routine and urgent cases appropriate to their needs.

- *Community pharmacists*: people with diabetes frequently take a number of different medications. Community pharmacists can be involved in care-planning, repeat prescriptions and medication review.

■ *Opticians*: as part of the systematic eye-screening process.

Planning should also encompass plans for the ongoing review of the diabetes service and the consideration of its evaluation and annual audit.

Organisation of the service

Clinics in primary care have traditionally been nurse led with GP support. New ways of working are, however, evolving, and the National Service Framework for Diabetes (Department of Health, 2002) suggests that people with diabetes should be involved in the design of the service.

Any primary care team providing a service acceptable to people with diabetes should consider the following:

■ *How to prevent duplication*:
   ◆ Is it possible to combine clinics for those with concomitant disorders, for example coronary heart disease or hypertension?

■ *Time*:
   ◆ Is there set aside time for a clinic with protected time for the nurse and/or GP running it? The session will need to be longer than a normal nursing appointment in order to provide a comprehensive approach to diabetes care involving the person with diabetes in that service.
   ◆ Is the appointment time long enough to fulfil the needs of the patient for effective education, including agreed goals and targets?
   ◆ Is the clinic set at a time suitable to most people? How will the service be provided for those who cannot attend the clinic?

■ *Flexibility*:
   ◆ Is there provision for frequent sessions for those who are newly diagnosed and those going through times of change?
   ◆ Are systems in place to allow telephone support so that people with diabetes can access routine advice?
   ◆ Can equity of care be offered to those who are in care or

housebound, and those with limited understanding or language barriers?

- ■ *Personnel*:
    - ◆ Who are the most appropriate members of the team? Are there protocols in place to ensure that each understands his or her place in the service? Do shared care or referral pathways exist or need to be formed? Who is the 'named contact' for people with diabetes?

Who might be offered the practice diabetes service?

It is to be hoped that every district will have agreed pathways between specialist teams and GPs on the arrangements for diabetes care provision and the suggested criteria for referral and sharing care.

The primary care service could be offered to the following groups of people:

- ■ those with type 2 diabetes who do not have major complications;
- ■ people with well-controlled type 1 diabetes;
- ■ people with diabetes who wish to attend the practice for their care;
- ■ those who are very elderly or frail, for whom hospital care is inappropriate unless absolutely essential;
- ■ those who are housebound;
- ■ individuals discharged from hospital care or for whom no care provision has been identified;
- ■ those attending hospital for other conditions, for whom diabetes care, education and surveillance are not provided by other specialists.

Those treated with diet alone and those who are housebound are more difficult to identify as they may not collect their prescriptions or need, or even be able, to attend the surgery for healthcare services. It is worth having a practice policy on the correct identification and registration of those with diabetes as it appears that those people whose diabetes is inappropriately thought of as 'mild' are receiving less-structured care (Hippisley-Cox and Pringle, 2004).

Who will be involved in the provision of the practice diabetes service?

In a moderate-to-large practice, a minimum team will consist of a receptionist/secretary, a nurse and a doctor. In a large practice, more than one receptionist/secretary and nurse may be required to keep the service and its administration running throughout the year. In a practice where many doctors may be in partnership, which doctor(s) will be involved needs to be clarified at an early stage. In some practices, all the medical practitioners wish to be involved in the total care of their own patients. This system is feasible as long as the person running the service (e.g. the nurse) communicates with each doctor about the care of each patient. The argument put forward in favour of this system is that all the medical practitioners retain their skill in the management of diabetes.

A disadvantage of this system is, however, that all the doctors may not be able to retain their knowledge and skills if they have very few patients with diabetes to manage. It is therefore probably best, in the interests of a high-quality service, for one doctor in the practice to take overall responsibility for diabetes care. Continuing education and the management of many patients will ensure a retention of knowledge and skills. This doctor can provide the necessary leadership for the diabetes service, at the same time communicating with colleagues about the service and the progress of their individual patients. Furthermore, the identified team will provide continuity and consistency of information – important in diabetes care where conflicting messages are often received by people with diabetes in their dealings with many health-care professionals.

The nurse's role as the linchpin is also important in continuity of care, in the support and education of clerks and reception staff, and in communicating with the doctors in the practice and other providers of care (NHS Modernisation Agency, 2002).

New ways of working are emerging to cope with increasing number of people with diabetes, and to achieve effective methods of providing them with care.

> If services are to cope, change will be needed within the specialist hospital team, within the primary care team and, perhaps most challenging of all, between the two, to provide the holy grail of 'seamless care' needed by people with diabetes. A creative approach to job redesign will also bring them to the fore as part of the care team.
>
> (NHS Modernisation Agency, 2002)

There are three reasons for implementing change:

1 in response to the views of people with diabetes and their carers;

2 to make the best use of limited resources;

3 to put individuals with diabetes at the centre of their care and to empower them to self-manage their condition.

Table 5.1 outlines a few examples of role redesign related to diabetes (for more, see NHS Modernisation Agency, 2002).

Table 5.1 Examples of role redesign	
Healthcare assistant in diabetes	■ Ensures appropriate call and recall from the diabetes register
	■ Ensures that necessary investigations are carried out 2 weeks before the clinic so that best use is made of trained nurse/GP and patient time
	■ As part of the clinic team, performs an examination (e.g. weight, blood pressure, urinalysis, foot health) prior to the health professional appointment
	■ Monitors vaccinations that are due, e.g. influenza, pneumonia
	■ Contacts those who do not attend to assess their reason and organise follow-up
	If indicated, may perform similar tasks as home visits
Ethnic support worker	■ Participates in the clinic to ensure that an appropriate translation is available
	■ Identifies appropriate learning materials relevant to the individual
	■ Understands local support groups and agencies relevant to the individual
	■ Works with the individual to agree a care plan appropriate to his or her needs
Expert patient	■ People with diabetes who have completed the Expert Patient programme could assist those with diabetes in terms of education and self-caring strategies
Practice educator	■ He or she is an appropriately trained person who can deliver group training sessions for individuals with diabetes

Frequency of clinics

In a large practice where the number of those with diabetes may be high (perhaps as a result of there being an older population) or the ethnic composition is high (e.g. Asians from the subcontinent of India or South Asians; those of African/Caribbean origin), it may be necessary to hold clinics every week. In a small practice, a clinic may only be required monthly or even bi-monthly. Alternatively, clinics could be held only during the spring or summer months when it is easiest for people to travel to the surgery.

Shared (integrated) care

Where care is 'shared' or 'integrated', it is important that each provider is aware of the others' roles, and that protocols and/or pathways are in place that enable the person with diabetes to understand the nature of the care provided by primary care and specialist teams.

In 'integrated' care, effective communication and record-keeping is fundamental to the service. Personally held records, as advocated by the National Service Framework (2002) for diabetes, should be agreed between all parties. To be useful, these records need to be kept up to date: they could hold GP system printouts and hospital clinic data in a form acceptable to the individual. They should form the basis for structured education and be a resource for people with diabetes in terms of achieving effective communication with their diabetes care team. Recommendations for the constituents of such a personally held record are given in Box 5.2.

Primary care teams should ideally ensure everyone on their practice register is receiving a planned programme of care from the provider most appropriate for them. Ignoring this principle encourages failures in the system, with the person with diabetes perhaps receiving no care at all.

Ideal facilities for the diabetes service

There are no special facilities necessary for diabetes care other than those which would be provided for all primary healthcare.

Flexible use of the waiting area should be considered, perhaps for periodic educational group sessions when discussions can be held and

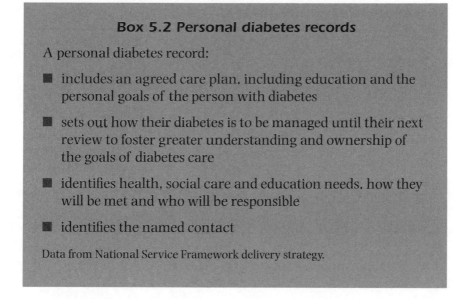

Box 5.2 Personal diabetes records

A personal diabetes record:

■ includes an agreed care plan, including education and the personal goals of the person with diabetes

■ sets out how their diabetes is to be managed until their next review to foster greater understanding and ownership of the goals of diabetes care

■ identifies health, social care and education needs, how they will be met and who will be responsible

■ identifies the named contact

Data from National Service Framework delivery strategy.

videos shown. This area may also be used for a display of literature about diabetes and information on relevant local services and facilities, along with other healthcare education material.

No particular clinical room facilities are necessary either. Visual acuity may be measured in the practice, but fundoscopy requires a completely darkened room and is not recommended for a primary care setting unless it is provided by a professional with specialised training as part of a centrally organised screening programme. If visual acuity is to be measured, a Snellen chart and a distance of 6 m are commonly used, although in a small surgery a 3 m chart can be obtained or a 6 m chart used with a mirror (see the section on testing for visual acuity in Chapter 13).

Who does what in which room is often a cause for debate! Where the nurse and doctor are setting up a new service, it may be helpful for both to work together in one room until confidence has been gained and each understands the other's role. Later on, the organisation may change so that clinical checks and education are provided by the nurse, with a review of these by the doctor and further medical checks, discussion and prescription to complete the periodic or annual review, follow-up care being decided appropriately.

It should be remembered that people with diabetes attending the surgery or medical centre may be elderly, visually impaired or disabled, and any facilities for diabetes care should accommodate these problems.

Essential equipment: general

- Hand-washing facilities with warm water, soap and paper towels; this is important for finger-prick tests to monitor blood glucose level and in terms of good hygiene.

- Weighing scales (metric or imperial),which should be checked and calibrated annually.

- A weight-conversion chart (kilograms to stones/pounds).

- An 'ideal' weight chart – the weight for height (i.e. the body mass index) of men and women.

- A tape measure as waist circumference is a good predictor of abdominal adiposity.

- A height gauge, correctly positioned to record the correct height.

- Equipment for the collection of laboratory samples, for example blood, urine, wound debris.

- A sphygmomanometer or electronic blood pressure machine with a standard cuff. Small and large cuffs should also be available, and these should be checked annually. A list of acceptable devices available on the British Hypertension Society website (see Appendix 4).

- Disposable gloves.

- A container for the disposal of 'sharps'and a shelf high enough to keep it out of reach of children.

Essential equipment: screening and monitoring

Glucose and albumin

- Glucose and albumin test strips. Microalbumin test strips are also available, albeit expensive. Check with your local laboratory or diabetes team for local advice on microalbuminuria testing.

- Cottonwool balls for drying the finger after the finger-prick test.

- Glucose 75 g for the oral glucose tolerance test. Note that the glucose concentration of Lucozade drink varies with the pack size and type. Check with your local laboratory for advice, and remember that low-calorie versions are unsuitable.

Glucose may be obtained on prescription if the patient is exempt from charges; otherwise, it is cheaper (than paying a prescription charge) to buy glucose ready measured from the pharmacy (see the section 'Oral glucose tolerance test' in Chapter 7).

Urine testing

For glucose in the urine (quantitative). Testing for glycosuria may be unreliable as a screening method owing to the individual having a high renal threshold and therefore not passing glucose in the urine until the level in the blood is higher than usual. A variety of companies produce strips; see the *British National Formulary* (BNF) for up-to-date lists.

For protein in the urine (quantitative). Protein-testing strips are available and should be used prior to microalbumin screening as, if protein is present, infection should be excluded and the test repeated before assessing microalbuminuria.

For ketones. Ketones can be detected in the urine using test strips or in the blood using specialist meters. See the BNF for up-to-date advice.

Finger-prick devices

To prevent cross-infection, any device or lancet used for finger-pricking must be for single-person use only or have every surface that is in contact with the person disposable. A guide to lancing devices on the UK market has been published by the Medicines and Health care projects Regulatory Agency (2005).

Test strips and meters for blood glucose measurement

Companies may provide meters free, with the test strips available on prescription. Health professionals should be aware that glucose meters should be subject to regular quality control procedures to ensure their accuracy. Check with your local specialist centre or laboratory for services in your area. If none exists, it is important to obtain the correct quality control solution from the company whose meter you use and to record the results. Blood glucose monitoring is considered further in Chapter 12.

Checking the at-risk foot

Monofilaments and neurotips are used for checking lower limb sensation. They normally bend on exerting 10 g of pressure on the foot, but local chiropodists/podiatrists will advise on local systems for foot-screening and referral. (See also Chapter 14.)

On no account should a needle be used as this may introduce infection and put the foot at further risk.

For emergency use: for the treatment of hypoglycaemia

These are listed in Table 5.2. See also Appendix 5.

Table 5.2 Equipment for the emergency treatment of hypoglycaemia

In the surgery	In the doctor's bag
Sugary drink/glucose/dextrosol tablets	GlucoGel (previously Hypostop Gel)
GlucoGel (previously Hypostop Gel) (available on form FP10 for people with diabetes)	Intramuscular injection of glucagon
	Intravenous dextrose
Intramuscular injection of glucagon (available on form FP10 for people with diabetes)	Blood glucose measuring strips and an up-to-date meter
Blood glucose measuring strips and an up-to-date meter	

Resources for diabetes education

Diabetes UK provides a wealth of non-promotional education material and resources, as well as a catalogue for people with diabetes. Primary care teams and other individuals can access this catalogue online (see Appendix 4); this includes many resources available for just the cost of the postage. Teams can also download information to print out in the practice. The local diabetes team can also help to recommend appropriate literature.

Companies involved in the field of diabetes can provide educational resources and materials too (see Appendix 4).

Structured education can be illustrated with recourse to a variety of different types of material (Table 5.3). The views of the person with diabetes are paramount in terms of which form of education is most appropriate for that individual (see also Chapter 16).

Table 5.3 Resources for education

Posters	Provide information. Useful as educational aids on specific topics. Helpful in providing waiting room alerts. Make sure they are from a reputable source and not just free advertising!
Information booklets/ leaflets	Must be provided in appropriate language and at appropriate level of understanding
Videos/DVDs	To reinforce education at home, where this is felt desirable
Self-monitoring diaries	Can be obtained from companies. These should be taught only as part of structured education and with clear guidelines for the action to be taken when results have been obtained
Identification	Cards from companies or Medic Alert information (see Appendix 4)
Personally held records	Developed locally. Discuss with your local specialist team or primary care organisation
Local information and contact numbers	Local contact number for out-of-hours advice Primary care team contact numbers Details for the local Diabetes UK branch and support groups Chiropody (podiatry) services Dietetic services (see Chapter 10) Dental services Pharmacy services Optician services Supporting/caring agencies/trusts Social services and benefits Rehabilitation services
Local initiatives	Details of local initiatives such as exercise on prescription schemes, smoking cessation classes, Expert Patient courses and structured education classes (see Chapter 16) Further resources should be identified through your local specialist team or primary care diabetes lead

Materials for organising and recording information

■ A diabetes register – normally on the GP computer system; EMIS, Vision, Torex systems for recording information.

- A recall sheet or card index.

- Appointment cards – for patient use.

- An appointment book or computer system – to record the appointments made.

- A standard letter – to use for new patients attending and recall.

- A card or leaflet with practice information and practice contact numbers.

- Laboratory forms.

- The individual's medical records – paper or computerised (sometimes a mixture of both).

- The diabetes personally held record.

References

Department of Health (2002). National Service Framework for Diabetes: Delivery Strategy. London: DoH.

Hippisley Cox J, Pringle M (2004). Prevalence, care and outcomes for patients with diet-controlled diabetes in general practice: cross sectional survey. *Lancet* **364**: 423–428.

Medicines and Health care Products Regulatory Agency (2005) *Guide to Lancing Devices*. London: MHRA.

NHS Modernisation Agency (2002). *Workforce Matters. A Guide to Role Redesign in Diabetes Care*. London: Modernisation Agency.

NHS Modernisation Agency (2004). *Protocol-based Care. Chronic Diseases – Some Case Studies and Examples*. London: Modernisation Agency.

Further reading

Department of Health (2001). National Service Framework for Diabetes. Standards.

Royal College of Nursing/UK Association of Diabetes Specialist Nurses (2005). *An Integrated Career and Competency Framework for Diabetes Nursing*. London: RCN.

Providing Diabetes Care in General Practice

6 The practice diabetes register and links with specialist services

Questions this chapter will help you answer

- How do I attract patients to the practice diabetes clinic?
- Do I have a system for non-attenders?
- What links do I have to specialist services?

> *. . . the re-shaping of primary care will have a direct impact on patterns of diabetes services in years to come.*
>
> Audit Commission (2000)

Advertising the practice diabetes service

Practices providing a diabetes clinic should advertise this in the waiting room to attract anyone who might be missing from the register (Figure 6.1). The poster needs to provide information on:

- time of day;
- day of the week;
- who is involved – including the dietitian and podiatrist (if available);
- how long is allowed for each appointment;
- how to get an appointment (with perhaps a note to speak to the nurse to arrange blood tests prior to the consultation).

A standard letter of invitation to attend the practice diabetes clinic can be produced and sent to those due for follow-up (Figure 6.2).

Diabetes Clinic

This practice offers a clinic for people with diabetes. Regular check-ups are important to tailor treatment to your health.

If you are not currently involved in regular reviews for your diabetes, please contact reception. It might be useful to have some tests done before your visit so that you can discuss the results at the clinic.

Monday afternoons 1.45pm to 5.45pm (other times may be available by arrangement).

20-minute appointments

Run by ____________ (Practice Nurse) & ____________ (GP)

Figure 6.1 Poster advertising the diabetes service

Diabetes registers

Prior to the 2004 General Medical Services contract (see Chapter 3), diabetes registers were organised in a variety of ways: through practices, district-wide or not at all. The new contract focused attention on providing care to all people with diabetes, and practice-based registers needed to be accurate to reflect the systematic approach advocated by National Service Frameworks and rewarded, financially, through the General Medical Services. District registers may still be used to facilitate services but can only be as up to date as the information provided by practices.

The advantages of registers are that they can help:

- to assess how many people in the practice have diabetes and compare this with national and regional figures;
- to ensure that care is available and provided for all people with diabetes in the practice;
- to achieve the targets set in the Quality and Outcomes Framework.

Practice Telephone No: 222333
The Medical Practice. Big Long Road, Ensleigh,
Wootton XX3 5XX

March _____

Mrs J Black
5 Short Road
Ensleigh
Wootton,
XX3 5YY

Dear Mrs Black

Re: Diabetes Clinic – Wednesday 2.30pm to 4.30pm

We would like to offer you a check-up for your diabetes. This will include a review of your treatment and an opportunity for you to discuss your situation with a nurse trained in diabetes and to agree a plan for the future.

The service will be provided in the practice (address above) every Wednesday afternoon, starting at 2.30pm (other times will be arranged if required). The appointment should only take about 20 minutes.

We have made an appointment for you to attend on Wednesday 19 April 2006 at 3pm. If that is not convenient, perhaps you could let us know (telephone number at top of letter) and we will arrange another time.

Please bring your personal record book with you, your blood glucose meter and results (if you use one) and a fresh urine sample. It would be very useful if you could have a blood test done two weeks before this appointment – a form is included for you to have this done. You can arrange a time to suit yourself for this test by contacting reception on _____. If you are on insulin, please contact us to discuss any changes to your injection that might be needed.

We look forward to seeing you.

Yours sincerely

Dr Andrew Sloop   Mrs Maggie Graham
General Practitioner   Practice Nurse

**Figure 6.2 Sample patient invitation letter
for practice diabetes clinic**

Additional elements on the register that help to organise systems of care are:

■ where care is provided (and by whom): primary care, shared care, specialist care;

■ which other members of the diabetes care team are involved.

The register is invaluable in 'tracking' people with diabetes who fail to attend or do not attend hospital or general practice for their care, or who may be 'lost' between the two. Nowadays, it is a 'virtual' register, being computer based and capable of instant updating when a new diagnosis is confirmed.

Those without an effective computer system should ensure that the following information is recorded – perhaps in a card index box. Recall can then be organised from that list. One person within the practice needs to be nominated to keep this paper system up to date.

Setting up the register

■ Collect the list of names of people identified with diabetes.

■ Take out their records – make a list of all the names (include those at branch surgeries).

■ Note the following:
  ◆ Name (and address if required)
  ◆ Date of birth
  ◆ Date of diagnosis and type of diabetes (not always possible to discern)
  ◆ Treatment – diet, diet and tablets, or diet and insulin
  ◆ Identified complications of the diabetes or important associated medical problems (this information should be recorded from hospital letters after clinic appointments)
    ● retinopathy
    ● neuropathy (peripheral/autonomic)
    ● nephropathy
    ● cardiovascular disease
    ● peripheral vascular disease.

■ Note who is providing care, for example a specialist diabetes physician, another hospital physician, a general practitioner, a combination of these or none. (The information regarding specialist and other physicians can be obtained by checking the letter heading and knowing who the specialist physicians are in the district, or from scanned files in the computer system.)

Links with specialist services

Anyone new to the practice diabetes team should acquaint themselves with local specialist services and how to liaise with them, refer to them and accept discharges from them.

Contact with the appropriate diabetes team should provide the following necessary information:

- The name(s) of the local diabetes physician(s) (diabetologists).

- The names of diabetes specialist nurses.

- Details of the hospital diabetes clinics (where and when clinics are held), including collaborative clinics, for example for foot, renal and antenatal care.

- The name(s) of paediatrician(s) with an interest in diabetes.

- The name of the diabetes specialist nurse caring for children (who may be separate or a part of the diabetes nurse team).

- Details of diabetes clinics for children, including collaborative clinics, such as those for teenagers and young people.

- Details of any community diabetes services, for example diabetes specialist nurses in primary care or available for home visits.

- Details of availability and access to diabetes centres – by both people with diabetes and the practice team.

- Local advice, information and materials that may be identified as being appropriate for the practice, such as agreed patient-held records and/or care plans and protocols, educational material for people with diabetes, and weight and exercise referral schemes.

- The availability of structured education sessions for people with diabetes.

- The availability of local training for primary care teams.

- Information regarding self-help groups for people with diabetes, for example local branches of Diabetes UK, that are aimed at adults and/or parents or children.

- The name of the contact for the national charity Diabetes UK.

... guidelines were often incomplete, out of date, or not used.

(Audit Commission, 2000)

Links with dietetic services

You should obtain information on the following:

- Is there a referral pathway or protocol for new patients and ongoing advice?

- What local information is available regarding dietetic advice (see also Chapter 10)?

- Who provides dietetic advice in the district and how can they be contacted?

- What dietetic advice is provided for people with diabetes who are seen in the general practice setting?

- Where and when are dietetic sessions available for people with diabetes who have been referred by the general practitioner?

Links with chiropody (podiatry) services

Information on the following should be available:

- Is there a referral pathway or protocol for referral to the chiropody/podiatry service?

- What local information is available regarding foot and shoe care?

- Who provides chiropody/podiatry services in the district and how can they be contacted?

- Where and when are chiropody/podiatry services available locally to the practice? Or are they already organised in the practice for the practice population? Alternatively, can people with diabetes be added in to an existing practice chiropody/ podiatry service?

■ Which private (state-registered) chiropodists/podiatrists are providing a service locally to the practice, and where? (If people with diabetes are attending these services privately, it cannot be assumed that a full neurological and vascular check has been performed unless there is a local arrangement for reporting on an individual's consultations.)

Links with other agencies

It may also be helpful to have available information on:

■ local support groups (for many general health problems, for example stroke support groups or Alcoholics Anonymous – addresses are available from local or central libraries);

■ social services;

■ environmental health practice in the local authority for the safe disposal of 'sharps';

■ prescription exemption and Disabled Living Allowance;

■ opticians/optometrists (local diabetes retinal screening services);

■ shoe-fitting services;

■ dentists;

■ care and after-care services (for walking sticks, frames, commodes, continence supplies, etc.);

■ translation services.

The diagnosis and symptoms of diabetes mellitus

Questions this chapter will help you answer

■ What are the diagnostic criteria for diabetes?

■ What is the difference between impaired fasting glycaemia and impaired glucose tolerance?

■ Who should be screened for diabetes?

■ How do I carry out an oral glucose tolerance test?

> *The initial diagnosis of my condition by my GP was quick and the care and attention I received at _____ Hospital, followed up subsequently at the diabetes centre, was nothing short of excellent. My rapid progress and control enabled me to modify my treatment from insulin down to tablets and now by diet alone. This must be attributed to the advice and care provided by all the medical staff concerned.*
>
> Audit Commission (2000)

The symptoms of diabetes are similar in both main types of the condition (Table 7.1) but may be absent or be just a general feeling of malaise. There are, however, certain differences between type 1 diabetes and type 2 diabetes (Table 7.2). In particular, the onset is rapid and can be dramatic in type 1 diabetes, whereas years may elapse before type 2 diabetes is identified.

Type 2 diabetes is strongly associated with insulin resistance. Reaven first described the role of insulin resistance in human disease in the Banting Lecture of 1988. In simple terms, he stated that type 2 diabetes might occur even though there are high circulating levels of insulin in the blood (hyperinsulinaemia; see Figure 24.1). There is an inability of the insulin to act on its target tissues (insulin resistance), so, with the insulin unable to act, blood sugar levels rise (hyperglycaemia). In

Table 7.1 Symptoms of diabetes as they occur in type 1 and type 2 diabetes, with the similarities and differences between the two types

Symptoms	Type 1 diabetes	Type 2 diabetes
Onset	**Fast (weeks)**	**Slow (months, years)**
Thirst	✔	✔
Polyuria/nocturia	✔	✔
Bed-wetting in children	✔	–
Tiredness/lethargy	✔	✔
Mood changes (irritability)	✔	✔
Weight loss	✔ + +	✔ + / –
Visual disturbances	✔	✔
Thrush infections (genital)	✔	✔
Recurrent infections (boils/ulcers)	✔	✔
Hunger	✔	✔
Tingling/pain/numbness (in the feet, legs, hands)	–	✔
Occasionally, abdominal pain	✔	–
Confusion	If advanced	Especially in the elderly
Incontinence	–	Especially in the elderly
Unexplained symptoms	✔	✔

Signs of diabetes
(things that can be observed/measured in practice)

Glycosuria	✔	May be absent (especially in the elderly or if there is a high renal threshold)
Ketones in urine or blood	May be present (ketoacidosis)	Usually absent
Blood glucose	See Box 7.1 later in the chapter	

Table 7.2 Differentiating features of diabetes

Type 1 (previously known as insulin-dependent diabetes)	Type 2 (previously known as non-insulin-dependent diabetes)
Rapid onset	Slow onset
The presenting symptoms in type 1 diabetes are obvious to the patient but may not always be recognised by the physician	Symptoms may be present in type 2 diabetes but go unrecognised by the patient or the physician
Age under 30 years at diagnosis (but can be older)	Age over 30 years at diagnosis (but can be younger)
A history of unplanned weight loss	Often overweight or obese
Beta-cell destruction	Beta-cell deterioration or insulin resistance
A positive family history in 10%	A positive family history in 30%
A 50% concordance rate in identical twins	Almost 100% concordance rate in identical twins
Insulin is essential in treatment	Healthy eating and keeping up activity levels are the key to control, with tablets and/or insulin to control blood glucose levels

response to this, more insulin is produced (compensatory hyper-insulinaemia) to combat the rise. This similarly fails to act, and eventually the output of insulin will diminish (hypoinsulinaemia) as the islet cells cease to be able to cope with the increasing demand and their function deteriorates.

Various methods of measuring insulin levels in the blood are described by Stout (1995), but suffice it to say that none is appropriate in primary care and practitioners need to be aware that many of their patients will suffer from this form of insulin insensitivity. And suffer from it they may – this is no 'mild' condition.

Reaven also described the correlation between this hyperinsulinaemia and its effect on hypertension and abnormal lipid levels. It is thought that many of the common complications of type 2 diabetes are linked to insulin resistance. Whether high levels of insulin itself are athero-genic is still under debate (Rett, 1999).

An increased awareness of diabetes in general practice has led to the earlier diagnosis of type 1 diabetes, possibly before the patient is acutely ill. This has, however, led to occasional misdiagnosis, with people being completely inappropriately treated as if they have type 2 diabetes, so that they are treated with diet alone and then given tablets, no insulin being started until the person is acutely ill. It cannot be emphasised enough that, if patient is under 35 years old and thin (particularly if he or she is athletic), then **think type 1 diabetes** even if the symptoms are not acute. Increased vigilance is required for slim individuals with type 2 diabetes at any age as type 1 diabetes can occur in older people and with a slower onset than is normally seen in the young.

Public awareness of diabetes

The signs and symptoms of type 1 diabetes (see Table 7.1 above) are usually acute and it is of paramount importance that the correct diagnosis is made, followed by urgent referral to the specialist team.

Conversely, many people ultimately diagnosed with type 2 diabetes will have lived with the condition for months or even years before a diagnosis is made. As many as 25% of these people will have complications at diagnosis – rising to around 50% if hypertension and erectile dysfunction (impotence) are included (King's Fund Centre 2, 1996).

The general public may well know 'something' about diabetes: this is often that diabetes is associated with 'sugar'. The nature of the association is, however, not necessarily understood. More importantly, the symptoms are not known or, because of their non-specific nature, are not related to the diagnosis of diabetes.

Symptoms of tiredness or lethargy may be explained away by 'I'm getting older', irritability by stress at work or in the home. Repeated infections may be treated by different doctors in a large practice and the significance of their frequency not realised. Symptoms may also occur or progress so slowly and in such a 'mild' way that they are not connected to type 2 diabetes.

Improving public awareness of diabetes

- All members of the public are (or should be) registered with a doctor. The primary care team in the practice should always have 'diabetes' in their thoughts when providing any health care.

- Posters (available from Diabetes UK; see Appendix 4) can be put up in surgeries and waiting areas showing the symptoms of diabetes.

- Health questionnaires used in routine screening or for patients new to the practice should contain questions about the symptoms of diabetes (as shown in the sample poster in Figure 7.1).

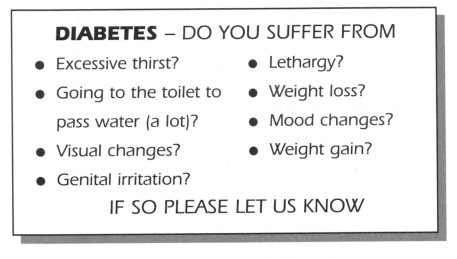

Figure 7.1 Poster showing symptoms of diabetes – for surgery use

Who should we screen?

The incidence of diabetes is rising, and it is largely type 2 diabetes that is responsible for this. Increasing sedentary lifestyles, at all ages, rising levels of obesity and the ability to live longer all contribute. Population screening for the detection of diabetes is the subject of research, and until a cost-effective system emerges, mass screening is not advocated.

It is wise to adopt a high level of suspicion in the following groups and screen them, normally with a laboratory blood test (Department of Health, 2002). An opportunistic, routine or 'on suspicion' approach should be adopted for several groups:

- All pregnant women.

Those presenting with the following symptoms:

- Thirst, polyuria and weight loss

- Nocturia, incontinence
- Recurrent infections, leg ulcers, thrush
- Neuropathic symptoms, for example pain, numbness and paraesthesia
- Visual changes such as blurring of vision
- Lassitude and general malaise
- Confusion – especially in the elderly.

Those already attending with;

- Hypertension
- Ischaemic heart disease
- Peripheral vascular disease
- Cerebrovascular disease.

When opportunities for screening (by the primary healthcare team) can present:

- During surgery
- In health-promotion clinics
- When new patients present to the practice
- During 'home' screening programmes, for example with elderly people
- At routine medical checks, such as for insurance purposes.

People who could be screened (those more likely to develop diabetes):

- People with a family history (of diabetes mellitus)
- Overweight people
- Elderly people
- Asians from Indian subcontinent and those of African/Caribbean origin
- Women with a relevant obstetric history (babies weighing over 4 kg; unexplained fetal loss)
- People with peripheral vascular disease
- People with cardiac problems
- People with circulatory problems.

Diagnosis of diabetes mellitus

Important notes

Confirmation of urine test – positive for glucose
Should a urine test reveal the presence of glucose, it is important that further tests are carried out for fasting and/or random blood glucose levels (or by oral glucose tolerance test (OGTT)), as glycosuria may be the result of a low renal threshold.

Conversely, the diagnosis of diabetes may be missed in an older person with a *high* renal threshold (the urine test may show a negative result, where the blood glucose level is 13 mmol/1 or more).

The renal threshold
The renal threshold (Figure 7.2) is the level at which glucose spills over into the urine as blood glucose levels rise. A normal renal threshold is about 10 mmol/l; i.e. when the blood glucose level is measured, it is 10 mmol/l and glycosuria is detectable. The renal threshold usually rises with age so that high blood glucose levels are present in the absence of glycosuria. The renal threshold may be low in some people and particularly during pregnancy.

Informing the patient
Once glycosuria has been found, the individual should be informed and advised that further tests are required before any diagnosis can be confirmed:

- The person may not have diabetes but may have a low renal threshold (e.g. in pregnancy).

- The person may have diabetes but a blood test is needed to exclude or confirm the diagnosis. (If the individual is pregnant, think of gestational diabetes.)

- The person may have impaired glucose tolerance (IGT) or impaired fasting glycaemia.

Reassuring the patient is important, and the diagnosis should be confirmed as quickly as possible so that appropriate treatment, support and education can begin. Preconceived ideas, fear and anxiety surround a diagnosis of diabetes. Firm evidence and careful explanation are therefore essential, whether or not the diagnosis is confirmed.

1. Normal renal threshold

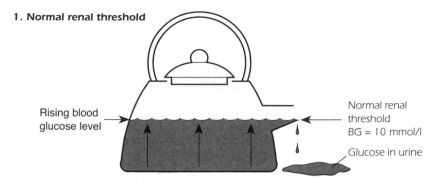

Rising blood glucose level → Normal renal threshold BG = 10 mmol/l

Glucose in urine

Rising blood glucose levels cause glucose to spill into urine at 10 mmol/l.

2. High renal threshold

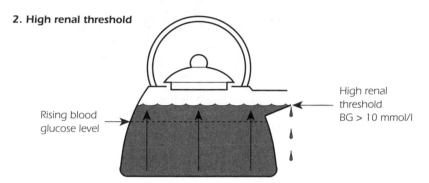

Rising blood glucose level → High renal threshold BG > 10 mmol/l

Rising blood glucose levels may not show in urine.

3. Low renal threshold

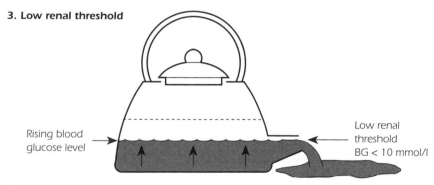

Rising blood glucose level → Low renal threshold BG < 10 mmol/l

Rising blood glucose level may show in urine below 10 mmol/l.

Figure 7.2 The renal threshold

BG, blood glucose

Confirming the diagnosis

It has never been easy to classify and diagnose diabetes mellitus because its very heterogeneity and characteristics have rendered most attempts at subdivision not entirely accurate and unable to reflect its underlying nature. There were anomalies in the earliest classification by age of onset, and the replacement by pathogenic mechanism (type 1 or type 2 diabetes, IGT), which was linked to treatment, also caused confusion and uncertainty. Diabetes UK advises the levels outlined in Box 7.1.

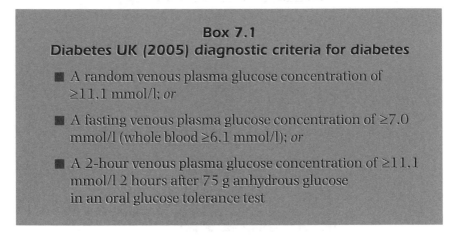

Box 7.1
Diabetes UK (2005) diagnostic criteria for diabetes

- A random venous plasma glucose concentration of ≥11.1 mmol/l; *or*

- A fasting venous plasma glucose concentration of ≥7.0 mmol/l (whole blood ≥6.1 mmol/l); *or*

- A 2-hour venous plasma glucose concentration of ≥11.1 mmol/l 2 hours after 75 g anhydrous glucose in an oral glucose tolerance test

If the individual is symptomatic and his or her blood sugar result is in the diabetic range, a diagnosis can be confirmed. For those without symptoms, a further check, on a subsequent day, should be performed to confirm the diagnosis. This can be either fasting, from a random sample or from the 2-hour OGTT. If the fasting or random values are not diagnostic, the 2-hour value should be used. A finger-prick test is not sufficient for diagnosis.

Any child in whom a diagnosis is suspected should be referred urgently by telephone to a hospital paediatric department, where the diagnosis can be confirmed.

Oral glucose tolerance test

There are local variations in performing these tests.

- A true OGTT relies on a fasting sample followed by a 75 g glucose load and another blood test 2 hours later. A person undergoing an OGTT starts fasting, after at least 3 days of eating a normal diet containing carbohydrates, when the first blood test is taken. A 75 g glucose load (seek advice on this from your local laboratory) is taken by the patient and the test repeated after 2 hours. Smoking is not permitted during the test; failure to adhere to this should be recorded. Patients should rest for the 2 hours after the glucose load to ensure an accurate result. (75 g anhydrous glucose is equivalent to 82.5 g glucose monohydrate.)

■ Some areas send patients 75 g glucose and ask them just to attend for the 2-hour test. This has limitations in that the fasting state is not known, impaired fasting glucose may be missed and the 2-hour deadline may not be feasible.

■ A random test can be taken at any time, as the name suggests, with the length of time from last meal recorded (just to make sure that the patient has not fasted for any other reason).

■ Fasting means overnight – 10–12 hours during which only water should be drunk.

Note: The glucose concentration of the drink Lucozade varies with pack size and type so check with your local laboratory for advice. Low-calorie versions are unsuitable.

Glucose may be obtained on prescription if the patient is exempt from charges; otherwise it is cheaper to buy it ready measured from the pharmacy rather than pay a prescription charge.

Some people have abnormal glucose results without these developing to the stage at which they would constitute diabetes. These people are at increased risk of developing diabetes and cardiovascular disease so should be offered lifestyle advice to suit. Type 2 diabetes is largely preventable, and changes to lifestyle, where indicated, can do much to reduce the incidence of diabetes (Diabetes UK, 2005).

Impaired glucose tolerance

IGT is indicated by a fasting plasma glucose of less than 7.0 mmol/l. Confirmation of IGT is made by carrying out an OGTT: the 2-hour value will be 7.8 mmol/l or more but under 11.1 mmol/l (Diabetes UK, 2005).

Impaired fasting glycaemia

The term 'impaired fasting glycaemia' has been introduced to classify individuals who have fasting glucose values above the normal range but below those diagnostic of diabetes; this means a fasting plasma glucose level of 6.1 mmol/l or more but below 7.0 mmol/l. Diabetes UK

(2005) recommends that all those with impaired fasting glucose should have an OGTT to exclude the diagnosis of diabetes.

Blood glucose meters
Blood glucose meters, even if subject to internal and external quality assurance (see Chapter 12) are not appropriate for confirmation of diagnosis.

Identification of people with diabetes mellitus

Details of people newly diagnosed with diabetes should be noted on a register (computer or written), as should those identified with diabetes and new to the practice. People attending the practice who have already been diagnosed with diabetes can be identified through records and prescriptions, and at surgery attendance. A comparison with other practices in the area may confirm the number of people identified with diabetes to be as expected. Figures will be lower in higher socioeconomic districts and higher in areas with poverty and/or a high ethnic mix.

References

Department of Health (2002). *National Service Framework for Diabetes; Delivery Strategy*. London: DoH.

Diabetes UK (2005) *Recommendations for the Provision of Services in Primary Care for People with Diabetes*. London: Diabetes UK.

King's Fund Centre (1996). *Counting the Cost of Type 2 Diabetes*. London: King's Fund Centre/British Diabetic Association.

Reaven GM (1988). Role of insulin resistance in human disease. *Diabetes* **37**: 1595–1607.

Rett K (1999). The relation between insulin resistance and cardiovascular complications of the insulin resistance syndrome. *Diabetes, Obesity and Metabolism* **1**: S8–S16.

Stout R (1995). Ageing and glucose tolerance In Finucane P, Sinclair A (eds) *Diabetes in Old Age*. Chichester: John Wiley & Sons, pp. 21–45.

Providing the service

Questions this chapter will help you answer

- What care should a person with diabetes expect at diagnosis?
- What investigations are recommended?
- How do I know when to refer?
- Am I aiming at the correct targets for metabolic control?
- Should I screen for microalbuminuria?

> *Diabetes services are often not well-planned and few places are making provision for future increases in demands.*
>
> Audit Commission (2000)

Diabetes UK, in its excellent *Recommendations for the Provision of Services in Primary Care for People with Diabetes* (2005), confirms that all people with diabetes should be fully assessed at diagnosis and any need for referral identified. In type 1 diabetes, this will be urgent, whereas in type 2 disease, it may be necessary to manage complications.

Children and young people presenting with signs and/or symptoms suggestive of diabetes should always be referred urgently on the same day by telephone (or by fax or email where these referral systems are in place) to a specialist paediatric team experienced in the management of childhood diabetes so that the child can be admitted to hospital for the initiation of insulin therapy.

Adults who are clearly unwell, and/or who have ketones in their urine, and/or who have a blood glucose level of over 25.0 mmol/l should also be referred urgently on the same day by telephone (or by fax or email where such referral systems are in place) to a specialist diabetes team. Those who present with diabetic ketoacidosis or diabetic hyperosmolar non-ketotic syndrome will require immediate treatment in hospital to correct these abnormal metabolic states.

Young adults (aged under 30 years) should also be referred to a specialist diabetes team. The majority will require insulin therapy, the

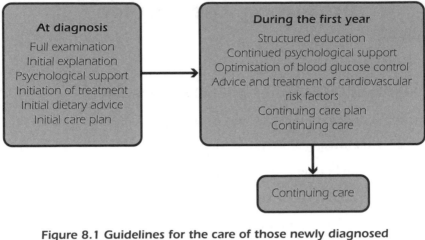

Figure 8.1 Guidelines for the care of those newly diagnosed with diabetes
(From Department of Health, 2002, with permission)

initiation of which can usually be undertaken on an outpatient basis, although some young adults will also require urgent specialist care.

People with newly presenting diabetes not included in the above categories may be managed within primary care (if knowledge and skills permit).

Diabetes UK has kindly allowed reproduction of care plans from *Recommendations for the Provision of Services in Primary Care for People with Diabetes* (2005). For further information, contact Diabetes UK (see Appendix 4).

Suggested guidelines for the initial care of people with newly diagnosed diabetes are set out in Figure 8.1 – the tasks performed and those responsible will vary according to local circumstances.

Initial explanation of diabetes and provision of psychological support

Once the diagnosis of diabetes has been confirmed, the nature of the condition and its management should be sensitively explained in a way that is tailored to the emotional and psychological state of the person and takes account of their social and cultural background. The impact of becoming diagnosed with a long-term condition should not be underestimated.

All those with newly diagnosed diabetes should be offered the opportunity to share any initial anxieties and concerns about the diagnosis and the implications for their future lifestyle. The possible effects of diabetes on occupation, driving and insurance should be discussed – if those concerned are drivers, they should be advised to inform the Driver and Vehicle Licensing Agency (DVLA) and their car insurance company. They should also be advised that they are exempt from prescription charges if started on medication for their diabetes.

Information about diabetes and its management in the form of leaflets, audiocassettes and/or videocassettes, in an appropriate language, should be provided for the individual to take away. It is recommended that this should include written information about Diabetes UK and details of the local Diabetes UK voluntary group (see Appendix 4). The psychological impact of the diagnosis should be assessed and any sources of immediate support (e.g. family/carers/friends) identified. Additional support should be provided as and when necessary.

Clinical examination and investigations

A clinical examination and investigations should be undertaken to:

- exclude any underlying causes of diabetes requiring specific treatment;
- identify any long-term complications of diabetes already present;
- assess cardiovascular risk;
- identify other conditions that may be associated with diabetes, such as other endocrine conditions.

Initial treatment and care

Treatment should be discussed with the person with diabetes and commenced as soon as possible.

1 Insulin may be required at diagnosis (Box 8.1).

2 People aged under 40 years with diabetes who are asymptomatic and who are overweight (body mass index (BMI) 25–30 kg/m^2) or obese (BMI>30 kg/m^2) should be advised to increase their physical activity levels, adopt a balanced diet and

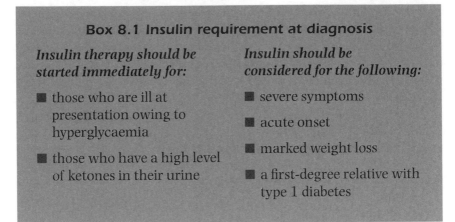

Box 8.1 Insulin requirement at diagnosis

Insulin therapy should be started immediately for:

- those who are ill at presentation owing to hyperglycaemia
- those who have a high level of ketones in their urine

Insulin should be considered for the following:

- severe symptoms
- acute onset
- marked weight loss
- a first-degree relative with type 1 diabetes

aim to reduce their calorie intake. Oral therapy or insulin may be necessary depending on glucose levels and symptoms. A high level of suspicion should be the norm in the slim person presenting with diabetes in this age group – he or she may require insulin more rapidly.

3 People aged over 40 with diabetes who are asymptomatic should initially be treated with diet, weight control and increased physical activity. They should be advised to increase their physical activity levels, adopt a balanced diet and, if they are overweight or obese, aim to reduce their calorie intake. If blood glucose control is not achieved within 3 months, treatment with oral hypoglycaemic agents should be commenced but may be indicated earlier if the individual is symptomatic or complications are present. Insulin treatment should be considered if blood glucose control is not achieved with diet, increased physical activity and combined drug therapy.

The majority of those with newly diagnosed diabetes will also need to make some changes to their eating habits. All should therefore receive culturally appropriate dietary advice. This should include advice on the distribution of meals in order to ensure a regular intake of carbohydrate across the day and the need to restrict the intake of fat, particularly saturated fat, and sugar. Those who are overweight or obese should be advised and supported to adopt a balanced diet as well as aiming to reduce their calorie intake.

All people with diabetes should also be advised of the benefits of increasing their physical activity level. All those with diabetes should be advised of the adverse effects of smoking and, where required, offered advice on how to stop smoking, as well as support to enable them to stop, including access to smoking cessation services. They should also be offered advice and treatment for any other cardiovascular risk factors.

The initial care plan should be discussed and agreed with the person with newly diagnosed diabetes. In addition, a named contact should be identified who will be responsible for providing support and information. The date of the next appointment should be agreed – regular reviews will initially be required.

Protocol

See Figures 8.2 and 8.3.

1 Enter the individual's details on the practice diabetes register or electronic record/template.

2 Discuss the general aspects of diabetes, and enquire about any family history and history of illness leading to diagnosis.

3 Listen and respond to preconceived ideas and anxieties. Establish the individual's existing knowledge of diabetes.

4 Discuss the person's general health.

5 Weigh the person and measure his or her height. Calculate the BMI and agree a target for ideal body weight as well as goals. BMI is calculated as:

Weight in kilograms / $(\text{Height in metres})^2$.

Waist measurement is a good predictor of metabolic control and is increasing in importance, central adiposity being responsible for many of the detrimental effects associated with diabetes.

6 Test the urine for glucose, ketones (if the person is unwell or the blood glucose level is over 15 mmol/l) and protein.

7 Measure the blood pressure and record this reading.

8 Test the blood for glucose, renal function and glycated haemoglobin (HbA_{1c}).

9 Arrange fasting cholesterol and triglyceride levels. These should ideally be measured after a period of glucose-lowering treatment because initial high triglyceride levels will fall to normal levels when the blood glucose is better controlled.

10 Practices should carry out the following tests on diagnosis and annually if indicated:

   a full blood count;

   b ECG;

   c microalbuminuria (by the locally agreed testing method; see Chapter 24);

   d liver function tests (especially if the person is on statins, angiotensin-converting enzyme inhibitors or glitazones);

   e renal function tests;

   f blood glucose level;

   g thyroid function tests.

11 Give a simple explanation of diabetes, and discuss any fears that the individual with diabetes may have.

12 Discuss lifestyle in relation to diabetes. Record levels of drinking and smoking, and advise strongly against the latter. If the person is ready to change, provide strategies for doing so.

13 Examine for complications of diabetes:

   a Examine the lower limbs.

   b Check the peripheral pulses and sensation.

   c Refer to the local diabetes retinal screening services.

   d If protein positive, take a mid-stream urine (MSU) specimen, to exclude infection.

14 Discuss food and meal-planning, and agree a healthy eating plan.

15 Record information in the practice records/electronic template and in the patient-held record (where these are available).

16 Arrange a prescription (if required) and the next appointment – regular and early reviews will be necessary until the person has a good understanding of diabetes and metabolic control has been achieved.

17 Notify the information to the district diabetes register (if one is in place).

18 It is important to note that individuals must be informed if data are held on a register outside the practice.

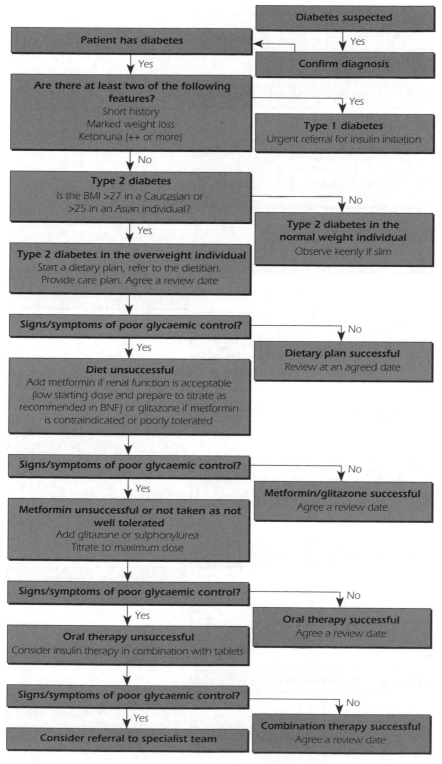

Figure 8.2 A scheme for managing people
with type 2 diabetes who are overweight

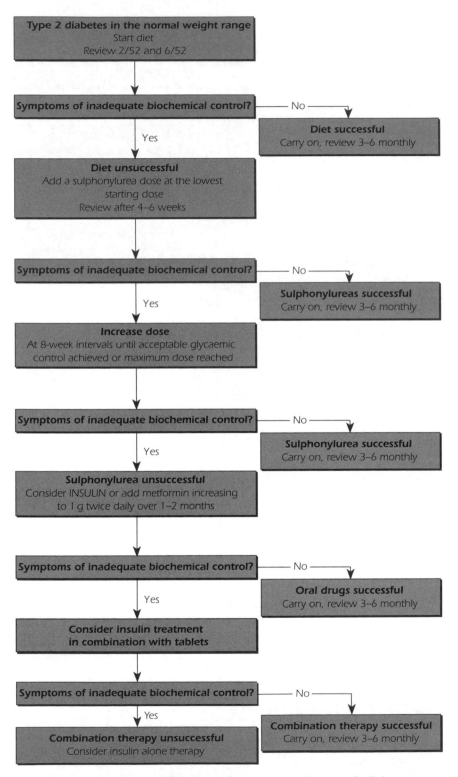

Figure 8.3 A scheme for managing people with type 2 diabetes who are of normal weight

Example of criteria for specialist referral

Referral is required in the following situations.

Urgent (telephone referral within 24 hours)

- For protracted vomiting – an emergency referral is required.
- For moderate or heavy ketonuria.
- For an acutely infected or ischaemic foot.
- In those who are newly diagnosed (type 1 diabetes).
- With an unplanned pregnancy.
- For unexplained loss of vision.

Routine

- If a pregnancy is planned.
- If insulin treatment is required (referral should be urgent in the newly diagnosed person) and there is no health professional in the practice with the knowledge and skills to initiate insulin therapy.
- If there are problems in patient management, for example if targets for control are not being met.
- If complications are detected, for example:
  - ◆ persistent proteinuria
  - ◆ raised serum creatinine
  - ◆ retinopathy
  - ◆ painful neuropathy, mononeuropathy, amyotrophy
  - ◆ deteriorating condition of the feet
  - ◆ uncontrolled hypertension
  - ◆ erectile dysfunction (impotence).
- Psychological problems complicating diabetes, for example:
  - ◆ failure to accept the diagnosis
  - ◆ a morbid fear of complications
  - ◆ family difficulties.

Sample protocol for performing a routine review

You should ensure that those with established diabetes are included on the diabetes register and are booked for regular appointments. A system for identifying and recalling defaulters should be organised and a policy agreed for the frequency of follow-up of people with diabetes. For routine visits where the management and understanding of the condition are established and uncomplicated, these may be required only two or three times a year.

Protocol

Organise blood test 2 weeks prior to review for:

- HbA_{1c} level
- fasting lipids
- renal function

and, if indicated:

- liver function
- thyroid function
- full blood count.

At the clinic appointment:

1 Weigh the person and agree goals for further management (keep the weight confidential, i.e. between the individual and the healthcare professional). Waist measurement is a good predictor of metabolic syndrome and is increasing in importance, central adiposity being responsible for many of the detrimental effects associated with diabetes.

2 Test the urine for glucose, ketones (if the person is unwell and there is poor glycaemic control) and protein. Send an MSU if protein is present, in order to exclude infection.

3 Check the individual's blood glucose meter technique (if used), including washing the hands prior to doing the test – this is often neglected.

4 Discuss the blood test results and agree therapy options.

5 Discuss the individual's general progress and well-being, and enquire about any problems (life changes, diet, etc.). If treatment is with insulin, check the injection sites.

6 Identify and discuss any weak spots in the individual's knowledge of diabetes and self-management skills. Check whether he or she is involved in a structured education plan.

7 Perform foot assessment according to local protocols if this is due or refer the person to the chiropodist/podiatrist.

8 Discuss and agree targets with the individual (see Chapters 12 and 17).

9 Record all the details on the diabetes record card and/or diabetes computer record/template.

10 Update the hand-held record or provide a printout of the relevant information.

11 Arrange the next appointment.

Sample protocol for performing an annual review

1 Weigh the person with diabetes and agree goals for further management (keep the weight confidential, i.e. between the individual and the healthcare professional).

2 Waist measurement is a good predictor of metabolic syndrome and is increasing in importance, central adiposity being responsible for many of the detrimental effects associated with diabetes.

3 Test the urine for glucose, ketones (if the person is unwell and there is poor glycaemic control) and protein. Send an MSU if protein is present, in order to exclude infection. Screen for microalbuminuria following local laboratory advice.

4 Enquire about:
   a claudication and possible circulatory problems (ask how the person sleeps at night and where. Claudication may lead to pain causing wakefulness, walking in the night to relieve it and/or sleeping in a chair);
   b changes in the eyes and feet;
   c symptoms of neuropathy, impotence;
   d chest pain, shortness of breath.

Examine the following to detect complications of diabetes:

a blood pressure;

   b peripheral pulses and sensation;

   c the lower limbs.

6 Visual acuity. Check that retinal screening has been performed by someone in the past year and refresh advice on dilated pupils: that the individual should not drive afterwards, and should take sunglasses if bright light is likely to dazzle them after the test.

7 Discuss the individual's general progress and well-being, enquiring about any problems relating to diabetes and whether any supplies are needed. If treatment is with insulin, check the injection sites.

8 Check the individual's blood glucose meter technique (if used), including washing the hands prior to doing test – this is often neglected.

9 Identify and discuss any weak spots in the knowledge of diabetes and self-management skills. Check whether the individual is involved in a structured education plan.

10 Discuss and agree targets with the person concerned (Table 8.1).

11 Record all the details on the diabetes record card and/or diabetes computer record/template.

12 Update the hand-held record or provide a printout of the relevant information.

13 Arrange any prescriptions needed and the next appointment.

14 Notify information to the district diabetes register (if one is in place).

Recall and follow-up

People with diabetes (whether those new to the practice or those who are newly diagnosed) need to understand how the diabetes service is organised, so the system of recall and follow-up should be explained. Should an individual have a problem regarding attendance (caused by employment shifts or family commitments), it is important that these problems are identified early on. The practice diabetes service should

Table 8.1 Targets to be discussed with the person with diabetes

	Desirable targets for people with type 1 diabetes	Desirable targets for people with type 2 diabetes
HbA$_{1c}$	≤6.5% (but ≤7.5% for those at risk of severe hypoglycaemia)	

SELF-MONITORED BLOOD GLUCOSE (mmol/l)		
Fasting preprandial	5.1–6.5 (Whole blood) 5.7–7.3 (Plasma)	<5.5 (Whole blood) <6.2 (Plasma)
Postprandial (2 hours after food)	7.6–9.0 (Whole blood) 8.5–10.1 (Plasma)	>7.5 (Whole blood) <8.4 (Plasma)
Before going to bed	6.0–7.5 (Whole blood) 6.7–8.4 (Plasma)	

BLOOD PRESSURE (mmHg)		
Normal albumin excretion rate	<130/80	<130/80
Abnormal albumin excretion rate	<120/70	<120/70

LIPIDS		
	Diabetes UK/NICE	Joint British Societies
Total cholesterol	<5.0 mmol/l	<4 mmol/l or 25% reduction
LDL cholesterol	<2.6 mmol/l	<2.0 mmol/l or 30% reduction
HDL cholesterol	≥1.0 mmol/l for men ≥1.2 mmol/l for women	Must be taken into consideration along with the above
Triglycerides	≤2.3 mmol/l	Must be taken into consideration along with the above

BODY MASS INDEX (kg/m^2)
<25.0 for Caucasians
<23.0 for those from an Asian background

Data from Diabetes UK (2005) and Joint British Societies (2005)
HbA$_{1c}$, glycated haemoglobin; HDL, high-density lipoprotein; LDL, low-density lipoprotein

be sufficiently flexible to accommodate certain particular difficulties and incorporate visits for surveillance to the housebound who are receiving no other healthcare (see Chapter 2).

Where no system is in existence, the following procedure is recommended:

1 Note the telephone number on the records.

2 Use a standard letter (see Chapter 6) inviting new patients to attend.

3 Agree a follow-up appointment at the end of each visit and record it in the hand-held record, or provide an appointment card with the agreed date and time and give it to the individual before his or her departure.

4 Keep a record of reviews and arrange recall by date of birth rather than by name. This allows people with diabetes to recognise that their annual review will be in the month of their birth.

5 Allow enough time for each person: 20 minutes for a routine follow-up visit, 30 minutes for an initial visit or an annual review.

6 Allow 5 minutes between consultations and 15 minutes (or more) at the end of each session for recording information and dealing with follow-up work (such as organising dietitian appointments, referral letters, chiropody/podiatry, etc.).

7 Allow for a little leeway in each session, if possible, for a person with diabetes requesting an unexpected or urgent visit or telephone advice.

Frequency of recall and follow-up

Note: it is not necessary, except in unusual circumstances, for people with diabetes to attend the practice every week or month to check their blood glucose level. A scheme such as this provides no benefit, promotes diabetes as an illness and discourages self-management.

Frequency of recall and follow-up may depend on the following:

■ The age, status and needs of the person with diabetes; this may relate to:
  ◆ being newly diagnosed
  ◆ being new to the practice

- being discharged from specialist care
- needing help with losing weight
- feet at risk
- impaired vision
- mobility problems
- glycaemic control
- other medical problems (which may affect diabetes)
- education requirements
- support (emotional) (family/other problems).

■ Realistic recall targets relating to the number to be seen in the practice cared for only by the practice team and those receiving shared care.

■ Frequency of specialist appointments where care is shared.

■ Available transport.

■ Doctor/nurse time allocated or available.

■ Time of year, which relates to practice workload and annual leave on the part of key team members.

In a small practice, diabetes sessions may only be required monthly or even bi-monthly. A larger practice or a practice with a large number of people with diabetes (e.g. where there is a high ethnic composition) may require weekly sessions.

Specific sessions may be allocated for the annual review as well as for appointments involving other health professionals such as the dietitian or podiatrist, or for structured education sessions.

The number of appointments for diabetes sessions or surgery visits should not be excessive if sufficient time has been spent on clinical care and education. Urgent or costly treatment may be avoided for the same reason:

■ Every person with diabetes should be seen at least twice a year (every 6 months).

■ People newly diagnosed with diabetes or those experiencing problems may need weekly visits for a while in order to achieve short-term goals and targets and so that they can become involved in structured education.

Notes

- Older people with diabetes are more likely to suffer with complications and concomitant conditions, so a more flexible approach involving other team members such as district nurses may need to be implemented.

- It is important to ensure that time, cost and travel are not proving too great a burden and are truly beneficial to each person concerned.

- The recall and follow-up system should be flexible and responsive to the needs of each person, reflecting organised, individualised care.

Screening for microalbuminuria

See Chapter 24.

References

Department of Health (2002). *National Service Framework for Diabetes. Supplementary Information.* London: DoH.

Diabetes UK (2005). *Recommendations for the Provision of Services in Primary Care for People with Diabetes.* London: Diabetes UK.

Joint British Societies (2005). Guidelines on prevention of cardiovascular disease in clinical practice. *Heart* **91**: 1–52.

9 Nurse prescribing in diabetes

Questions this chapter will help you answer

- What items can a nurse prescribe?

- What is the difference between a clinical management plan and a patient group direction?

- If I need a clinical management plan, what information does it need to contain?

- How do I get up-to-date information?

> *Services are finding it hard to cope with current demands ... and demands for support, treatments and specialist staff will increase.*
>
> Audit Commission (2000)

The background

- In 1986, the Cumberlege Report (Department of Health and Social Security, 1986) recommended allowing district nurses and health visitors to prescribe.

- In 1989, the first Crown Report (Department of Health, 1989) recommended the rapid implementation of this concept.

- In 1992, nurse prescribing pilots involving district nurses and health visitors were set up.

- In 1999, the Review of Prescribing, Supply and Administration of Medicines report (Department of Health, 1999) proposed:
  - the introduction of a new framework of prescribing, supply and administration of medicines whereby the majority of patients would continue to receive medicines on an individual patient-specific basis;

- ◆ that the prescribing authority of doctors, dentists and district nurses and health visitors would continue;
- ◆ that prescribing authority would be extended to include new groups of healthcare professionals; independent prescribers and dependent (now known as *supplementary*) prescribers.

■ In 2001, *extended formulary nurse prescribing* was introduced.

■ In 2002 came *supplementary prescribing*, defined as:

> a voluntary prescribing partnership between an independent prescriber and a supplementary prescriber, to implement an agreed patient-specific clinical management plan with the patient's agreement.

> (National Prescribing Centre, 2003)

■ In 2006, nurse independent prescribing became possible for those who had undertaken new training courses in England. Independent prescribing is defined (Department of Health, 2006) as:

> prescribing by a practitioner (e.g. doctor, dentist, nurse, pharmacist) responsible and accountable for the assessment of patients with undiagnosed or diagnosed conditions and for decisions about the clinical management required, including prescribing. Within medicines legislation the term used is 'appropriate practitioner'.

In partnership with an individual with diabetes, independent prescribing is one element of that person's clinical management. It requires an initial patient assessment, an interpretation of that assessment, a decision on safe and appropriate therapy, and a process for ongoing monitoring. The independent prescriber is responsible and accountable for at least this element of a person's care. Prescribing is usually carried out in the context of practice within a multidisciplinary healthcare team, either in a hospital or in a community setting, and within a single, accessible healthcare record. Scotland, Wales and Northern Ireland have formed local systems along the same lines.

Supplementary prescribing through a clinical management plan (CMP) for existing supplementary nurse prescribers will continue.

Types of nurse prescriber

Nurses have their own prescribing pads: form FP10P for National Health Service patients in England, form HS21(N) in Northern Ireland and form GP10(N2) in Scotland.

Qualified nurse independent prescribers and pharmacist independent prescribers are able to prescribe any licensed medicine for any medical condition – with the exception of some controlled drugs – as long as it is within their skills, knowledge and competence.

This extension to the role means that specialist nurses running diabetes and coronary heart disease clinics will be able to prescribe independently for those under their care. Pharmacists will be able to prescribe independently for the local community, for example for controlling high blood pressure, smoking cessation, diabetes, etc. This is intended to take the pressure off GPs, allowing them to focus on more complex cases and improving the availability of patient care. Nurses and pharmacists will have to have completed the relevant course.

Supplementary prescribers (previously known as 'dependent prescribers') are able to prescribe from the *British National Formulary* (BNF) as long as they possess the skills, knowledge and competencies to do so and have an agreed CMP with a doctor or dentist and the patient themselves.

Examples of possible diabetes-related prescriptions include:

- insulin – all licensed types
- oral hypoglycaemic agents
- anti-hypertensives
- lipid-lowering therapy
- anti-obesity therapy
- aspirin
- blood glucose testing strips
- glucagon injection.

A full list is provided in the current BNF.

Remember that the most expensive treatment is one that doesn't work or isn't taken.

At the time of writing, supplementary prescribers cannot prescribe controlled drugs and unlicensed drugs (unless they are part of a clinical trial that has a clinical trial certificate or exemption), but changes to legislation are occurring rapidly. Any nurse prescriber should adhere to seven principles of good prescribing (Box 9.1).

Box 9.1 Seven principles of good prescribing

1 Examine the holistic needs of the individual. Is a prescription necessary?

2 Consider the appropriate strategy

3 Consider the choice of product

4 Negotiate a 'contract' and achieve concordance with the individual

5 Review the individual on a regular basis

6 Ensure that record-keeping is both accurate and up to date

7 Reflect on your prescribing.

Supplementary prescribing

Key features of supplementary prescribing

The key features are:

- the importance of communication between the prescribing partners;

- the need for access to shared patient records;

- the fact that patients are treated as partners in their care and are involved at all stages in decision-making, including whether part of their care is delivered via supplementary prescribing.

Why adopt supplementary prescribing?

Supplementary prescribing:

- is intended to provide patients with quicker and more efficient access to medicines;

- will make the best use of the skills of trained nurses and pharmacists;

- is likely to reduce doctors' workloads, freeing up their time to concentrate on patients with more complicated conditions and more complex treatments.

Name of Patient:			Patient medication sensitivities/allergies:		
Patient identification e.g. ID number, date of birth:					
Independent Prescriber(s):			Supplementary Prescriber(s)		
Condition(s) to be treated			Aim of treatment		
Medicines that may be prescribed by SP:					
Preparation		Indication	Dose schedule		Specific indications for referral back to the IP
Guidelines or protocols supporting Clinical Management Plan:					
Frequency of review and monitoring by:					
Supplementary prescriber		Supplementary prescriber and independent prescriber			
Process for reporting ADRs:					
Shared record to be used by IP and SP:					
Agreed by independent prescriber(s)	Date	Agreed by supplementary prescriber(s)		Date	Date agreed with patient/carer

Figure 9.1 Department of Health suggested clinical management plan proforma for teams that have full co-terminus access to patient records

ADR, adverse drug reaction; IP, independent prescriber; SP, supplementary prescriber

Essential features

- An independent prescriber (normally a GP in diabetes in general practice) has diagnosed the condition.

- This person has made a full assessment of the patient.

- A CMP has been agreed (Figure 9.1).

- The supplementary prescriber nurse must work within the boundaries of the plan.

- There should be shared records between the nurse and the GP; if this is not possible, an alternative CMP should be used (Figure 9.2).

The clinical management plan

A CMP is required by law for supplementary prescribing to take place. It will be agreed between the patient, the doctor and the nurse prescriber (National Prescribing Centre, 2003). The CMP:

- is tailored to the individual;

- is agreed by the patient, GP and prescribing nurse;

- should be fairly simple and quick to complete. A toolkit is provided on the Nurse Prescriber website (see the list at the end of the chapter).

- does not need to duplicate medical information.

The CMP should contain enough detail to ensure patient safety and must contain the following:

- The name of the patient.

- The illness or conditions that may be treated.

- The date on which the plan is to take effect.

- The date for review by all parties concerned.

- Reference to the class or description of medicines or types of appliance that may be prescribed or administered under the plan; this does not need to relate to a specific medication, for example 'insulin', as an encompassing term, is acceptable rather than the specific insulin, such as 'NovoMix 30'.

- Any restrictions or limitations on the strength or dose of any medicine.

- The duration of use of the medication.

Name of Patient:	Patient medication sensitivities/allergies:
Patient identification e.g. ID number, date of birth:	
Current medication:	Medical history:
Independent prescriber(s) Contact details [tel/email address]	Supplementary prescriber(s) Contact details [tel/email address]
Condition(s) to be treated:	Aim of treatment:

Medicines that may be prescribed by SP:			
Preparation	Indication	Dose schedule	Specific indications for referral back to the IP

Guidelines or protocols supporting Clinical Management Plan:

Frequency of review and monitoring by:

Supplementary prescriber	Supplementary prescriber and independent prescriber

Process for reporting ADRs:

Shared record to be used by IP and SP:

Agreed by independent prescriber(s)	Date	Agreed by supplementary prescriber(s)	Date	Date agreed with patient/carer

Figure 9.2 Department of Health suggested clinical management plan proforma for teams in which the supplementary prescriber does not have co-terminus access to the medical record
ADR, adverse drug reaction; IP, independent prescriber; SP, supplementary prescriber

Note: The CMP may include a reference to published national or local guidelines. These must, however, clearly identify the range of the relevant medicinal products to be used in the treatment of the patient, and the CMP should draw attention to the relevant part of the guideline.

- Relevant warnings about known sensitivities of the patient to, or known difficulties of the patient with, particular medicines or appliances.

- The arrangements for notification of:

  - suspected or known reactions to any medicine that may be prescribed or administered under the plan, and suspected or known adverse reactions to any other medicine taken at the same time as any medicine prescribed or administered under the plan;

  - incidents occurring with the appliance that might lead, might have led or have led to the death or serious deterioration of state of health of the patient.

- The circumstances in which the supplementary prescriber should refer to, or seek the advice of, the doctor or dentist who is party to the plan.

Any guideline referred to also needs to be easily accessible.

Training

Nurses wishing to become prescribers must complete the relevant course. It is now possible to combine extended and supplementary nurse prescribing courses in many areas. Distance learning is becoming more available. Pharmacists are also able to undertake supplementary prescribing and may work more closely with primary care teams.

Patient group directions

Patient group directions are not to be confused with nurse prescribing (Table 9.1).

Table 9.1 Comparison between patient group directions and nurse prescribing

Patient group directions	Nurse prescribing
Groups	Individuals
Specific individuals are not identified	Specific individuals are named
Written instructions	Agreed clinical management plans

References

Department of Health (1986). *Neighbourhood Nursing: A Focus for Care* (Cumberlege Report). London: Department of Health and Social Security.

Department of Health (1989). *Report of the Advisory Group on Nursing Prescribing* (Crown Report). London: DoH.

Department of Health (1999). *Final Report on the Review of Prescribing, Supply and Administration of Medicines.* London: DoH.

Department of Health (2006). *Improving Patients' Access to Medicines: A Guide to Implementing Nurse and Pharmacist Independent Prescribing within the NHS in England.* London: DoH.

National Prescribing Centre (2003). *Supplementary Prescribing: A Resource to Help Healthcare Professionals to Understand the Framework and Opportunities.* Liverpool: NPC.

Further reading

Department of Health (2004). *Management of Medicines: A Resource To Support Implementation of the Wider Aspects of Medicines Management for the National Service Frameworks for Diabetes, Renal Services and Long-Term Conditions.* London: DoH.

Websites

Nurse prescriber: www.nurse-prescriber.co.uk
National Prescribing Centre: www.npc.co.uk
Prodigy: www.prodigy.nhs.uk

10 Non-medical treatment of diabetes

Questions this chapter will help you answer

- What first-line advice do I need to discuss with people with diabetes?

- Do I understand up-to-date dietary advice?

- Is 'glycaemic index' useful to patients?

- How do I tackle other lifestyle issues?

- Am I involving people with diabetes in agreed goals and care plans?

> *...the incidence of Type 2 diabetes could be reduced by lifestyle changes in the broader community.*
>
> Audit Commission (2000)

Aims of treatment

- To relieve symptoms.

- To ensure a satisfactory lifestyle.

- To prevent unwanted effects of treatment (i.e. hypoglycaemia, side effects of drugs).

- To reduce the risks of acute complications (hypoglycaemia, hyperglycaemia).

- To reduce the risks of long-term complications.

Relieving symptoms

Treatment should aim first of all to relieve symptoms. A holistic approach is essential here: the focus should not be on glycaemic control alone but on the management of hypertension, dyslipidaemia and lifestyle factors, all of which may impact on the person's life.

Ensuring a satisfactory lifestyle

People with diabetes and their families need sufficient information to make any lifestyle adjustments required by their treatment and monitoring, and to enable independence in their management of the condition. It is important that activity, exercise, eating habits, family and social life, and work are all considered in relation to the suggested treatment.

Preventing unwanted effects of treatment

The person with diabetes and his or her carers should be part of the care team, involved in the decision-making process and agreeing goals and targets. They need education on self-management and the prevention of problems arising from drug therapy, for example hypoglycaemic attacks caused by sulphonylureas or insulin, as well as on the benefits of taking their medication as prescribed.

Reducing the risks of acute complications

Information is required on the importance of:

- regular eating;
- regular activity suitable to mobility;
- the sufficient consumption of carbohydrate;
- monitoring of weight and/or waist measurement (by the person themselves and/or the practice) as a reduction in weight or girth may indicate a need for therapy review;
- noting and reporting symptoms of hypoglycaemia (see Chapter 12);
- advice regarding the prevention of hypoglycaemia (see Chapter 12);
- the side effects of drugs prescribed (the symptoms and the fact that these should be reported to the care team);
- cardiovascular risk prevention, for example stopping smoking, blood pressure management.

Preventing and reducing the risk of diabetes complications (types 1 and 2 diabetes)

See Chapter 24.

Starting treatment (type 2 diabetes)

Note: It is anticipated that people with type 1 diabetes will have their treatment started through the specialist diabetes team. The following therefore only considers type 2 diabetes.

Some important points

■ Assess preconceived ideas and knowledge about diabetes and its treatment. Reassurance, support and information are needed. People with diabetes, newly diagnosed, are often concerned that they will be on a 'strict diet' for the rest of their lives or are frightened that they will be 'on the needle'.

■ Explain that there are three types of treatment for diabetes:

◆ A healthy eating plan for life in combination with regular activity.

◆ A healthy eating plan, regular activity and oral medication.

◆ A healthy eating plan, regular activity and insulin with or without oral medication.

■ Explain that treatment is ongoing and that it may be changed if symptoms persist and blood glucose levels remain high.

■ Emphasise that, should a change in treatment become necessary, this does not mean failure on the part of the person with diabetes. Type 2 diabetes is progressive, and treatment options have to be tailored to this.

■ Explain that the treatment is individually prescribed and that the treatment and its effects are particular to each person.

■ Emphasise that lifestyle changes can reduce the need for medication and promote well-being.

■ People with diabetes themselves may not be an accurate source of information.

The treatment

■ The treatment prescribed will depend on the age, weight, lifestyle and any other medical conditions of the person concerned (being of particular importance in elderly people).

■ WARNING! Patients should not be started on treatment with drugs before a full assessment of their weight, dietary habits, activity levels and self-care targets has been discussed.

■ WARNING! No treatment should be started before the diagnosis has been confirmed.

■ A healthy eating plan is the first line of treatment in almost all cases, combined with regular activity.

■ It is important, when planning treatment, to distinguish between people with diabetes who are of normal weight and those who are overweight with type 2 diabetes.

■ It is usually clinically obvious that the person concerned is overweight. However, a body mass index (BMI) of greater than 25 indicates this condition – the formula for calculating the BMI is given in Chapter 8. A tape measure can also be deployed – a measurement taken round the waist (not under or over the belly!) of over 35 inches (89 cm) for a woman and over 40 inches (102 cm) for a man increases the risk.

Examples of treatment schemes are shown in Figures 8.2 and 8.3.

Dietary and lifestyle support for people with diabetes

Diabetes UK (2005) recommends that all people with newly diagnosed diabetes should be assessed by a registered dietitian, who will provide a tailored and individualised dietary care plan based on the latest evidence of effectiveness.

Issues that should be addressed include the need for people with diabetes to:

■ eat regular meals planned around wholegrain, starchy foods, such as bread, chapattis, potatoes, yam, plantain, rice, pasta, dhal and wholegrain cereals;

■ eat at least five portions of fruit and vegetables each day;

■ reduce their calorie intake if overweight or obese, and increase their physical activity;

■ achieve and maintain a healthy weight;

- reduce their dietary intake of fat, particularly saturated fat;

- reduce their sucrose intake;

- aim to include more foods with a low glycaemic index (GI);

- reduce their dietary salt intake;

- drink alcohol in moderation (less than 14 units per week for women and less than 21 units per week for men) – excess alcohol can cause weight gain, high blood pressure and dyslipdaemia, and in those taking sulphonylurea drugs or insulin can make hypoglycaemia more severe. If alcohol is consumed, this should be with or after food. Alcohol also can mask awareness of the symptoms of hypoglycaemia;

- be advised that special diabetic foods are not necessary – they can be expensive and are often high in fat and calories.

People taking hypoglycaemic drugs and insulin will need further advice on dietary management to balance their food intake and physical activity levels with their medication.

Dietary changes need to be agreed at a pace suited to the individual – monthly follow-up appointments are recommended in the initial stages after diagnosis or at times of transition, such as when medication is changed.

People with diabetes who present with possible eating disorders (e.g. bingeing) should be referred to a clinical psychologist and dietitian for a joint programme of care.

Reducing cardiovascular risk

The following dietary changes particularly aim to reduce the risk of heart disease:

- Choose monounsaturated fat – found in olive oil, rapeseed oil and groundnut oil.

- Aim to eat two portions of oil-rich fish each week to boost the intake of omega-3 oils. For strict vegetarians, alternative sources include flaxseed oil, rapeseed oil, walnuts and tofu.

- Reduce dietary saturated fat, which is found mainly in animal products such as meat fat, cheese, butter, ghee and cream.

- Also limit the intake of hydrogenated vegetable oils and *trans* fatty acids – found in some margarines, biscuits, pastries and processed foods.

- Have only a moderate intake of polyunsaturated fat, such as sunflower oil/spreads.

- Include some low-fat dairy foods, such as semi-skimmed or skimmed milk and low-fat or virtually fat-free yoghurt, to provide calcium.

- A 125 ml glass of wine equals 1.5 units of alcohol, and half a pint of 3.5% beer equals 1 unit. Units of alcohol should be kept under the recommended level.

- Eat more fruit and vegetables: aim for at least five helpings per day. Fresh, frozen, tinned in natural juice or dried is fine.

- Eat more pulses, such as beans and lentils.

- Increase the use of fresh rather than processed foods.

Recommended dietary changes for people with hypertension and/or early renal problems

In addition, the following dietary changes are needed to address hypertension and/or early renal problems:

- Tackle obesity.

- Reduce salt intake by not adding it at the table and avoiding obviously salty foods such as crisps, bombay mix, salted nuts and cured meats and fish.

- Reduce the portion sizes of protein foods such as meat, fish, poultry and cheese.

- Keep alcohol intake within healthy limits.

Tackling obesity

Measurements of waist circumference provide a useful guide to the need for an individual to lose weight: a waist circumference of more than 40 inches (102 cm) in Caucasian men and 35 inches (89 cm) in Caucasian women, or more than 35 inches (89 cm) in South Asian men and 31.5 inches (80 cm) in South Asian women, is associated with a substantially increased risk to health (Stuhldreher et al, 1994).

A 10 kg weight loss can result in (Goldstein, 1992):

- a 30% fall in the number of diabetes-related deaths;

- a 10 mmHg reduction in systolic blood pressure;

- a 20 mmHg reduction in diastolic blood pressure;
- a 50% reduction in fasting glucose in people with newly diagnosed diabetes;
- a 10% reduction in total cholesterol level;
- a 13% reduction in low-density lipoprotein (LDL) cholesterol;
- a 30% reduction in triglyceride concentration;
- an 8% increase in high-density lipoprotein (HDL) cholesterol.

Even if patients are unable to lose weight, it is still worthwhile for them to set a goal to maintain their weight, without gaining weight, which can improve diabetes control and reduce their risk of developing heart disease.

When helping a person with diabetes to lose weight:

- establish their readiness to make dietary and lifestyle changes and explore behavioural and/or social barriers to change;
- agree a realistic weight loss goal – aim for a reduction of 5–10 kg or 10% of body weight;
- agree dietary changes at a pace suitable to the person with diabetes – this may only be two or three changes, but ensure that there is no risk of hypoglycaemia;
- encourage them to start an exercise plan and to aim to undertake moderate physical activity for 30 minutes every day;
- provide regular and ongoing support, to maintain the patient's motivation.

Remember that the type and dose of insulin, and of medication, may need to be adjusted if carbohydrate intake is reduced and/or physical activity is increased.

- 'Stop-gap' advice, backed up with written information, is acceptable initially.
- The practice nurse or other designated member(s) of the primary care team can give dietary advice if he or she is appropriately trained to do so.
- Access to a dietitian should be provided if there is no trained member of the primary care team able to provide the initial dietary advice.
- Ongoing support will be needed.

Healthy eating and diabetes

■ Modification of food intake is almost always the first line of treatment.

■ The diet for a person with diabetes is not 'special': it is a healthy way of eating, recommended for everyone.

■ It is important that an adequate and balanced nutritional intake is maintained (particularly in an older person, who may have a diminished appetite).

■ It is important to remember the social aspects of meal-planning, shopping, cooking and meal time in relation to family life. If there is a family life change (e.g. retirement, bereavement of a partner), this can have a profound effect on eating habits.

■ 'Healthy eating' for diabetes is of benefit to all family members, and dietary advice should emphasise this point.

■ No 'special' arrangements are required: adaptations to the usual food eaten are all that is needed.

■ Diabetes UK produces the booklets *Eating Well with Diabetes, Weight Creeping up on You?: Diabetes and Weight Management* and *Food Choices and Diabetes*. These booklets provide general dietary advice.

Dietary recommendations for people with diabetes

A combination of up-to-date research and the Diabetes UK's dietary recommendations for people with diabetes (Figure 10.1) has seen many changes in the advice. Advice is summarised in this section.

■ The concept of the GI (see later in the chapter) has allowed more flexibility in dietary intake and shows that certain types of starchy carbohydrate foods help to control blood glucose levels more effectively.

■ Rapidly absorbed carbohydrate foods (e.g. sweets, chocolates, sweet drinks) should be kept for special occasions and situations such as illness, or as a snack before strenuous activity.

Healthy eating is important to help control your diabetes. It is best to make small but permanent changes to your diet and lifestyle. Short-term dramatic changes that you cannot keep up for long are not as effective as smaller changes you can continue.

What are the important rules for management of diabetes?

■ Eat at regular times, including some breakfast, a lunchtime meal or snack, and an early evening meal

■ Include starchy foods, particularly the wholegrain varieties, at each meal e.g. bread, rice, pasta, pulses, potatoes, porridge, breakfast cereals

■ Aim for 5 portions (servings) of fruit and/or vegetables every day. (Don't count potatoes as one of the 5)

■ It is best to avoid foods high in sugar. Swap high sugar foods for fruit or low calorie puddings or low calorie snack items. It is not necessary to buy "diabetic" foods

■ A reduction in fats, oil, and fatty food will help with weight control. This does not apply to oily fish. Moderate portions of mackerel, herring, sardines or other oily fish should be taken twice weekly

■ Be careful not to use too much salt

■ Drink plenty of fluid – at least 8–10 cups per day (1 cup = 300ml). Include a variety of fluids e.g. water, low calorie squash, tea, coffee, but limit fruit juice to one small glass per day and avoid drinks containing added sugar. Alcohol may be taken in moderation

■ Try to increase your exercise or activity levels. Even small changes are beneficial, but aim for a 30 minute walk at least 5 times a week

■ Make sure that you achieve and maintain a sensible weight. If you are overweight ask about a referral to a weight management programme

**Figure 10.1 Dietary recommendations
from West Surrey State Registered Dietitians**
(Reproduced with permission)

So what can I eat?

A sample menu is shown overleaf. Remember that snacks, puddings, cakes and biscuits should only be eaten in small quantities, even when choosing low-fat or low-sugar varieties.

Instead of . . .	Try these . . .
White bread, sugar-coated breakfast cereals, croissants	Granary or wholemeal bread, porridge, wholegrain breakfast cereals
Sugar for sweetening drinks, fruit or custard	Artificial sweetener e.g. Canderel, Sweetex, Hermesetas, Splenda
Squashes and fizzy drinks	Low-calorie versions with no added sugar
Desserts & puddings, milk puddings, jellies, canned fruits in syrup	Canned fruit in juice, low-calorie/diet yoghurts, fresh fruit or sugar-free jelly or low-calorie instant whip or mousses
Cakes, biscuits, crisps	Fresh fruit, rice cake or a plain biscuit (oat biscuit, Rich Tea, garibaldi or low-fat digestive). A scone or plain tea cake is acceptable if you are not overweight
Jam, marmalade or honey	Reduced sugar jam. Marmite or peanut butter in small amounts
Fried & fatty foods	Use only small amounts of oil in cooking. Choose lean meats & remove any visible fat. Choose lower fat ready prepared meals
Butter, lard, ghee, hard margarine	Choose a margarine or low-fat spread labelled 'high in mono or polyunsaturates'. Use sparingly
Full-fat milk and cheeses	Semi-skimmed or skimmed milk, Lower fat cheeses such as Edam, Camembert, cottage cheese or reduced fat cheddar

Figure 10.1 (continued) **Dietary recommendations from West Surrey State Registered Dietitians**
(Reproduced with permission)

```
                           Sample Menu

Breakfast:              Porridge or wholegrain cereal
                        Wholemeal toast with low-fat spread
                        Fruit or small fruit juice

Snack Meal:             Granary or wholemeal bread or roll
                        Mixed salad vegetables
                        Lean meat or fish or beans
                        or egg or low-fat cheese
                        Fresh fruit or low calorie yoghurt

Main Meal:              Potatoes or rice or pasta
                        Large serving of vegetables or salad
                        Lean meat or fish or pulses or vegetarian dish
                        Fruit or low calorie dessert

Between Meals:          Fruit or a plain biscuit if required
                        Water, low calorie squash, tea, coffee
```

Figure 10.1 (continued) **Dietary recommendations
from West Surrey State Registered Dietitians**
(Reproduced with permission)

■ Hypoglycaemic attacks should be treated with rapidly absorbed carbohydrate, for example glucose tablets, ordinary fizzy drinks or ordinary Lucozade or glucose drinks. They should not be treated with chocolate, cakes or biscuits as these do not allow a quick enough increase in blood glucose level to help. Quick-acting carbohydrate should be followed up with longer-acting food to maintain blood glucose levels over the longer term; this could be a sandwich, or a meal if this has been delayed.

■ Fibre has proved not to be as beneficial in controlling blood glucose levels as was once thought. Only 'soluble fibre', for example pulses, oats, pasta, fruit and vegetables, helps to control blood glucose levels. Having insoluble fibre in 'wholemeal' versions does not actually help to control blood glucose levels any more than do the 'white' versions. Fibre does, however, have other health benefits, such as reducing the risk of bowel cancer, diverticular disease and constipation. Plenty of fluids are needed to help this type of fibre to work properly.

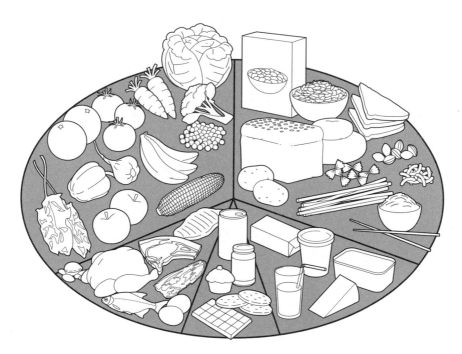

Figure 10.2 The balance of good health

■ Foods lower in energy content than their sweetened equivalents, such as low-calorie squashes, diet fizzy drinks, diet yoghurts, fruit tinned in natural juice and artificial sweeteners, may be used (but not to treat hypoglycaemic attacks).

■ Figure 10.2 is a useful tool for menu planning. You can enlarge this figure by photocopying and give it to your patients, or you can obtain coloured posters from Diabetes UK. It is useful to demonstrate quantities of different foods and the proportion recommended of each in a plate model.

■ The recommended portion sizes need to be adjusted according to the individual's weight, but the balance will still be the same.

Fat

■ Monounsaturated fats should be used if fat is needed in cooking. These have the added benefit of lowering fasting plasma triglyceride and very-low-density lipoprotein (VLDL) cholesterol concentrations, and increasing HDL cholesterol, with no change in LDL cholesterol level. Monounsaturated fats include olive oil and pure vegetable oil made from rapeseed.

- Eat less fatty meat and fewer meat products; choose smaller portions of meat, fish and poultry.

- Cut down on high-fat diary products such as cheese, butter and cream.

- Use a low-fat spread instead of butter or margarine.

- Use skimmed or semi-skimmed milk instead of whole milk. Skimmed milk has fewer calories, but some people find that semi-skimmed milk is initially more palatable when changing from full-fat milk.

Salt

Reduce salt intake by:

- eating fewer salty foods, such as precooked meats, smoked fish or cheese;

- adding less salt during cooking;

- cutting down on salt added at the table.

Alcohol

- A maximum of three 'units' for men and two for women per day is recommended, after consultation with a physician.

- 1 'unit' = half pint of ordinary beer or lager, or a single measure of spirits (whisky, gin, rum, vodka, etc.), or a glass of wine, or a measure of vermouth or aperitif.

- It is better to drink less alcohol. If weight is a problem, consumption should be limited to one drink per day.

- The patient should aim to have at least two or three alcohol-free days each week.

- Low-carbohydrate beers and lagers should be avoided as these are high in both calories and alcohol.

- High-alcohol beers, special brews and 'Pils'-type alcohol should be avoided. Just stick to ordinary beers and lagers, and spirits with a low sugar content.

- Alcohol lowers the blood sugar so it is important not to drink on an empty stomach. Meals or snacks should **not** be replaced with alcohol.

- Mixers should be 'diet' or low calorie.

Special diabetic foods

■ These are not recommended: they may contain more fat or energy than other foods and may be low in fibre.

■ Sorbitol is used to sweeten them, and this may cause diarrhoea.

■ Fructose may also be used in diabetic products. This has the same energy value as sugar. No more than 25 g/day should be taken.

■ A small piece of ordinary (sweetened) cake or chocolate on the odd occasion, preferably taken at the end of a meal, is not likely to be harmful. Remember that these foods may add weight if they are eaten too often.

■ Diabetic squashes are no better than the low-calorie squashes found in most supermarkets. Use 'low-calorie', 'diet' or 'sugar-free' drinks.

Important:

■ Diabetic foods are expensive and unnecessary.

■ Remember Diabetes UK's recommendations regarding the use of sugar: if the person with diabetes is not overweight and follows a high-starchy carbohydrate, high-fibre, low-fat diet, up to 25 g of sugar can be used each day. This should be spread throughout the day and used in combination with high-fibre foods where possible. Sugar should not be used in drinks or on cereals where artificial sweeteners can be used.

Further helpful hints, recipes and cooking tips are available from local dietitians and Diabetes UK. These include special cultural modifications, for example for the South Asian (i.e. from the Indian subcontinent) or African/Caribbean person with diabetes. For more information on the eating patterns and advice to give African/Caribbean individuals and people from South Asia, see Chapter 15.

Schedule of dietary treatment for people with type 2 diabetes who are overweight

■ Assess food and alcohol intake (the types of food and alcohol enjoyed and the amounts taken during the day).

- Assess any activity or exercise taken (on a daily basis).

- Agree targets for weight loss – both short and long term. These targets should be realistic, possible and desired by the person with diabetes.

- Provide appropriate support.

- Monitor and support regularly, for example monthly if weight loss is not seen within 3 months and the blood sugar level remains elevated.

- Aim for a slow weight loss by reducing food intake and not skipping meals. Aim to support the patient in losing 0.5–1.0 kg (1–2 pounds) per week.

Schedule of dietary treatment for people with type 2 diabetes who are of normal weight

- Assess food and alcohol intake (the types of food and alcohol enjoyed and the amounts taken during the day).

- Assess activity or exercise taken (on a daily basis).

- Discuss targets for maintaining weight – both short and long term.

- Provide appropriate support.

- Encourage regular activity and exercise.

- Monitor at regular intervals to check on weight regulation and blood sugar level control.

- Observe for unplanned weight loss as insulin may be required. *Note:* This is very important as it is often missed in primary care, even by good practices.

Activity for health

- Physical activity will help with weight loss, regulate blood glucose level and improve insulin sensitivity.

- Advice about healthy activity levels should be realistic and possible, and should include information on the local facilities available (e.g. swimming pools, health clubs). It is important to find out what the person with diabetes enjoys doing.

- The information provided should include costs, which may be prohibitive for some people.

- Advice regarding increased activity (particularly for those not used to it) should be given only in association with a medical examination and advice.

- Recommendations from the Department of Health (2004) are given in Box 10.1.

- It is important to build any activity levels slowly. Ideally, the pace should make you breathe a little more quickly but not be so out of breath that you cannot talk. The recommended 30 minutes can be spread throughout the day in 5–10-minute slots.

Glycaemic index

GI is very much in vogue, and you may be approached by people with diabetes asking you about it. The British Dietetic Association (2004) suggests this is the latest in a long line of food fads for diets. Research shows, however, that it can be useful in diabetes control.

In this concept, foods are ranked on how quickly they raise the blood glucose level. Foods that are digested quickly raise the blood glucose level quickly and vice versa, but there are some confusing anomalies.

- *High GI (>70)*: glucose, baked potatoes, cornflakes, digestive biscuits, fizzy high-sugar drinks. Fatty foods high in GI are high in saturated fats too: pies, pastries, croissants.

- *Intermediate GI (55–70)*: basmati rice, taco shells, bananas.

- *Low GI (<55)*: Pasta, whole-grain breads, porridge, reduced-sugar muesli, bran-based breakfast cereals, plain sponge cake, lentils, Rich Tea biscuits, sweet potatoes and new boiled potatoes in their skins, nuts (limit to a small handful – 28 g (1 oz) a day), some fruits (apple yes; melon and grapes no), vegetables (raw or lightly cooked), salads (choose low-fat dressings) and basmati rice.

Many healthy foods such as vegetables have a low GI, but so may high fat content meals. Just because a food has a low GI doesn't make it healthy. As always, a holistic approach needs to be borne in mind. Remember that a low GI does not necessarily encourage a low lipid profile.

Box 10.1 Recommendations for active living throughout the life course

- Children and young people should achieve a total of at least 60 minutes of at least moderate intensity physical activity each day. At least twice a week this should include activities to improve bone health (activities that produce high physical stresses on the bones), muscle strength and flexibility.

- For general health benefit, adults should achieve a total of at least 30 minutes a day of at least moderate intensity physical activity on 5 or more days of the week.

- The recommended levels of activity can be achieved either by doing all the daily activity in one session, or through several shorter bouts of activity of 10 minutes or more. The activity can be lifestyle activity [activity that is performed as part of everyday life, such as climbing stairs or brisk walking] or structured exercise or sport, or a combination of these.

- More specific activity recommendations for adults are made for beneficial effects for individual diseases and conditions. *All* movement contributes to energy expenditure and is important for weight management. It is likely that, for many people, 45–60 minutes of moderate intensity physical activity a day is necessary to prevent obesity. For bone health, activities that produce high physical stresses on the bones are necessary.

- The recommendations for adults are also appropriate for older adults. Older people should take particular care to keep moving and retain their mobility through daily activity. Additionally, specific activities that promote improved strength, co-ordination and balance are particularly beneficial for older people.

The principle is that regulating fluctuations in blood glucose levels may stave off hunger, allowing the individual to feel full for longer. Evidence shows that foods with a low GI create a slow rise in blood sugars, leading to a better overall control of blood sugars – a benefit to people with diabetes. Other positive aspects of GI are a reduction in cardiac risk factors, benefits in terms of insulin resistance and a fall in

Box 10.2 Healthy eating and diabetes

■ Eat regular meals and do not miss meals. If you get hungry in between meals, choose healthy snacks such as fresh fruit, vegetable sticks, diet yoghurt, two Rich Tea biscuits or a slice of bread.

■ Eat starchy carbohydrate foods with each meal, for example bread, potatoes, oats, cereals, basmati rice, sweet potato, chapatti, yam or couscous.

■ Cut down on fried and fatty foods, such as butter, margarine, oil, cheese, fatty meats and pastries/pies. If you need to use fat, choose olive- or rapeseed-based oils and margarines. Use semi-skimmed/skimmed milk and margarines labelled 'low-fat spread'. Choose lean meats and cut away all visible fat. Try to grill, bake, steam or cook with very little oil instead. Look for foods labelled 'low/reduced fat', but make sure that they are also low in sugar.

■ Aim to eat at least five portions of fruit or vegetables each day, such as apples, oranges, bananas that are not too ripe and any vegetables you like.

■ Aim to reduce your sugar intake. Cut down on sugar, cakes, confectionery and sugar in drinks. If you need some sweetness in drinks, use sweeteners. You can also choose diet pop and no-added-sugar squash, which taste sweet but contain no sugar. Similarly, choose reduced sugar jam/marmalade, sugar-free desserts and sugar-free jelly. Avoid sweets, biscuits, cakes and all foods labelled 'Diabetic'.

■ Check whether you need to lose weight. Choose a realistic target and lose weight slowly (0.5–1 kg (1–2 pounds) per week).

■ Be careful not to add too much salt in cooking and at the table. Give yourself time to get used to the taste of less salt.

■ Be careful not to drink too much alcohol. It is best to avoid drinking on an empty stomach.

■ Avoid foods labelled 'Diabetic'. They are expensive and do not help you control your diabetes.

the risk of type 2 diabetes. Studies published on GI point to improved glycaemic control, and having a low-GI meal actually helps in glycaemic control of the next meal.

Eating foods with a low GI can reduce the risk of hypoglycaemic episodes. It is no longer good practice to advise eating chocolate when someone has a 'hypo' because the GI of chocolate is not high enough to increase the blood sugar quickly enough. Everyone digests foods at a different rate, so the GI concept is not the answer for everyone. Home monitoring helps the individual to see whether dietary changes make a difference. GI can only assist with weight reduction if combined with a reduced calorie intake and the maintenance of a regular activity level (see above).

It is worthwhile advising people with diabetes of local initiatives, such as Weight Watchers or Exercise on Prescription, to help them achieve their personal goals.

Box 10.2 summarises recommendations for healthy eating for people with diabetes.

References

British Dietetic Association (2004). *Glycaemic Index. Is it Just Hype?* London: BDA.

Department of Health (2004). *At Least Five a Week. Evidence on the Impact of Physical Activity and its Relationship to Health. A Report from the Chief Medical Officer.* London: DoH.

Diabetes UK (2005). *Recommendations for the Provision of Services in Primary Care for People with Diabetes.* London: Diabetes UK.

Goldstein DJ (1992). Beneficial health effects of modest weight loss. *International Journal of Obesity and Related Metabolic Disorders* **16**: 397–415.

Stuhldreher WL, Becker DJ, Drash AL et al (1994). The association of waist/hip ratio with diabetes complications in an adult IDDM population. *Journal of Clinical Epidemiology* **47**: 447–456.

Further reading

Bradley C, Todd C, Gorton T, Symonds E, Martin A, Plowright R (1999). The development of an individualised questionnaire measure of perceived impact of diabetes on quality of life: the ADDQoL. *Quality of Life Research* **8**: 79–91.

Jarvis S, Rubin AL (2003) *Diabetes for Dummies.* Chichester: John Wiley & Sons.

King's Fund Centre (1996) *Counting the Cost of Type 2 Diabetes.* London: King's Fund Centre/British Diabetic Association.

Drug and insulin therapy

Questions this chapter will help you answer

- How do the different oral therapies for diabetes work?

- Are my patients taking their medication appropriately?

- How do I involve the person with diabetes in their choice of medication?

- What are the common side effects of oral hypoglycaemic agents that people with diabetes need to be aware of?

- When should I consider insulin in a person with type 2 diabetes?

> *... more routine care will need to be provided by primary care teams in the future.*
>
> Audit Commission (2000)

Oral medication

See also Chapter 9.

As new medications become available, readers would do well to acquaint themselves with up-to-date information from the *British National Formulary* (BNF).

Healthy eating through a modification of food intake plus regular activity may be sufficient to achieve the aims of treatment in the early stages of type 2 diabetes, but research has shown that people treated with diet and exercise alone may be at risk of poorer care and less systematic review (Hippisley-Cox and Pringle, 2004). All avenues of lifestyle change should be discussed with those with diabetes and their carers before considering starting medication.

If symptoms persist and blood glucose levels remain elevated, oral medication may be required in addition to the dietary recommendations suggested. Traditionally, this has been via a stepwise approach, yet evidence suggests that a significant number of patients do not increase their medication rapidly enough and fail to achieve their target. Expert groups such as the International Diabetes Federation 'Control to Goal' partnership (Global Partnership for Effective Diabetes Management, 2005) are now recommending an approach involving combinations of glucose-lowering agents at an earlier stage in therapy.

Many people do not take their medication as prescribed so check on this before considering further titration. The higher the number of pills to be taken, the less likely it is that medical advice will be followed. A simple review of the individual's repeat prescriptions will demonstrate any anomalies. People with diabetes need to be fully involved in structured education related to their medication if they are to be expected to understand why they are taking it.

Information regarding oral medication should include:

- the name of the drug;

- the dose to be taken and in what form, for example tablet or injection;

- when to take the drug (i.e. before or at meal times);

- how the drug works;

- the hypoglycaemic effect of the drug (sulphonylureas);

- the side effects of the drug;

- possible interactions with other drugs taken;

- what to do if problems occur (i.e. contact the doctor or practice nurse);

- how to obtain a prescription exemption (form FP92A, to be signed by a doctor).

Oral hypoglycaemic agents

There are five groups of oral agent used in the treatment of type 2 diabetes:

1 biguanides;

2 glitazones (insulin-sensitisers);

3 sulphonylureas;

4 postprandial glucose regulators;

5 alpha-glucosidase inhibitors.

Biguanides

Metformin is the only biguanide in use in the UK. Its mode of action is not entirely clear, but it works predominantly by decreasing glucose output from the liver (gluconeogenesis) and to a lesser extent by increasing the peripheral utilisation of glucose by muscle and fat. Insulin has to be present in sufficient quantities for metformin to work effectively, and the drug is most effective in overweight patients with hyperinsulinaemia and insulin resistance.

Note: It is important to understand gluconeogenesis when supporting people with diabetes in glycaemic control. It is the process of making glucose from its own breakdown products or from the breakdown products of lipids or proteins. Gluconeogenesis occurs mainly in cells of the liver or kidney.

Metformin is the first choice of drug in overweight people with type 2 diabetes after dietary and activity measures have been implemented. It does not have the disadvantage of weight gain and is very unlikely to cause hypoglycaemia, unless combined with sulphonylureas or insulin.

Contraindications

- Even mild renal impairment (creatinine >130 mmol/l) as it may provoke lactic acidosis. Estimated glomerular filtration rate is an accurate method of assessing renal impairment (see Chapter 24).

- Significant impairment of liver function.

- Ketoacidosis.

- Use of iodine-containing X-ray contrast media: the Royal College of Radiologists advises that intramuscular contrast media should not be given to people taking metformin, and thus that this medication should not be given for 24 hours before such a procedure. It can be restarted when renal function returns to normal.

- General anaesthesia (metformin should be suspended 2 days beforehand and restarted when renal function returns to normal).

- Pregnancy and breastfeeding.

Side effects

- Gastrointestinal upsets. The most commonly reported side effect of metformin is wind and diarrhoea, but other

Table 11.1 Metformin

Drug	Proprietary brands	Normal dose	Price as at March 2006
Metformin	Glucophage Plus prolonged release Glucophage SR Also available in combination with rosiglitazone and pioglitazone	500 mg–3 g (2 g being the normally accepted maximum dose) Take with food Start on a low dose and titrate up according to blood blood glucose results and toleration of the drug	Non-proprietary 500 mg × 28 = £1.31, 850 mg × 56 = £1.88 Glucophage SR 500 mg × 28 = £2.67

Note: Metformin may also be used in patients with polycystic ovary syndrome, although this is an unlicensed indication

gastrointestinal side effects are common. These can be minimised by starting the drug at a low dose and slowly titrating, in response to blood glucose levels. Side effects are usually transient but may appear at dosage increases. Patients should be advised about this. Glucophage SR (sustained-release metformin) may be better tolerated and be more acceptable as up to 2 g can be taken in a single dose with the main meal.

■ Anorexia.

■ A metallic taste.

■ Decreased vitamin B_{12} absorption.

■ Rarely, lactic acidosis (in which case withdraw the drug immediately).

Note:

■ Metformin should be taken with food to minimise the side effects (Table 11.1), which may affect up to 30% of those treated with the drug.

■ Metformin should not be used in:

◆ renal failure: measure the serum creatinine before treatment and once or twice annually during treatment;

◆ hepatic failure;

◆ heart failure;

- alcoholism;
- pregnancy;
- breastfeeding.

Glitazones (insulin-sensitisers)

The thiazolidinediones, also and more easily known as insulin-sensitisers or glitazones, reduce peripheral insulin resistance, allowing endogenous insulin to work more effectively. They work in a different way from metformin. They may be especially useful in combination with metformin for overweight and obese patients, or as monotherapy in those for whom metformin is not suitable (Table 11.2).

Table 11.2 Glitazones

Drug	Proprietary brands	Normal dose	Price as at March 2006
Rosiglitazone	Avandia Also available in combination with metformin as Avandamet	4 mg daily if used alone or in combination with metformin, may increase to 8 mg daily (in one or two divided doses)	Proprietary 4 mg × 28 = £24.74 8 mg × 28 = £50.78
Pioglitazone	Actos Also available in combination with metformin as Competact	15–45 mg once daily	15 mg × 28 = £24.14 30 mg × 28 = £33.54 45 mg × 28 = £36.96

Contraindications

- Hepatic impairment (liver function tests are required before and periodically during treatment)
- A history of heart failure
- Combination with insulin
- Pregnancy and breastfeeding.

Side effects

These are shown in Table 11.3.

Table 11.3 Side effects of glitazones

Rosiglitazone	Pioglitazone
Gastrointestinal disturbances	Gastrointestinal disturbances
Headache	Weight gain/oedema
Anaemia	Anaemia
Altered blood lipids	Headache
Weight gain/oedema	Visual disturbances/dizziness
Less commonly: increased appetite, heart failure, fatigue, paraesthesia, alopecia, dyspnoea	Arthralgia, hypoaesthesia, haematuria, impotence
	Less commonly: fatigue, insomnia, vertigo, sweating, altered blood lipids, proteinuria

See the current BNF for rare side effects and precautions

Note:

■ Combining glitazones with metformin is preferable to combining them with a sulphonylurea, especially in those who are overweight and obese. A poor response to a combination of metformin and sulphonylurea may suggest a diminishing output of endogenous insulin from beta-cells, and insulin may be required.

■ Glitazones are not licensed to treat impaired glucose tolerance or fasting hyperglycaemia. However, a recent study with rosiglitazone (the DREAM trial) showed a reduction in the development of diabetes with this group.

■ By improving insulin action, these agents have a number of other potentially beneficial effects. Studies have shown positive effects on a number of cardiac risk factors, such as blood pressure, and a delay in progression to insulin in patients taking glitazones.

■ Not all the side effects listed apply to both drugs.

Sulphonylureas

These act mainly by augmenting insulin secretion and will therefore only work where some beta-cell function has been retained. Owing to this increased secretion of insulin, hypoglycaemia can be a side effect. Hypoglycaemia caused by sulphonylureas can be protracted, particularly with the longer-acting preparations (chlorpropamide – which is

Table 11.4 Sulphonylurea preparations

Drug	Proprietary brands	Normal dose	Price as at March 2006
Glibenclamide Can cause protracted hypoglycaemia	Daonil, Semi-Daonil, Euglucon	2.5 mg (older people) – 15 mg daily Take with breakfast Divide higher doses	Non-proprietary 2.5 mg × 28 = £0.78 5 mg × 28 = £0.95
Gliclazide Can be used in renal insufficiency	Diamicron Plus Modified Release (MR)	40–320 mg daily Take with breakfast Divide higher doses Maximum dose 120 mg	Non-proprietary 80 mg × 28 = £1.62
Glimepiride Once a day – may help with concordance	Amaryl	1–4 mg daily Take with the first main meal	Proprietary 1 mg × 30 = £4.51 2 mg × 30 = £7.42 3 mg × 30 = £11.19 4 mg × 30 = £14.82
Glipizide	Glibenese Minodiab	2.5–20 mg daily Take before breakfast or lunch Up to 15 mg as a single dose; divide higher doses	Non-proprietary 5 mg × 56 = £3.94
Gliquidone	Glurenorm	15–180 mg daily Take before breakfast Maximum single dose 60 mg, maximum daily dose 180 mg	Proprietary 30 mg × 100 = £17.54
Tolbutamide Large tablets, may be difficult to swallow		500 mg – 2 g Take with breakfast Divide higher doses	Non-proprietary 500 mg × 28 = £1.70

no longer recommended – and glibenclamide), and may necessitate admission to hospital.

Sulphonylureas are considered for patients who are not overweight or in whom metformin is contraindicated or not tolerated. There are several sulphonylureas in use in the UK (Table 11.4), the choice being determined by the duration of action, the frequency of taking the drug across the day, and the patient's age and renal function. Sulphonylureas increase appetite and may encourage weight gain.

Tolbutamide, which is short acting, may be used in renal impairment, as may gliquidone and gliclazide as they are principally metabolised in the liver. The lowest possible dose to achieve glycaemic control should be chosen and careful monitoring of levels adopted.

Contraindications

- Sulphonylureas should be avoided in severe hepatic and renal impairment.
- They should be discontinued during pregnancy and breastfeeding.

Side effects

These are generally mild and the drug is normally well tolerated:

- slight gastrointestinal disturbances;
- weight gain;
- hypoglycaemia (see above);
- hypersensitivity skin reactions (rashes).

Note: Rarely:

- sulphonylureas can cause liver damage leading to jaundice, hepatitis and, ultimately, liver failure;
- blood disorders (rare), for example thrombocytopenia, agranulocytosis and aplastic anaemia.

Postprandial glucose regulators

These drugs work in a similar way to sulphonylureas but have a very short duration of action and are usually taken before each meal (Table 11.5). As such, they are of use to people who are well motivated to take medication more than once a day and shift-workers who vary their meal times. There are two in use in the UK: nateglinide and repaglinide.

Contraindications

- Ketoacidosis
- Severe hepatic impairment
- Pregnancy
- Breastfeeding.

Table 11.3 Postprandial glucose regulators

Drug	Proprietary brands	Normal dose	Price as at March 2006
Repaglinide Monotherapy or combination with metformin	NovoNorm	500 µg – 16 mg Take within 30 minutes before main meals Up to 4 mg as a single dose	Proprietary 500 µg × 30 = £3.92 2 mg × 90 = £11.76
Nateglinide In combination with metformin	Starlix Amino acid derivative	60–180 mg three times daily Take within 30 minutes before main meals	Proprietary 60 mg × 84 = £19.75 120 mg × 84 = £22.50 180 mg × 84 = £22.50

Side effects

- Gastrointestinal disturbances
- Hypoglycaemia (rarely)
- Hypersensitivity (pruritis, rashes, vasculitis, urticaria)
- Visual disturbances.

Alpha-glucosidase inhibitors

Acarbose (Table 11.6) is the only inhibitor of intestinal alpha-glucosidases in use in the UK. It delays the digestion and absorption of starch and sucrose thereby reducing glucose entering the blood.

Contraindications

- Pregnancy and breastfeeding
- Inflammatory bowel disease (e.g. ulcerative colitis, Crohn's disease)
- Partial intestinal obstruction (or predisposition)
- Hepatic impairment
- Severe renal impairment
- Hernia
- History of abdominal surgery or hernia.

Table 11.6 Alpha-glucosidase inhibitor			
Drug	Proprietary brands	Normal dose	Price as at March 2006
Acarbose Glucose needed to treat hypo- glycaemic attacks if used in combination with sulphonylureas or insulin	Glucobay	50–600 mg Titrate slowly in response to blood glucose levels and tolerability Split large doses	Proprietary 50 mg × 90 = £6.60 100 mg × 90 = £12.51

Side effects

■ Flatulence and diarrhoea (may need to reduce the dose or withdraw)

■ Abdominal distension and pain.

Rarely, the following occur:

■ nausea

■ abnormal liver function tests

■ skin reactions.

Note:

■ Antacids are unlikely to be of use in treating side effects.

■ If acarbose is used in combination with sulphonylureas or insulin, patients should be advised to carry glucose for the treatment of hypoglycaemia. Sucrose absorption is affected by acarbose.

Emerging therapies

Historically, people with type 2 diabetes have been treated in a stepwise approach: diet and exercise, one oral agent, combination therapy, and then, as the condition progresses, an increasing number of people requiring insulin. The burden of managing these therapies and their side effects falls on people with diabetes, their carers and the health service. New therapies are in development that may shape the future of diabetes care.

Glucagon-like peptide-1

Glucagon-like peptide-1 (GLP-1) agonists (exenatide, liraglutide) will be available in the near future. GLP-1 is a naturally occurring gut hormone (incretin) released after food consumption. It reduces the secretion of glugacon, preventing it stimulating the liver to convert glycogen to glucose, with a subsequent increase in blood glucose. GLP-1 is injectable, carrying a low risk of hypoglycaemia, and has the following actions; it:

- stimulates insulin secretion;

- reduces appetite;

- inhibits the release of glucagon after meals;

- slows gastric emptying;

- increases beta-cell mass (as long as there is some mass there to increase, but studies are ongoing in this area).

Dipeptidyl peptidase IV inhibitors

Dipeptidyl peptidase IV (DPP-IV) is an enzyme that breaks down GLP-1. DPP-IV inhibitors (stagliptin, vildagliptin) are expected to have advantages similar to those of GLP-1 but will be available as oral therapy. Studies on these medications are in progress.

Combination therapy

Combination therapy can mean combinations of different oral hypoglycaemic agents (i.e. different tablets) or combinations of tablets and insulin. The National Institute for Health and Clinical Excellence guidance on blood glucose control published in 2002 will be updated to take account of new therapy options available.

- As type 2 diabetes is a progressive disease, people with diabetes need increasing doses of tablets, extra medication and eventually insulin to maintain good glucose control.

- The progressive nature of type 2 diabetes encourages a 'stepwise' approach to treatment.

- Metformin is the first drug of choice for the overweight. It can be combined with:
  - glitazones – generally if the person is overweight;
  - sulphonylureas – where there is capability for increased beta-cell secretion of insulin;
  - postprandial glucose regulators;

- ◆ acarbose – although gastrointestinal side effects from both may not encourage people to take the medication;
- ◆ insulin.

■ Sulphonylureas may be chosen for those of normal or slim build. They can be combined with:

- ◆ metformin – if it is thought that insulin resistance is present. Frequent review will be necessary as deteriorating beta-cell function may be the cause of poor glycaemic control and insulin therapy may be required;
- ◆ glitazones if additional metformin is not suitable;
- ◆ acarbose – patients must carry glucose for potential hypoglycaemia treatment;
- ◆ insulin – not as common as metformin with insulin. Weight gain could be an issue;

■ Triple therapy with metformin, glitazones and sulphonylureas is licensed in the UK.

■ People with diabetes often have other risk factors, such as hypertension or raised lipids, and need to take additional tablets to reduce these risks.

■ The UKPDS (Gray et al, 2002) demonstrated the importance of tight blood glucose and blood pressure control. Thus, patients with a glycated haemoglobin (HbA$_{1c}$) level of over 7.5% on a combination of tablets should discuss the possible need for insulin with their diabetes care team. A tighter target is advisable for those at increased risk.

■ Tablet boxes to organise daily medication are available from chemists (at a cost).

Combination therapy can also include insulin and tablets:

■ Traditionally, people with type 2 diabetes have been treated with tablets for as long as possible and then changed over to insulin.

■ An acceptable approach is combination therapy with tablets and insulin. This allows the treatment of insulin resistance through metformin while addressing the progressive loss of pancreatic output of insulin.

■ The regime should be chosen in discussion with the patient. Once-daily insulin in the evening, twice-daily mixtures or basal bolus regimens are all possible.

- Start by adding a long-acting insulin at bedtime, following the manufacturer's recommendations on dosage, and monitoring the early morning glucose.

- The target is to maintain the blood glucose level at between 4 and 8 mmol/l throughout the day, but this will not be achievable for all.

- The dose of insulin should be adjusted continuously to maintain the target and limit hypoglycaemia.

- Sulphonylureas and/or metformin should be continued at the previous dose, which should be more effective if the fasting glucose is well controlled (National Institute for Health and Clinical Excellence, 2002).

- As the beta-cells in the pancreas continue to deteriorate, daytime blood glucose levels will creep up, with a rise in HbA_{1c}.

- At some stage, tablets may become less effective, and increasing amounts of insulin may be required.

Note:

- Glitazones may be effective in combination with insulin but are currently contraindicated for such use in the UK; they should be stopped prior to initiating insulin.

- People with type 2 diabetes may be treated with insulin. It does not make them into a person with type 1 diabetes: they still have insulin resistance that needs to be addressed with oral agents.

Potential interactions between oral hypoglycaemic agents are shown in Table 11.7.

Insulin therapy

Evidence suggests that although general practitioners (GPs) recognise the importance of preventing complications, they may well decide to do what they think their patient would want (Freeman and Sweeney, 2001). This, combined with patients' fairly natural reluctance to convert to insulin injections, may delay the initiation of insulin therapy.

- Health professionals may be reluctant to start a patient on insulin.

Table 11.7 Oral hypoglycaemic agents – drug interactions

Drug affected	Drug interacting	Effect
Sulphonylureas	ACE inhibitors, chloramphenicol, cimetidine, MAOIs	Hypoglycaemic effect may be increased
	Corticosteroids, bumetanide, furosemide (frusemide) phenothiazines, thiazides, oral contraceptives	Hyperglycaemic effect increased (antagonistic)
	Lithium	May impair glucose tolerance
	Fibrates	May improve glucose tolerance
Gliquidone, tolbutamide	Rifampicin	Reduced effect
Metformin	Alcohol	Increased risk of lactic acidosis
	Cimetidine	Increased plasma concentration of metformin
	ACE inhibitors, MAOIs	Hypoglycaemic effects possibly enhanced
Postprandial glucose regulators (repaglinide, nateglinide)	ACE inhibitors, anabolic steroids, beta-blockers, monoamine oxidase inhibitors, NSAIDs, oral contraceptives, salicylates, sympathomimetics, thiazides, corticosteroids, thyroid hormones	Interactions are not significant Plasma concentration of nateglinide reduced by rifampicin Increased risk of severe hypoglycaemia when repaglinide given with gemfibrozil – avoid concomitant use
Thiazolidinediones (rosiglitazone, pioglitazone)	Insulin – not licensed for combination with insulin use in the UK	

ACE, angiotensin-converting enzyme; MAOI, monoamine oxidase inhibitor;
NSAID, non-steroidal anti-inflammatory drug
For updated drug information, see BNF online at www.bnf.org

- People with diabetes may not understand the benefit of tight glycaemic control.

- Hypoglycaemic attacks are a significant risk, causing anxiety.

- Weight gain is a risk to overweight patients. This can be due to improved control lessening weight loss through glucosuria or increased appetite. This should be included in patients' education.

Overall, health professionals and people with diabetes should work more closely together to agree a management plan incorporating lifestyle issues and, when necessary, increases in therapy.

Type 2 diabetes is progressive, but the good news is that people are living longer and in better health than previously. This good news has a barb in the tail – the beta-cell production of insulin may deteriorate over time, encouraging blood glucose levels to rise steadily. Unless individuals can do something to increase their insulin sensitivity – weight loss and regular exercise will help most people – additional insulin will be required. Needless to say, to obtain the best outcome, a healthy lifestyle should be adopted lifelong regardless of the therapy taken.

There are several reasons to consider initiation of insulin in type 2 diabetes:

- clear signs of inadequate endogenous insulin production – persistently high HbA_{1c} and blood glucose levels on maximal oral therapy;

- people with diabetes who are slim at presentation and may have diminished insulin production;

- continuing weight loss (which may be gradual);

- persistent or recurrent ketonuria;

- in the presence of intercurrent illness such as a cardiovascular event;

- diabetes-related complications;

- pregnancy.

When insulin is obviously needed, symptoms persist, blood glucose levels are high, weight loss has continued and ketonuria persists, the decision is clear. The introduction of insulin therapy will almost always relieve symptoms, lower blood glucose levels and improve well-being.

If intercurrent illness occurs, insulin may be required for the following reasons (and others) but may be administered in the short term:

- *infections* – when oral agents cannot control the rise in blood glucose associated with infection;

- *increased insulin resistance* – perhaps due to other drugs;

- *deteriorating blood glucose control* – perhaps due to a reduction in physical activity;

- *steroid therapy* (increasing doses) – which have a hyperglycaemic effect;

- *myocardial infarction* – studies (Malmberg et al, 2001) show that insulin improves morbidity.

Note: After recovery, therapy may be stepped down and insulin may be withdrawn, although it is generally continued for at least 3 months.

Trial of insulin

Some people with type 2 diabetes are extremely reluctant to start insulin therapy. Suggesting a short trial to allay their fears may be appropriate for some, but it should be made clear that reverting to tablet-only therapy is likely to be against medical advice. Once started on insulin, very few people choose to stop it. People treated with insulin following the DIGAMI protocol may be on short-term insulin for 6 months to 1 year (Malmberg et al, 1995).

Aims for therapy

In younger people with type 2 diabetes
The aim of treatment should be near-normal blood glucose levels in order to reduce the risks of long-term complications.

In older people with type 2 diabetes (especially elderly people)
The aim of treatment should be to reduce any symptoms and improve quality of life, health and well-being.

Starting insulin therapy for people with type 2 diabetes

- The person concerned will require considerable support, education and careful management.

- Specialist help (the hospital team) may be required if the primary care team does not possess the necessary knowledge and skills in starting insulin therapy.

- An individual programme is required for stabilisation and continuing education.

- Blood glucose monitoring is almost always required if insulin therapy is commenced.

- Assessment of the capability, lifestyle and wishes of the patient is important when starting insulin, so that the insulin regimen allows a desired and appropriate lifestyle.

- The regime should be tailored to the individual: once daily, twice daily or multiple injections.

- Visual aids and 'automatic' injectors may be required; if so, the specialist team may need to be consulted.

- Insulin pens, needles and 'sharps' boxes are available on prescription.

Insulin sources

- Human insulin and the analogues are made by recombinant technology in the yeast *Saccharomyces cerevisiae*. They do not come from humans!

- Animal insulin is still available in a few different preparations (see the current BNF for up-to-date information).

- Inhaled insulin is available.

About insulin

- Insulin plays a key role in the body's regulation of carbohydrate, fat and protein metabolism.

- Insulin is inactivated by gastrointestinal enzymes and must therefore be given by injection.

- It is usually injected into the upper arms, thighs, buttocks or abdomen (note that there may be increased absorption from a limb site after strenuous exercise).

- Insulin is usually administered subcutaneously using a syringe and needle or pen device.

- Portable injection devices (e.g. NovoPen, Autopen, HumaPen Luxura, OptiClik) hold insulin in cartridge form. The dose can be selected and shown on a dial. Disposable pen injection devices are also readily available (Figure 11.1).

- Pen devices allow greater flexibility of lifestyle although more injections are required where a multiple-dose regimen is used.

- Alternatives to pen devices are available but may have a restricted range of insulins, for example Innolet from NovoNordisk.

- Insulin can be given by continuous subcutaneous infusion (an insulin pump).

- Minor allergic reactions at injection sites during the first few weeks of treatment are uncommon, usually transient and require no treatment.

- Rotation of injection sites lessens the chances of lipohypertrophy/lipoatrophy (Figure 11.2). Certain sites may become 'favoured' as their continued use lessens the discomfort of the injection.

- Insulin doses are determined on an individual basis (about 0.5–0.8 unit/kg body weight initially) and titrated to the effective dose to suit the patient.

- Initial doses are small and gradually increased to avoid hypoglycaemia.

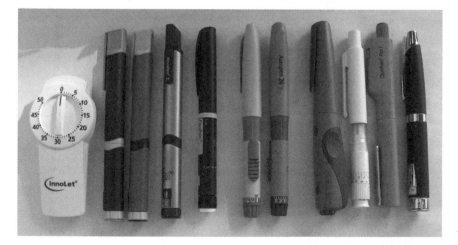

Figure 11.1 Some insulin injection devices: (Left to right) NovoNordisk Innolet, NovePen Fun Blue, NovoPen Fun Red, NovoPen Classic, FlexPen, Autopen 24 1–21 units, Autopen 24 2–42 units, OptiClik, OptiSet, OptiPen Pro and HumaPen Luxura

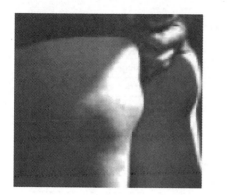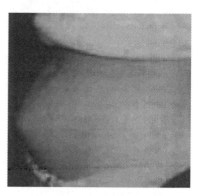

Figure 11.2 Examples of lipohypertrophy
(© Becton, Dickinson and Company. Reproduced with permission)

■ People with type 2 diabetes generally need higher doses of insulin, owing to insulin resistance, than do those with type 1 diabetes.

There are five main types of injected insulin preparation (Table 11.8) plus inhaled insulin (check the BNF for updated information):

1 rapid-acting;

2 short-acting – previously called soluble or clear;

3 intermediate acting – also called isophane insulin;

4 fixed mixtures of rapid or short-acting and intermediate-acting insulin;

5 long-acting – newer preparations, for example glargine (Lantus) and detemir (Levemir).

Note: Different people respond to insulin differently and have different needs. Treatment should be individualised and regularly adjusted. The monthly MIMS Index contains a chart giving the onset, peak activity and duration of action of insulins. GP practices may have this publication.

Management of the side effects of insulin

■ Hypoglycaemia may not be regarded as a side effect of insulin, because its hypoglycaemic action is therapeutic and normoglycaemia is the goal of treatment.

■ Although hypoglycaemia may be defined as a blood glucose level of less than 4 mmol/l, symptoms of hypoglycaemia may

Name of insulin	Manufacturer	Source	Vial, cartridge or prefilled pen
Rapid acting analogue			
Humalog	Lilly	Analogue	Vial, cartridge and prefilled pen
NovoRapid	Novo Nordisk	Analogue	Vial, cartridge and prefilled pen
Apidra	Sanofi-Aventis	Analogue	Vial, cartridge and prefilled pen
Short-acting			
Actrapid	Novo Nordisk	Human	Vial
Human Velosulin	Novo Nordisk	Human	Vial
Pork Actrapid	Novo Nordisk	Pork	Vial
Humulin S	Lilly	Human	Vial and cartridge
Hypurin Bovine Neutral	Wockhardt UK	Beef	Vial and cartridge
Hypurin Porcine Neutral	Wockhardt UK	Pork	Vial and cartridge
Insuman Rapid	Sanofi-Aventis	Human	Cartridge and prefilled pen
Medium- and long-acting			
Humulin 1	Lilly	Human	Vial, cartridge and prefilled pen
Insulatard	Novo Nordisk	Human	Vial, cartridge and prefilled pen
Insulatard Penfill	Novo Nordisk	Human	Cartridge
Pork Insulatard	Novo Nordisk	Pork	Vial
Hypurin Bovine Isophane	Wockhardt UK	Beef	Vial and cartridge
Hypurin Bovine Lente	Wockhardt UK	Beef	Vial
Hypurin Bovine PZ1	Wockhardt UK	Beef	Vial
Hypurin Porcine Isophane	Wockhardt UK	Pork	Vial and cartridge
Insuman Basal	Sanofi-Aventis	Human	Vial, cartridge and prefilled pen
Analogue mixtures			
Humalog Mix 25	Lilly	Analogue	Cartridge and prefilled pen
Humalog Mix 50	Lilly	Analogue	Prefilled pen
NovoMix 30	Novo Nordisk	Analogue	Cartridge and prefilled pen
Mixtures			
Humulin M3	Lilly	Human	Vial, cartridge and prefilled pen
Mixtard 30	Novo Nordisk	Human	Vial, cartridge and prefilled pen
Mixtard 10, 20. 40, 50	Novo Nordisk	Human	Cartridge; discontinued Dec. 2007
Pork Mixtard 30	Novo Nordisk	Pork	Vial
Hypurin Porcine 30/70 mix	Wockhardt UK	Pork	Vial and cartridge
Insuman Comb 15	Sanofi-Aventis	Human	Prefilled pen
Insuman Comb 25	Sanofi-Aventis	Human	Vial, cartridge and prefilled pen
Insuman Comb 50	Sanofi-Aventis	Human	Cartridge and prefilled pen
Long-acting analogue			
Lantus	Sanofi-Aventis	Analogue	Vial, cartridge and prefilled pen
Levemir	Novo Nordisk	Analogue	Cartridge and prefilled pen

Table 11.8 The five main types of insulin preparation

Taken	Onset, peak and duration
	2 4 6 8 10 12 14 16 18 20 22 24 26 28 30 32 34
Just before/with/just after	
Just before/with/just after	
Just before/with/just after	
30 mins before food	
15 – 30 mins before food	
30 mins before food	
20 – 45 mins before food	
15 – 30 mins before food	
15 – 30 mins before food	
15 – 30 mins before food	
About 30 mins before food or bed	
About 30 mins before food or bed	
About 30 mins before food or bed	
About 30 mins before food or bed	
About 30 mins before food or bed	
About 30 mins before food or bed	
About 30 mins before food or bed	
About 30 mins before food or bed	
About 45 – 60 mins before food or bed	
Just before/with/just after food	
Just before/with/just after food	
Just before/with/just after food	
20 – 45 mins before food	
30 mins before food	
30 mins before food	
15 – 30 mins before food	
20 – 45 mins before food	
30 – 45 mins before food	
30 – 45 mins before food	
20 – 30 mins before food	
1 a day, anytime (but at same time daily)	
Once or twice a day	

Onset Peak

Duration

Onset:
The time taken for the insulin to start having an effect

Peak action:
This is the time when the insulin is working at greatest effect

be experienced when blood glucose levels are higher than this. Symptoms of hunger, light-headedness and tingling may be experienced as blood glucose levels are falling (from previously high levels), for example from 28 to 11 mmol/l.

■ People on insulin need structured education on the effects of physical activity on their blood glucose levels.

■ Weight gain can be a problem, and specific dietary advice, tailored to the individual, will be required.

Prevention of hypoglycaemia in an effort to achieve normoglycaemia includes the following in clinical management.

Insulin species

■ Changing species of insulin may cause problems. If people have been treated with animal (porcine and bovine) insulin for many years, and then changed over to 'human' insulin, the daily dose requires reduction by 10% or more. Human insulin can have a profound hypoglycaemic action when used by some people. Although this has not yet been proven scientifically, subjective changes should not be taken lightly. Likewise, it is reported by some people with diabetes that the warning signs of hypoglycaemia may be 'reduced' when their species of insulin is changed from 'animal' or 'natural' (porcine and bovine) to 'human'.

■ If the person with diabetes expresses a wish to return to 'animal' insulin owing to hypoglycaemia or a loss of warning signs, those wishes should be respected and the nearest equivalent chosen. Close blood glucose monitoring is essential when any change of insulin is made.

■ A choice of insulin species is available for people with diabetes. This choice is included in the insulin delivery systems that accompany the insulins in use, i.e. pens, syringes, needles, vials and cartridges of insulin. Note that syringes, insulin vials and cartridges, pen needles and most pens are available on prescription.

■ It is important that the species of insulin is recorded and that any change of insulin species is recorded. The person with diabetes should know his or her own insulin species.

Insulin type

When discussing the introduction of insulin, several factors should be explained:

- The choice of insulin will depend on many factors, especially how it will fit into the person's life. The onset, rise, peak, fall and duration of insulin effect are considered when insulin is prescribed (Figure 11.3). The prescription will relate to the person's glycaemic state, lifestyle (eating habits, activity levels) and medical state. Close blood glucose monitoring is required when any change in insulin type is made.

- It is important that the type of insulin is recorded and that any change in insulin type is recorded. The person with diabetes should know his or her own insulin type(s).

- Insulin analogues: rapid-acting insulin analogues have a short-duration effect and can be injected at or just before meal times. This effect deals with the postprandial glucose peak. This insulin can also be taken after meals, but this is not generally recommended on a regular basis.

- Inhaled insulin: inhaled insulin (Exubera) is now a therapeutic option. It provides short-acting mealtime doses – longer-acting basal injected insulin is, however, still required. Inhaled insulin is suitable for individuals who have a severe needle phobia or those in whom other intensive forms of injected insulin have failed to achieve acceptable control. The initiation of this type of insulin is advised to be undertaken through specialist centres.

Insulin dose

- This will vary after stabilisation and will relate to the glycaemic state, lifestyle (eating habits and activity levels), medical state and insulin regimen desired by the person with diabetes. In addition HbA_{1c} levels and day-to-day glucose levels are discussed with the person concerned. In this way, the person with diabetes is engaged in all discussions and decisions relating to his or her own diabetes control and care.

- It is important that the dose of insulin is recorded and that any change in insulin dose is recorded. The person with diabetes should also know his or her own insulin dose.

Note: For further information regarding the detection, prevention and treatment of hypoglycaemia, see Chapter 12.

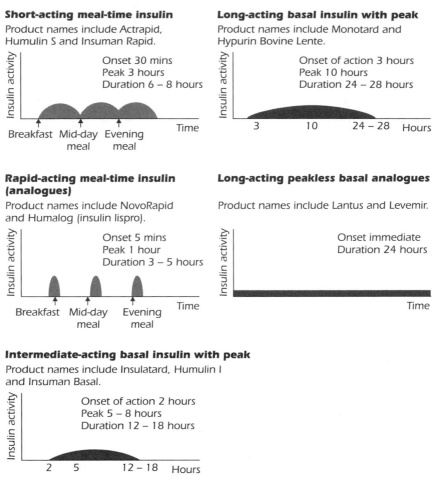

Short-acting meal-time insulin

Product names include Actrapid, Humulin S and Insuman Rapid.

Onset 30 mins
Peak 3 hours
Duration 6 – 8 hours

Insulin activity

Breakfast Mid-day Evening Time
           meal   meal

Long-acting basal insulin with peak

Product names include Monotard and Hypurin Bovine Lente.

Onset of action 3 hours
Peak 10 hours
Duration 24 – 28 hours

Insulin activity

3   10   24 – 28 Hours

Rapid-acting meal-time insulin (analogues)

Product names include NovoRapid and Humalog (insulin lispro).

Onset 5 mins
Peak 1 hour
Duration 3 – 5 hours

Insulin activity

Breakfast Mid-day Evening Time
           meal   meal

Long-acting peakless basal analogues

Product names include Lantus and Levemir.

Onset immediate
Duration 24 hours

Insulin activity

Time

Intermediate-acting basal insulin with peak

Product names include Insulatard, Humulin I and Insuman Basal.

Onset of action 2 hours
Peak 5 – 8 hours
Duration 12 – 18 hours

Insulin activity

2   5   12 – 18   Hours

Figure 11.3 Type 2 diabetes and insulin
(Reproduced with kind permission of the Royal College of Nursing, from **Starting insulin treatment in adults with Type 2 diabetes** [2004, updated 2006])

Guideline for teaching self-administration of insulin

Ideally, people with diabetes requiring insulin therapy should have access to someone with specialist knowledge and skills. The latter should also have experience of different teaching methods and methods of assessing learning.

Considerable time, support, education, telephone contact and/or home visiting will be required initially and in a staged, continuing process until confidence has been gained and blood glucose levels have stabilised.

The following steps are required:

1 Assessment of the person with diabetes

2 Preparation and support

3 Understanding the equipment

4 Drawing up insulin

5 Giving the injection

6 Care of equipment

7 Prevention of hypoglycaemia

8 Treatment of hypoglycaemia

9 Contact telephone number

10 Identification

11 Anticipation of problems and questions

12 Evaluating learning

13 Agreeing a care plan

14 Driving and insurance.

Assessment

Language	For communication
Literacy	Understanding written material
Culture	
Home, work, social conditions	Lifestyle
Hearing	
Sight	
Other medical problems	
Physical state	Physical ability
Mobility	
Dexterity	
Mental state	
Intellect	
Preconceived ideas	Mental and emotional state
Fear factor	

Preparation and support required

It is important to take into account preconceived ideas and fears (particularly of needles). Emphasise the benefits of insulin and improved well-being, and stress that support is available.

The benefits of insulin are:

- feeling better;
- an improved lifestyle;
- lower blood glucose levels;
- a reduced risk of complications;
- possibly fewer tablets (if on combination oral hypoglycaemic therapy);
- weight gain (which is, in those who are underweight, a benefit).

Experience of a 'dummy' injection assisted by the nurse or doctor but done by the person with diabetes can be useful. No insulin need be injected at this stage, but 2 units can be delivered safely without fear of hypoglycaemia. Many people imagine the needle to be large and think that it is to be inserted into a vein. It may be helpful for the person concerned to meet another patient who has successfully transferred to insulin treatment.

An optimistic, helpful and positive approach is essential.

Understanding the equipment

The equipment includes insulin (bottle or cartridges), syringes, injection devices, needles, cottonwool, a needle-clipper and a 'sharps' bin, as well as educational material (leaflets on drawing up and giving insulin).

Insulin bottle or cartridges

Teach:

- the name, species and type;
- the action – peak and duration;
- the dose;
- the expiry date;
- storage. Insulin will last up to 1 month at normal room temperatures (not in the car or on a windowsill). Devices in use may be kept out of the fridge, but back-up supplies should be stored in the fridge (not touching any freezer parts);
- prescription (check exemption).

Syringes, pen devices and needles
Teach:

- how to take these devices to pieces;
- how they work;
- the types of syringe/markings (50 units – 0.5 ml; 100 units – 1 ml);
- a demonstration of the pen device/needle – correctly fitting it together and following the manufacturer's printed advice;
- how to expel air bubbles;
- how to fit and dispose of needles safely;
- observe the person with diabetes copying your demonstration and answer any queries;
- prescription (required).

Cottonwool
Teach:

- that there is no need for alcohol wipes;
- that tissues may be used at home.

Needle-clipper (if used)
Teach:

- demonstration of use;
- disposal;
- replacement (obtained from the GP or specialist clinic on prescription);
- prescription (required).

Disposal of 'sharps'
Guidance entitled the *Safe Disposal of Clinical Waste* (Health Services Advisory Committee, 1999) contains the following advice on 'sharps' disposal:

> Sharps (Group B) should be placed in an appropriate sharps container as outlined earlier in this document. On no account should soft drink cans, plastic bottles or similar containers be used for the disposal of needles, since these could present serious hazards to staff if they were disposed of in domestic waste.

Health professionals have lengthy processes to follow to ensure safety from 'sharps'. If you are treating someone in their own home, the disposal of these becomes your responsibility.

Teach:

- the safe disposal of all 'sharps' – lancets, needles, syringes, pen devices;

- to keep out of the reach of children;

- to fill the container no more than two-thirds full;

- to dispose of the bin safely – return it to the GP practice (if it is licensed and accepts these) or provide contact details for the local authority responsible (remembering that they may make a reasonable charge for this service). Section 45(3)(b) of the Environmental Protection Act 1990 says that local authorities are obliged to collect clinical waste such as 'sharps' boxes from householders on request.

These are generally accepted guidelines in England and Wales, but there may be local variations in practice in other areas.

Further information is available from the National Diabetes Support Team (2004).

Educational material:

- written leaflets;

- pictorial information;

- websites, for example the Diabetes UK website (see Appendix 4).

Drawing up insulin

Teach:

- the correct dose (write this down leaving room for future adjustments);

- how to draw up insulin correctly;

- how to expel air bubbles;

- when to give injections (20–30 minutes before a meal for human insulins; just before, or even after, a meal for analogues);

- that written leaflets are available (see Appendix 4).

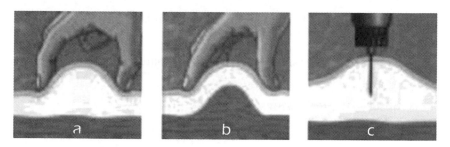

Figure 11.4 Insulin injection: (a) correctly lifted skin fold;
(b) incorrectly lifted skin fold; (c) lifted skin fold
(© Becton, Dickinson and Company. Reproduced with permission)

Giving the injection
Teach:

- the angle of injection (Figure 11.4);

- check dexterity (right or left handed; use of hands);

- sites and rotation (insulin is absorbed more quickly from abdominal sites or into the limbs following exercise) (Figure 11.5);

- that the site for injection needs to be relaxed;

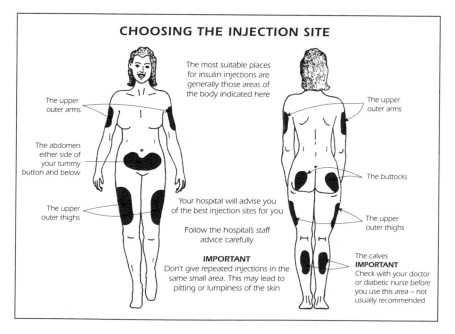

Figure 11.5 Site rotation chart

- that quick needle insertion is better (as it is less uncomfortable);

- that the plunger should be depressed steadily when injecting insulin;

- observe the technique;

- give written and illustrated leaflets (see Appendix 4);

- discuss the effects of too many injections in one small area of injection site, for example poor absorption, reduced insulin effectiveness resulting from lipohypertrophy (human insulin) and lipoatrophy (animal insulin).

Care of equipment
Teach:

- to keep everything together (with other equipment, e.g. for monitoring);

- always have a spare insulin bottle or cartridges or pen (kept in the fridge);

- to keep equipment away from children;

- to list the equipment required before attending the surgery or hospital clinic – check insulin species, name, types of syringe used;

- the re-use of syringes (pen device needles);

- correct disposal (syringe/pen device needles, insulin vials and cartridges).

Prevention of hypoglycaemia
See Chapter 12 for patient information.
Teach:

- that exercise, alcohol and sexual activity may lower blood glucose levels sufficiently to cause hypoglycaemia;

- to eat regularly (meals and snacks);

- not to delay or miss meals;

- check dietary advice (refer to a dietitian);

- to take the correct dose of insulin at the correct time;

- to eat more carbohydrate or reduce insulin if activity increases;

- that less insulin may be needed (if strenuous activity is anticipated);

- always to carry glucose tablets or sweets (keep these in the car if driving);

- to inform the Driver and Vehicle Licensing Agency (DVLA) if a driver is new to insulin;

- to carry identification (necklace, bracelet or card) (see Appendix 4).

Note: monitoring and education are required for the self-adjustment of insulin.

Contact telephone number
Teach:

- the surgery telephone number;

- the hospital diabetes centre/clinic telephone number;

- the out-of-hours telephone number;

- the name of the person to contact;

- the Diabetes UK Careline number (see Appendix 4).

Identification
Teach:

- the importance of personal identity;

- the availability and source of necklaces or bracelets (try the local jewellers or see Appendix 4);

- about identification cards (Diabetes UK or insulin companies; see Appendix 4).

Anticipation of problems and questions
Examples are given below:

Human insulin – does it come from humans?

- Reassure the person that this is not so. This may reflect concerns about AIDS (see 'About insulin' earlier in this chapter).

'Forgetting' the injection: what should I do?

■ Assess which insulin the person is on.

◆ If this is a multiple (basal bolus) regimen and a short-acting insulin has been forgotten, wait until the next one is due to prevent possible hypoglycaemic episodes from having two injections close together.

◆ If it is a twice-a-day regimen, the same applies.

◆ If the insulin is longer acting, for example Lantus, and not too long has passed, it may still be feasible to take a reduced dose.

■ Only provide this advice if you have the knowledge and skills to do so. Otherwise, refer the person to the specialist team.

Giving the wrong dose (too much or too little)?

■ Explain the action, peak and duration of insulin.

■ Explain the effects of too much insulin – hypoglycaemia – and its recognition and treatment.

■ Explain the effects of taking too little insulin – hyperglycaemia; correct this at the next dose, or seek medical advice if the blood glucose level is high (a dose of a quick-acting insulin may be required).

Spirit for cleaning the skin?

■ This is not required.

■ It makes injections uncomfortable.

■ It also toughens injection sites.

Bleeding after injection?

■ Reassure that this is nothing to worry about.

■ Check the injection technique.

■ Apply gentle pressure to site if bleeding occurs.

Evaluating learning

■ At each stage after demonstration and teaching, the person with diabetes and/or their carer should demonstrate understanding.

- Practical skills should be demonstrated and observed.

- Understanding can be evaluated by appropriate questions and in discussion.

- Follow-up appointments or home visits should be made at regular intervals until confidence has been gained.

- Monitoring is important once insulin therapy is commenced, in order to adjust the insulin dose slowly to the appropriate level required for control of blood glucose level, symptom relief and improved well-being.

- Monitoring techniques require education and evaluation after the start of insulin therapy.

References

Freeman AC, Sweeney K (2001). Why general practitioners do not implement evidence: qualitative study. *British Medical Journal* **323**: 1–5.

Global Partnership for Effective Diabetes Management (2005). Control to Goal Factsheets. International Diabetes Federation/Federation of European Nurses in Diabetes. www.idf.org.

Gray A, Clarke P, Farmer A, Holman R (UKPDS Group) (2002). Implementing intensive control of blood glucose concentration and blood pressure in type 2 diabetes in England: cost analysis (UKPDS 63). *British Medical Journal* **325**: 860–863.

Health Services Advisory Committee (1999). *Safe Disposal of Clinical Waste.* Health Services Advisory Committee.

Hippisley-Cox J, Pringle M (2004). Prevalence, care, and outcomes for patients with diet controlled diabetes in general practice: cross sectional survey. *Lancet* **364**: 423–425.

Malmberg K, Ryden L, Hamsten A, Herlitz J, Waldenstrom A, Wedel H, Welin L (1995). Randomized trial of insulin-glucose infusion followed by subcutaneous insulin treatment in diabetic patients with acute myocardial infarction (DIGAMI study): effects on mortality at 1 year. *Journal of the American College of Cardiology* **26**: 56–65.

Malmberg K, Norhammar A, Ryden L (2001). Insulin treatment post myocardial infarction: the DIGAMI study. *Advances in Experimental and Medical Biology* **498**: 279–284.

National Diabetes Support Team (2004). *Disposing of Used Syringes and Other Sharp Clinical Waste.* Factsheet No. 2. London: NDST.

National Institute for Health and Clinical Excellence (2002). *Management of Type 2 Diabetes. Management of Blood Glucose.* Inherited Guideline G. London: NICE.

Further reading

Airey M, Williams R (2000). Hypoglycaemia induced by exogenous insulin 'human' and animal insulin compared. *Diabetic Medicine* **17**: 416–432.

DCCT Research Group (1993). The effect of intensive treatment of diabetes on the development of long term complications in insulin-dependent diabetes mellitus. *New England Journal of Medicine* **329**: 977–986.

DECODE Study Group (1999). Glucose tolerance and mortality: comparison of WHO and American Diabetes Association diagnostic criteria. *Lancet* **354**: 617–621.

Royal College of Nursing (2004). *Starting Insulin Treatment in Adults with Type 2 Diabetes*. London: RCN.

UKPDS Study Group (1998). Intensive blood-glucose control with sulphonylureas or insulin compared with conventional treatment and risk of complications in patients with type 2 diabetes (UKPDS 33). *Lancet* **352**: 837–853.

12 Monitoring and control

Questions this chapter will help you answer

- What measures should I be considering in monitoring to achieve holistic care?
- What is an HbA_{1c}?
- What are the symptoms of hyperglycaemia, and what should I advise patients?
- What are the symptoms of hypoglycaemia (a 'hypo'), and what should I advise patients?
- When should a person with diabetes self-monitor?
- What are 'sick day rules'?

> *I have no idea whatsoever why I do daily blood-checks . . . I have not the remotest idea what I am keeping the record for.*
>
> Audit Commission (2002)

Monitoring metabolic control is fundamental to the care of people with diabetes.

Blood glucose control is only part of the holistic care people with diabetes deserve.

The benefits of monitoring

Monitoring in this instance refers to more than blood glucose monitoring, which is discussed later in this chapter.

- *Weight*: to agree goals and targets to include in the patient's individual management plan. Successful weight reduction will almost always improve blood glucose levels in type 2 diabetes. Waist measurement may be a better predictor of risk (see Chapter 10).

- *Physical activity*: to assess and agree goals and targets to include in the individual management plan.

- *Dietary assessment* and possible referral to a dietitian and/or structured education.

- *Glycated haemoglobin (HbA$_{1c}$) level*: to assess long-term control, but this should be combined with a review of home blood or urine glucose monitoring (if done) and with a discussion of general well-being. The frequency of tests should be dictated by glycaemic control, with more frequent tests in times of change or to assess the need to alter medication.

- *Blood pressure*: to assess cardiovascular and renal risk, and to discuss this with the patient.

- *Lipids*: to assess cardiovascular risk; discuss this with the patient.

- *Renal function*: to detect any deterioration in function and adjust therapy and education to suit.

- *Thyroid function*: there is a higher than normal rate of abnormal thyroid function in diabetes. Hypothyroidism makes it more difficult to lose weight and affects general well-being. Screening can confirm that there is no problem or indicate whether therapy would be beneficial.

- *Liver function*: a high percentage of people with type 2 diabetes have dyslipidaemia requiring treatment with a statin. Liver function needs to be checked if statins or glitazones are indicated.

- *Proteinuria and microalbuminuria*: to assess cardiovascular and renal risk, and consider the need for angiotensin-converting enzyme inhibitor therapy (see Chapter 24).

- *Eye screening*: to detect and treat any early retinopathy (see Chapter 13).

- *Foot assessment*: to detect and treat the 'at-risk' foot and provide education to the patient on the importance of foot care (see Chapter 14).

When appropriate, after diagnosis and if they are able, people with diabetes should become accustomed to monitoring their own health. In a broad sense, this includes general health and well-being, diabetes control, eyesight, weight, dental care, care of the feet and footwear.

In order to promote health and reduce the risk of complications, monitoring diabetes control (blood glucose levels) requires particular attention and involves careful assessment and education by the care team. Self-monitoring allows the person with diabetes to check his or her own control, take responsibility for his or her own condition and (as far as possible) maintain independence.

Blood glucose control

The importance of blood glucose control in preventing complications of diabetes has been well established (Diabetes Control and Complications Trial Research Group, 1993; UK Prospective Diabetes Study Group, 1998).

- The monitoring of the person with diabetes by the primary care team should support and check self-monitoring as well as ascertain the effectiveness of treatment.

- Targets for control should be negotiated and realistic.

- Long-term control can be confirmed by annual HbA_{1c} readings or, less usually except in pregnancy, serum fructosamine tests.

Glycated haemoglobin

HbA_{1c} concentration is widely accepted as an objective and quantitative index of blood glucose levels during the preceding 6–10 weeks. According to the National Institute for Health and Clinical Excellence, 2002), it should be performed 2–6-monthly as part of the routine review and structured education involving the patient. The frequency of HbA_{1c} measurement should be dictated by glycaemic control. If good, HbA_{1c} readings may be indicated 6-monthly to assess any progression in the condition. At times of change or poor control, or with those who cannot self-monitor, it should be performed more often, and the person with diabetes informed of the result and its implications.

It should be remembered that the HbA_{1c} test does not represent individual peaks and troughs in blood glucose level. A low HbA_{1c} level or a result within the normal range may suggest good glycaemic control, although not reflecting levels of hypoglycaemia. Individual home blood glucose monitoring results are important and should always be discussed in any review of blood glucose control.

Serum fructosamine measurement

This is an objective and quantitative test reflecting blood glucose control over the preceding 2–3 weeks only. This test is thus less useful for most people, although it may be of benefit in gestational diabetes because of its shorter time span.

Sick day rules

See sections below, Figure 12.1, Boxes 12.1 and 12.2, and Appendix 5.

High blood glucose levels (hyperglycaemia)

In people without diabetes, the blood glucose normally ranges from 4 to 8 mmol/l, generally being slightly higher postprandially (after eating) and lower after physical activity or fasting. In order to prevent the complications caused by hyperglycaemia, targets within this range are desirable. This is certainly correct in a younger person with diabetes. For women who are pregnant, blood glucose levels should not rise above 7 mmol/l even after meals. In older people, however, especially if weight

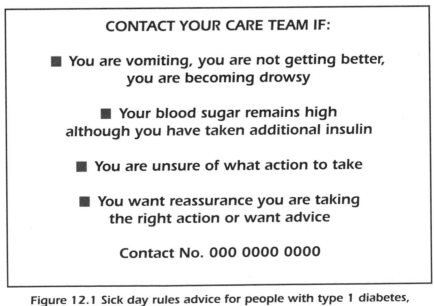

CONTACT YOUR CARE TEAM IF:

■ You are vomiting, you are not getting better,
you are becoming drowsy

■ Your blood sugar remains high
although you have taken additional insulin

■ You are unsure of what action to take

■ You want reassurance you are taking
the right action or want advice

Contact No. 000 0000 0000

Figure 12.1 Sick day rules advice for people with type 1 diabetes,
to be included in their care plan

is a problem, blood glucose levels may be higher than 10 mmol/l and the target needs to be tailored to the individual. It is important that levels are discussed and that the person is symptom-free.

Hyperglycaemia may be caused by:

- untreated diabetes
- too much food ⎫ these may occur
- the wrong type of food ⎭ on special occasions
- insufficient medication (incorrect dose)
- insufficient insulin (incorrect dose)
- the overuse of particular injection sites
- a poor injection technique
- reduction in activity
- decreased mobility
- infections/illness
- an increase in concurrent medication affecting glycaemic control (e.g. steroid therapy)
- stress – life changes (retirement, bereavement)
- weight increase.

Note:

- Apparent hyperglycaemia can be caused through neglecting to wash the hands prior to performing home blood glucose monitoring so that something containing glucose sticks to the fingers, for example juice from peeling an orange, some hand creams or biscuit crumbs.
- Apparent hyperglycaemia can occur if the blood glucose meter is set to units other than mmol/l.

Symptoms of hyperglycaemia need to be explained, for example thirst, polyuria, nocturia (incontinence, in older people), lethargy, irritability and visual changes. Hyperglycaemia encourages infections, and infection raises the blood glucose level.

Suggested changes and action to be taken are as follows. If the person with diabetes is self-monitoring, it should be explained that occasional 'high' tests need not be acted upon. However, should hyperglycaemia persist, adjustments may be required (according to identified causes of the high blood sugar levels) regarding food, activity, medication and/or insulin. Particular action should be taken if an infection or illness disturbs blood glucose control.

Guidelines for management of hyperglycaemia (by the primary care team)

A blood glucose meter used in the practice or from a doctor's bag should be subject to internal quality control and the results recorded. All *in vitro* devices are subject to Medicines and Healthcare products Regulatory Agency (2002) guidance.

Short-acting insulin (e.g. NovoRapid; kept in the surgery and in the doctor's bag) may be useful to lower the blood glucose level in acute illness.

- Review therapy, check blood glucose levels and the presence or absence of ketones, and treat intercurrent illness. Ketonuria is unlikely in type 2 diabetes, but protracted hyperglycaemia can lead to hyperosmolar non-ketotic coma (HONK).

- Consider short-term insulin therapy (for people usually treated with diet and oral hypoglycaemic agents).

- Refer the person to hospital if vomiting, hyperglycaemia or ketosis persists.

- Blood glucose control may deteriorate rapidly during an illness of any kind. People with diabetes require instructions on action to be taken during any intercurrent illness (Boxes 12.1 and 12.2; see also Appendix 5). It is helpful if the relative or carer is also aware of these instructions in case the person with diabetes is unable to carry them out.

- The relative or carer should be able to draw up and give insulin if necessary and be able to monitor blood or urine glucose levels (if this is possible and appropriate).

- The person with diabetes and/or their relative should have an emergency contact telephone number (Figure 12.1).

When people feel nauseous, it helps to find out what they would prefer to eat. The composition of foods is usually described on the packet. You are aiming to replace the carbohydrate in the food that people would normally eat during the day. For example, some people find that foods such as rice cakes are useful if they feel nauseous.

Box 12.1
Sick day rules for a person with type 2 diabetes

■ A minor illness, such as a cold, may cause your blood sugar levels to rise

■ Be prepared – have the right equipment and information readily available

■ Your local diabetes care team may have printed advice sheets

■ Sugar-free cough remedies are available from your local pharmacist

■ Blood sugar levels will return to normal once the infection is over, so your usual treatment can then be resumed

■ If you test your blood, you may need to increase the frequency to three or four times a day – especially if you use insulin to manage your diabetes

CONSULT YOUR DOCTOR

■ Consult your doctor if the illness persists, if you have symptoms of high sugar levels or if you have high test results

■ Vomiting may result in you being unable to keep tablets down – consult your doctor

■ Vomiting and diarrhoea may result in you losing a lot of fluid – consult your doctor

IMPORTANT RULES

■ NEVER stop taking your tablets or insulin. You may need an increase in medication during the illness. Discuss this with your diabetes care team

■ Ensure that you drink plenty of liquid (water, tea, etc.) – regular sips if larger amounts are not tolerated

■ If you are not hungry, substitute meals with a liquid or light diet (soup, ice cream, glucose drinks, milk; see Box 12.3 for an emergency exchange list)

Consult your diabetes care team in good time

Box 12.2
Sick day rules for a person with type 1 diabetes

■ A minor illness, such as a cold, may cause your blood sugar levels to rise

■ Sugar levels may continue to rise even though you are off your food

■ Even if you are off your food or vomiting, you may need additional insulin

NEVER STOP YOUR INSULIN

■ Be prepared – have blood glucose testing and ketone testing equipment handy

■ If you test your blood, you may need to increase the frequency to three or four times a day – especially if you use insulin to manage your diabetes

■ Test for ketones if you are unwell and your blood sugar levels are high

■ Drink plenty of sugar-free fluids

■ Contact your local diabetes care team

■ Sugar-free cough remedies are available from your local pharmacist

■ Blood sugar levels will return to normal once the infection is over, so your usual treatment can then be resumed

CONSULT YOUR DOCTOR

■ Consult your doctor if the illness persists, if you have symptoms of high sugar levels or if you have high test results

■ Vomiting may result in escalating blood sugar levels – consult your doctor

■ Vomiting and diarrhoea may result in you losing a lot of fluid – consult your doctor

- NEVER stop taking your insulin. You may need an increase in medication during the illness. Discuss this with your diabetes care team

- Ensure that you drink plenty of liquid (water, tea, etc.) – regular sips if larger amounts are not tolerated

- If you are not hungry, substitute meals with a liquid or light diet (soup, ice cream, glucose drinks, milk; see Box 12.3 for an emergency exchange list)

Consult your diabetes care team in good time

Low blood glucose levels (hypoglycaemia, 'hypo')

- Hypoglycaemia (see also Appendix 5) is generally regarded to exist when the blood glucose level is are below 4 mmol/l ('four is the floor').

- It is important to remember that symptoms of hypoglycaemia may be experienced at blood glucose levels higher than 4 mmol/l, in particular where blood glucose levels have been high for a period of time (e.g. after diagnosis).

- People with diabetes who strictly control their blood glucose levels are at greater risk of hypoglycaemia.

- Hypoglycaemia can be delayed (for many hours after extra activity).

- People on metformin and/or glitazones without other diabetes medication are unlikely to have hypoglycaemic episodes.

- Hypoglycaemic episodes can be protracted on sulphonylureas, for example glibenclamide (which is contraindicated in the elderly).

Hypoglycaemia may be caused by:

- too little food (especially in elderly people);

- delayed or missed meals;

- increased medication or insulin;

Box 12.3
Food/fluids to substitute for portions when you are off your food

If you are ill and do not feel like eating, replace your normal food portions (which used to be called 'exchanges') with fluids such as milk, fruit juice or Lucozade. The list below gives you an idea of suitable substitutes. You should also aim to drink plenty of sugar-free liquids (at least 5 pints (3 litres) each day).

Substitutes to provide 10 g carbohydrate (i.e one exchange or portion)	Quantity (approximate)
Milk	1 cup (200 ml/7 fl oz)
Fruit juice (unsweetened)	1 small glass (100 ml/4 fl oz)
Lucozade	50 ml/2 fl oz
Coca Cola (not diet)	1 wine glass (150 ml/6 fl oz)
Lemonade (fizzy/sweetened)	1 wine glass (150 ml/6 fl oz)
Ice cream	1 briquette or 1 scoop
Jelly (ordinary)	2 tablespoons
Yoghurt (fruit)	½ small carton (60 g)
Yoghurt (plain)	1 small carton (120 g)
Soup (thickened, creamed, e.g. chicken)	1 cup (200 ml/7 fl oz)
Soup (tomato, tinned)	1 small glass (100 ml/4 fl oz)

- increased activity (exercise);
- increased mobility;
- a decrease in concurrent medication affecting glycaemic control;
- stress – life changes;
- hot weather (insulin being absorbed more rapidly);
- a change of injection site (where one site has been used repeatedly followed by the use of a new site);
- a decrease in weight (particularly in elderly people);
- the presence of renal failure;
- alcohol use (as it prevents the release of glucose from the liver in response to lowering blood glucose levels).

People with diabetes need to be aware of this.

An explanation of the symptoms of hypoglycaemia should be included in individuals' care plans, with printed information on how to avoid them and the action to be taken if symptoms develop.

Symptoms of hypoglycaemia

- Sweating
- Pallor
- Headache
- Tingling of the lips
- Pounding heart
- Blurred vision
- Irritability
- Lack of concentration (confusion).

Note: The person having the hypoglycaemic episode may be mistaken as drunk. It is important for them to carry identification.

Diminished warning signs of hypoglycaemia

Warning signs may not occur:

- in the presence of autonomic neuropathy, where diabetes has been diagnosed for many years (over 10 years);
- where strict blood glucose control exists;
- where repeated attacks of hypoglycaemia reduce significant symptoms;
- if the individual is on beta-blockers.

Self-monitoring of blood glucose

Used effectively, the self-monitoring of blood glucose encourages empowerment and the ability for those with diabetes to take appropriate action to control their blood glucose levels. Used ineffectively, however, it is a wasteful use of a costly resource. There is evidence to support the use of self blood glucose monitoring (Welschen et al, 2005; Karter et al, 2006) when it is included in care plans and structured education. Some trusts have limited the prescription of testing strips on the basis of cost, but if patients are motivated and engaged in the process, this should not be the case (Diabetes UK, 2003).

In 2004 and 2005, a group of specialists in diabetes care, comprising consultants, general practitioners and nurses among others, provided a Consensus Statement that was published in the journal *Diabetes and Primary Care* (Owens et al, 2004, 2005). The table of recommendations is reproduced as Box 12.4.

Why monitor?

■ To involve individuals with diabetes in their own care and education.

■ To allow the individual to alter his or her medication to suit blood glucose levels.

■ To indicate a deterioration of diabetes control, so that an appropriate treatment review can take place.

■ To indicate an improvement in diabetes control after a weight, dietary, medication or insulin change or adjustment.

■ To appreciate the reasons for self-monitoring, the person with diabetes needs to understand the factors affecting the rise and fall of blood glucose levels, including the associated symptoms, possible reasons, changes to be made and actions to be taken.

■ Targets for testing and control should be appropriate and individually negotiated.

Urine testing for glucose is little used nowadays and is an ineffective measure of current blood glucose levels. There is little evidence of its efficacy.

Blood testing technique

■ It is essential that the hands are washed (by the person testing), preferably in warm water to encourage blood flow to the fingertips and to ensure that the test is uncontaminated.

■ Spirit swabs should not be used to clean the skin as the spirit may affect the results.

■ The side of the tips of fingers should be used (as this is less painful).

■ Use a different finger at each test (to avoid discomfort).

Box 12.4
Advice on self-monitoring of blood glucose (SMBG)

- The most important principles for establishing SMBG in patients with type 1 or type 2 diabetes must be to improve the quality and stability of glycaemic control and the avoidance of hypoglycaemia

- In general, blood glucose concentrations fluctuate more widely in people with type 1 diabetes than those with type 2 diabetes

- Appropriate training and education is required so that people with diabetes can through SMBG understand their diabetes and safely adjust their lifestyle and insulin doses according to their SMBG results

- Good glycaemic control is essential to minimise the risk of short-term (hyper- and hypoglycaemia) and long-term (vascular) complications relating to diabetes

- Individual patients should be made aware of the importance of SMBG in recognition of the evidence emanating from the DCCT (type 1 diabetes) and UKPDS (type 2 diabetes)

- SMBG has an essential role to play in ensuring the safety and efficacy of blood glucose lowering therapies

- The provision of materials for SMBG is key to patient empowerment and to ensure the achievement of good glycaemic control safely

- Drivers with diabetes should SMBG before commencing any journey and at regular intervals on long journeys

- Depending on the treatment regimen, knowledge of actual pre-meal and/or post-meal blood glucose levels is needed to avoid hyperglycaemia and prevent hypoglycaemia

- Any change in blood glucose lowering therapy requires SMBG to ensure safety (avoidance of hypoglycaemia) while optimising effectiveness

- Reliance on subjective assessment of blood glucose levels is unhelpful

- Patients receiving terminal care will require monitoring to ensure that they avoid hypoglycaemia and/or periods of excessive hyperglycaemia

■ People with diabetes who are in coronary care units should be monitored using hospital laboratory facilities

■ All people with type 1 diabetes should have access to SMBG at least four times per day as required

■ People with type 2 diabetes have different SMBG requirements depending on their treatment regimen

■ In the absence of regular testing by the patient, more frequent SMBG measurements during the two weeks before a clinic visit may provide the patient and the clinician with more information to assess current glycaemic control

Diabetes type	Treatment group	Monitoring regime
Type 1 diabetes	All people with type 1 diabetes	• SMBG should be regarded as an integral part of treating all people with type 1 diabetes
		• People with type 1 diabetes should be educated to SMBG and adjust treatment appropriately
		• The majority of patients with type 1 diabetes should consider SMBG four or more times per day to prevent hypoglycaemia and control hyperglycaemia
		• To avoid metabolic emergencies such as diabetic ketoacidosis may require frequent SMBG
Diabetic pregnancy	Diabetic pregnancy	• Pregnant women with type 1 diabetes, plus those with type 2 diabetes requiring insulin and patients with gestational diabetes requiring insulin should SMBG at least four times per day to include both fasting and postmeal blood glucose measurements

Diabetes type	Treatment group	Monitoring regime
Diabetic pregnancy	Diabetic pregnancy	• In diet-treated patients it may be necessary to SMBG with the same frequency as insulin-treated patients to ensure strict glycaemic control • In insulin-treated patients increased frequency of testing may be necessary in the first trimester when the risk of hypoglycaemia is greatest
Type 2 diabetes	Intensive insulin therapy	• People who adopt intensive insulin therapies require regular feedback regarding SMBG levels • People with type 2 diabetes who use a multiple daily insulin regimen should SMBG in the same way as those with type 1 diabetes • Fasting blood glucose should be tested daily during basal insulin dose titration
Type 2 diabetes	Conventional insulin therapy	• People with type 2 diabetes who are using a conventional insulin regimen and who have stable control should SMBG two or three times a week • People with type 2 diabetes who are using a conventional insulin regimen and who have less stable control should SMBG at least once daily, varying the time of testing between fasting, premeal and postmeal • Fasting blood glucose should be tested daily during basal insulin dose titration

Diabetes type	Treatment group	Monitoring regime
Type 2 diabetes	Combined insulin and oral antidiabetic therapy	• Fasting blood glucose should be tested daily during basal insulin dose titration • People with type 2 diabetes who use insulin or oral hypoglycaemic agents should SMBG at least once daily, varying the time of testing between fasting, premeal and postmeal
Type 2 diabetes	Diet and exercise	• People with type 2 diabetes who have good control on diet and exercise, metformin or glitazone treatment do not need SMBG monitoring, unless they are destabilised by other factors • Glycaemic control managed through diet and exercise in people with type 2 diabetes is best monitored through HbA$_{1c}$ testing • Patients with type 2 diabetes managed only on diet and exercise do not normally require routine SMBG. Informed patients may choose SMBG as a means of monitoring lifestyle changes
Type 2 diabetes	Metformin (+/– glitazone)	As for diet and exercise
Type 2 diabetes	Glitazone (+/– metformin)	As for diet and exercise
Type 2 diabetes	Sulphonylurea alone (or in combination with other oral antidiabetic)	• Hypoglycaemia may be more common than assumed in people with type 2 diabetes on sulphonylureas and SMBG will reveal this situation

From Owens et al, 2005, with kind permission of SB Communications.
HbA$_{1c}$, glycated haemoglobin.

- If the drop of blood is difficult to collect, 'milking' the finger from the base up may help, as may lowering the finger.

- Finger-pricking lancets should be used only once and disposed of safely (see Chapter 11).

- Modern meters require very small amounts of blood and usually have strips that keep the blood away from the machine.

Note: Health professionals using blood glucose meters must ensure they are subject to quality-control procedures and that disposable devices, for example Unistix or Softclix Pro, are used to prick the finger.

Interpretation of results: action to take

- Blood tests taken before meals and before bedtime will indicate control.

- One blood test each day, taken at a different time, will provide a blood glucose profile over several days.

- Pre-meal tests are the most useful in type 1 diabetes to adjust insulin; those with type 2 diabetes should take a mixture of pre- and post-meal samples if their HbA_{1c} level is above 7.5%.

- A post-meal test can be useful in noting the effects of foods eaten.

- Blood tests should be carried out more frequently during the course of an infection or intercurrent illness (2–4-hourly).

- Should blood glucose levels be consistently high or low, the reasons for this should be examined and appropriate action taken.

- Occasional high tests should not be acted upon unless they consistently occur at the same time of day.

- Should lifestyle be different on weekdays or weekends, blood tests will demonstrate this. Adjustments in food, medication or insulin may be required.

- If extra activity is anticipated, blood glucose levels should be checked beforehand and extra carbohydrate taken or insulin reduced (or both).

- After extra activity or exercise, blood glucose levels should be checked soon afterwards and some hours later (in case of delayed hypoglycaemia). Strenuous physical activity may continue to have an effect into the next day.

- Talking meters are available, at a cost, for people with poor eyesight. Your local specialist team should be able to advise.

- Meters should be suggested only in association with education about their use.

- Blood monitoring strips are available free on prescription for people receiving medication for their diabetes – oral agents and insulin.

- Finger-pricking devices can be purchased by the individual. They are not available on FP10 prescription forms.

- Finger-pricking lancets should be checked for their compatibility with the selected device.

- Recording of blood tests should be taught and a testing diary provided. Many companies will provide these free (see Appendix 4).

References

Diabetes Control and Complications Trial (DCCT) Research Group (1993). The effect of intensive treatment of diabetes on the development and progression of long-term complications in insulin-dependent diabetes mellitus. *New England Journal of Medicine* **329**: 977–986.

Diabetes UK (2003). *Position Statement on Home Monitoring of Blood Glucose Levels*. London: Diabetes UK.

Karter A, Parker M, Moffet H et al (2006). Longitudinal study of new and prevalent use of self-monitoring of blood glucose. *Diabetes Care* **29**: 1757–1763.

Medicines and Healthcare products Regulatory Agency (2002). *Management and Use of IVD Point of Care Test Devices*. London: DoH.

National Institute for Health and Clinical Excellence (2002). *Management of Type 2 Diabetes. Management of Blood Glucose*. Inherited Guideline G. London: NICE.

Owens D, Barnett AJ, Pickup J et al (2004). Blood glucose self-monitoring in type 1 and type 2 diabetes: reaching a multidisciplinary consensus. *Diabetes and Primary Care* **6**: 8–16.

Owens D, Pickup J, Barnett A et al (2005). The continuing debate on self-monitoring of blood glucose in diabetes. *Diabetes and Primary Care* **7**: 9–21.

UK Prospective Diabetes Study Group (1998). Intensive blood-glucose control with sulphonylureas or insulin compared with conventional treatment and risk of complications in patients with type 2 diabetes (UKPDS 33). *Lancet* **352**: 837–853.

Welschen LMC, Bloemendal E, Nijpels G et al (2005). Self-monitoring of Blood Glucose in Patients with Type 2 Diabetes Mellitus Who Are Not Using Insulin. Cochrane Database of Systematic Reviews, Issue 2, Article CD005060, pub2.

Further reading

Diabetes UK leaflet: *Coping with Diabetes When You Are Ill*. London: Diabetes UK. (See Appendix 4)

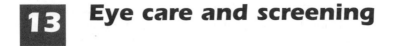

13 Eye care and screening

Questions this chapter will help you answer

- What targets are set for retinal screening?
- What is quality-assured retinal screening?
- Does everyone on my register have access to it?
- How do we ensure call and recall?
- When should eye drops not be used?
- What other eye conditions are more common in diabetes?

> *I did not realise how serious diabetes was at first.*
> *Perhaps I might have taken it more seriously*
> *if I knew then what I know now.*
>
> Audit Commission (2002)

Further information is contained in Chapter 24.

Critical diabetes-specific targets for eye screening were set in the National Service Framework for Diabetes in 2002:

> By 2006, a minimum of 80% of people with diabetes to be offered screening for the early detection (and treatment if needed) of diabetic retinopathy as part of a systematic programme that meets national standards, rising to 100% coverage of those at risk of retinopathy by end 2007.

In order to deliver this service, primary care organisations needed to put in place a systematic eye-screening and treatment programme, including recall. The system needed to be capable of quality assurance.

Scotland (National Services Division NHS Scotland, 2006) and Northern Ireland are developing their own systems. Scotland initiated the first national eye-screening programme in the world in 2002 but did not utilise digital camera screening. Neither did it fully address those who could not attend for screening, creating inequalities.

The recommendation across the UK is that there should be a nation-wide screening programme offering recall from diabetes registers, providing quality assurance on whichever system is used and being available to all people with diabetes.

The UK National Screening Committee provides information and updates on its website (see Appendix 4) and published a workbook in 2004 entitled *Essential Elements in Developing a Diabetic Retinopathy Screening Programme*, with the following recommendations:

- Assess current screening practice within the locality and involve the key stakeholders, for example commissioners, ophthalmologists, diabetologists, optometrists, nurses and IT representatives, in planning future developments, and ensure that each programme is based around at least 12 000 people with diabetes per 500 000 population base.

- Appoint an individual with responsibility for leading the diabetic retinopathy programme.

- Have a policy to involve people with diabetes and create public information and awareness.

- Set up a central administration structure for the service, including establishing a single collated patient list.

- Determine who is going to screen people with diabetes for retinopathy, and at what location, and what to do with patients who have poor-quality images.

- The screening appointment should produce two digital colour photographs of each eye after mydriasis by a trained and accredited screener.

- Set up a grading centre for grading images and for quality assurance purposes.

- Organise arbitration grading so that an ophthalmologist can view the images of people considered to be referable, and an ophthalmologist or other health professional experienced in this field can quality-assure a second full grading.

- At the eye clinic, set up measures to determine the number of false-positive results, report any false-negative presentations and collect data for standards relating to clinic appointments and treatment.

- Consider the IT requirements that will be needed in the light of local requirements (server size, software for managing the program, back-up of server and images after capture, number of users, number of sites and any upgrade to existing hardware and connections).

- Consider the local training requirements of the workforce in parallel with national initiatives.

- Strategic Health Authorities should take an active interest in the commissioning process of the primary care organisations to assess whether the essential elements contained in this document are addressed. Strategic Health Authorities should also ensure that what is included in the Local Development Plan adequately provides for both capital purchases such as cameras, software, trolleys and transport, and revenue workforce expenditures.

- According to National Service Framework targets, 80% of patients on the single collated list should have been offered screening appointments by the end of March 2006. In addition, all patients should have been offered screening appointments between April 2006 and the end of December 2007.

Features of an acceptable national programme: an integrated pattern of care

The main features of any acceptable national programme are:

- the systematic call and recall of all eligible patients;

- trained professionals;

- recorded outcomes;

- targets and standards;

- quality assurance;

- promotion of uptake of screening;

- efficient and appropriate follow-up of all those with retinopathy.

Organisation of diabetic eye screening in primary care

Maintain a practice register of all people with diabetes. Check that the numbers match the expected prevalence in the locality.

The role of the primary care team

It is important that all people with diabetes are aware of the importance of eye-screening and know why and how to access their local eye-screening programme. Although it is feasible to check visual acuity in general practice, fundoscopy requires a fully darkened room and, with the National Screening Committee's guidance, a digital retinal camera.

■ Ensure that individuals are aware of the significance of diabetes eye disease and the need for regular eye examination regardless of any absence of symptoms.

■ Make sure that they are aware of the local eye-screening programme and how to access it.

■ Explain that the National Health Service pays for diabetes eye-screening programmes (where available) and that there will be no charge to them.

■ Give people with diabetes written information explaining the local system for eye-screening.

■ Encourage them to attend.

■ Unless symptoms (of visual deterioration) are present, advise the patient not to have his or her visual acuity tested for 2–3 months immediately after diagnosis, because the lens may be affected by changes in blood glucose level.

■ Check that they have attended, that the results have been recorded and that referral or other action has been taken if indicated.

■ Note when the next annual eye examination is due.

■ Ensure that the recall and follow-up system is in place for the next annual sight test and eye-screening to take place (see the sample letter and form in Figures 13.1 and 13.2).

Sheffield Diabetes Eye Screening Programme
Royal Hallamshire Hospital
Glossop Road, Sheffield S10 2JF
Tel: 0114 271 1821 / Fax: 0114 271 1931

2 August 2001

Mrs P Johnston
The Tannery
Black Terrace
SHEFFIELD
S1 1XX

Dear Mrs Johnston

As part of your diabetes care, I would like to inform you that you are now due for a vision test and eye examination. Please follow the steps below:

1. Ensure that the details on the enclosed screening form are correct. If there are changes to be made, write them on the form. (There is no need to telephone the co-ordinator.)

2. Telephone one of the opticians named on the list attached, and state that you have received your screening form and need to make an appointment. Please ensure that the appointment is made with the person whose name is on the list.

Note: you DO NOT attend the hospital for this appointment.

3. Take the enclosed screening form with you to your appointment and give it to the optician on arrival.

Please avoid driving to this appointment.

Please note: If you attend the Eye Department or Diabetes Centre at the Royal Hallamshire Hospital or the Diabetes Centre at the Northern General Hospital, please contact the Eye Screening Office on the above telephone number BEFORE you make your appointment with the optician.

If you have any further queries please contact the screening department.

Yours sincerely

J Smith

Co-ordinator

Figure 13.1 Example of a local diabetes eye-screening programme recall letter (Sheffield)

When the eye-screening result is known

If the result is normal:

- record the result and confirm the next screening date;

- ensure that the person with diabetes is aware of the result.

If the result is abnormal:

- ensure that the findings and implications are explained to the individual;

- ensure an appropriate referral to ophthalmology if indicated;

- ensure that there is a general assessment of diabetes control and associated vascular risk factors, and treat further as necessary;

- refer to a specialist diabetes clinic as per your local arrangements;

- confirm the next screening date as indicated.

Audit: Points are awarded through the General Medical Services contract for achievement of clinical indicators.

Visual acuity

Visual acuity is a simple test indicating the acuteness of central vision for distance and near or reading vision.

- In the condition of diabetes, normal visual acuity may be shown even though diabetic retinopathy is demonstrated by fundoscopy.

- Visual acuity should be checked annually either separately or together with full retinal screening.

- If the pupils are dilated before visual acuity is checked, the patient will be unable to see the test chart.

- If visual acuity is checked in the practice and has deteriorated, the person with diabetes should be advised to visit an optometrist.

- Sight deterioration may be caused by a cataract, which (if mature) requires referral to an ophthalmologist for removal. (Remember that both eyes may be affected by cataracts.)

Patient Information	Diabetes Data	GP Information

Our Ref 123
NHS No. 22222
Surname SMITH
Forename MARGARET
Address 2 WHITE CLOSE
  SHEFFIELD
Postcode S100 2FT 25/12/48
DOB
	Duration
	Control: DIET/TABLETS/INSULIN
	
	Care For Follow Up Of Diabetes
	Specify: GP/RHH/NGH/SCH/Other
		Name DR F. BLOGGS
		Practice ACORN MEDICAL PRACT.
		Address OAKTREE ROAD
		  SHEFFIELD
		Postcode S100 2FF
		Previous Ophthal. Attend. Y / Ⓝ
		Consultant

Examination Date: ....

	R	L	FUNDUS	R	L	ACTION	Tick
			Normal			Routine Recall	
Visual Acuity (Best Corrected)			Background DR			Routine Recall	
Previous Visual Acuity Date:			Preproliferative DR			Early Referral	
PINHOLE ACUITY			Vitreous Haemorrhage			Urgent Referral	
CORNEA			Proliferation			Urgent Referral	
IRIS			Retinal Detachment			Urgent Referral	
LENS			Mild Maculopathy			Routine Recall	
VITREOUS			Moderate Maculopathy			Routine Referral	
IOP (pneumo/applan)			Severe Maculopathy			Early Referral	
			Previous Laser RX	Y / N	Y / N		
			Other			Specify	

Any Pre-Existing Pathology: ....

Any other Information / Referral / Sketches:

Stamp

Examiner: .... Signature: ....

CSUH Payment Slip   NHS No: 22222

Patient: Surname: ...... SMITH ....   Forename ...... MARGARET ......

Address: ...2 WHITE CLOSE
SHEFFIED S100 2FT

I have examined the above patient with a mydriatic and claim the agreed fee ☐

I have examined the above patient without a mydriatic for the following reasons ☐

GOC No: ....

Examiner: ....

Practice Address: ....

Address for Payment if Different ....

....

Stamp

Figure 13.2 Example of a local diabetes eye-screening programme multi-copy form (Sheffield). The top white form is retained by the optometrist, the green copy is for the person with diabetes, and the yellow or pink copy is returned to the diabetes eye-screening coordinator or sent to the GP

- If diabetic retinopathy is detected and is sight-threatening, urgent referral to an ophthalmologist is required.

- During the stabilisation of diabetes (after diagnosis or where medication or insulin has been introduced or adjusted), visual disturbances, such as blurred vision, may be experienced. These visual changes may vary from individual to individual and will improve with time.

- Possible visual changes such as these should be explained (they occur as a result of changes in glucose levels in the lens of the eye).

- The person concerned should be reassured and told that, once blood glucose levels settle, vision will almost certainly improve.

On diagnosis and if alterations in therapy are made (such as a change from medication to insulin), the person concerned should be advised not to visit an optician until visual changes have settled (which may be a period of 2–3 months).

Considerable inconvenience and expense (if new spectacles are advised) will be incurred by those with diabetes if they are not correctly informed of the possibility of visual changes.

Note: Annual eye tests (by an optician) are free for people with diabetes.

Opticians/optometrists

There are three types of optician:

1 *Optometrists* (also called ophthalmic opticians) carry out eye tests to check the quality of the individual's sight, look for signs of eye disease that may need treatment from a doctor or eye surgeon, and prescribe and fit glasses and contact lenses. These may work with general practices to perform fundoscopy where no central system is in place.

2 *Ophthalmic medical practitioners.* These are medical doctors who are also trained to carry out eye examinations and prescribe glasses.

3 *Dispensing opticians.* These professionals fit and sell glasses but do not test eyes. They can give advice on types of lens, such as single vision or bifocal, and help to choose frames. They are available on many high streets.

Note: Although they are experienced practitioners of ophthalmoscopy, ophthalmic opticians screening for diabetic retinopathy do not always dilate the pupils before fundoscopy examination. Dilatation of the pupils (by instilling mydriatic drops) is essential for the detection of diabetic retinopathy, especially peripheral maculopathy (retinopathy detected at the periphery of the retinal fundus and not uncommon in people with type 2 diabetes of long duration; this may also be present at diagnosis).

Fundoscopy should not be carried out in general practice unless as an emergency and only then if facilities exist, for example a fully darkened room and an approved ophthalmoscope.

Warning:

- If the patient has a lens implant in place after a cataract extraction, mydriatic drops should not be used.

- Mydriatic drops can precipitate closed-angle glaucoma in patients with shallow anterior chambers. The onset is rapid and painful. The eye becomes red with a hazy cornea and blurred vision. This is, however, very rare. Should it occur, immediate ophthalmic treatment is required.

- The possibility of precipitating acute glaucoma should not preclude the use of mydriatic drops and fundoscopy examination because this complication is so rare and, in the practice situation, can be quickly referred for treatment.

- People with diabetes should be advised not to drive for at least 2 hours after dilatation of the pupils and may benefit from sunglasses to prevent glare immediately afterwards.

- It is important that the retinas are screened annually for diabetic retinopathy.

Cataracts

- Cataracts are more common in older people.

- Studies suggest that cataracts occur more often and at an earlier age in people with diabetes.

- It is important that cataracts are monitored and extracted as soon as appropriate when found in people with diabetes, so that vision and independence are restored.

- Screening for diabetic retinopathy is facilitated once the cataracts have been removed.

Age-related macular degeneration

- Age-related macular degeneration is a common cause of visual loss in older people. There is no effective treatment for this condition.

Chronic glaucoma

- Chronic glaucoma (as well as cataract) is more common in people with diabetes.
- The development of chronic glaucoma is slow and painless.
- It is important that intraocular pressure is measured and recorded annually.
- The measurement of intraocular pressure may be carried out in general practice (with appropriate equipment, knowledge and skills), by an optometrist or in a screening programme.
- People with diabetes and individuals (aged 40 years and over) who are close relatives of known glaucoma patients are eligible for free National Health Service tests for the detection of glaucoma.
- Chronic glaucoma results in a gradual reduction in the peripheral field of vision so insidious that the patient is unaware, even at a late stage, when tunnel vision develops.
- Treatment consists of eye drops or oral agents. If these fail, surgical trabeculectomy or laser therapy is carried out.

Laser treatment/therapy

(Figure 13.3.)

- The risks of having laser treatment are far less than the risks of not having laser treatment.
- Laser therapy seals blood vessels that are leaking. It can appear very bright and may disturb the sight immediately after treatment. Individuals with diabetes should be advised that disturbances are usually transient. Night and colour vision may also be affected.

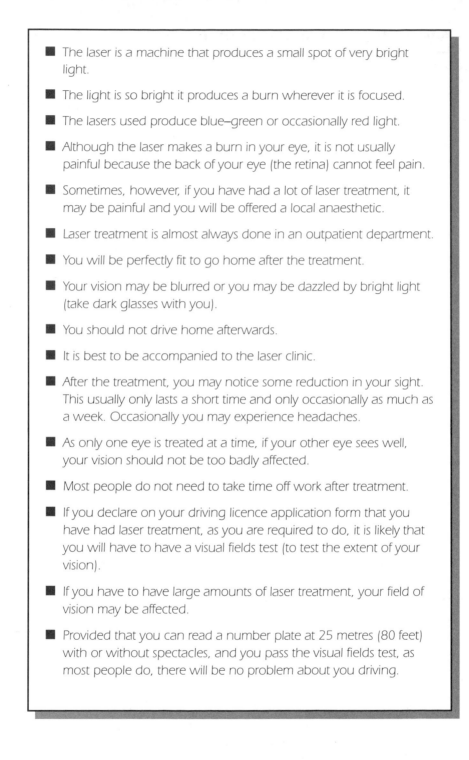

- The laser is a machine that produces a small spot of very bright light.

- The light is so bright it produces a burn wherever it is focused.

- The lasers used produce blue–green or occasionally red light.

- Although the laser makes a burn in your eye, it is not usually painful because the back of your eye (the retina) cannot feel pain.

- Sometimes, however, if you have had a lot of laser treatment, it may be painful and you will be offered a local anaesthetic.

- Laser treatment is almost always done in an outpatient department.

- You will be perfectly fit to go home after the treatment.

- Your vision may be blurred or you may be dazzled by bright light (take dark glasses with you).

- You should not drive home afterwards.

- It is best to be accompanied to the laser clinic.

- After the treatment, you may notice some reduction in your sight. This usually only lasts a short time and only occasionally as much as a week. Occasionally you may experience headaches.

- As only one eye is treated at a time, if your other eye sees well, your vision should not be too badly affected.

- Most people do not need to take time off work after treatment.

- If you declare on your driving licence application form that you have had laser treatment, as you are required to do, it is likely that you will have to have a visual fields test (to test the extent of your vision).

- If you have to have large amounts of laser treatment, your field of vision may be affected.

- Provided that you can read a number plate at 25 metres (80 feet) with or without spectacles, and you pass the visual fields test, as most people do, there will be no problem about you driving.

Figure 13.3 Laser therapy: patient information sheet

- It is fairly common to lose some peripheral vision after laser treatment. Patients should be advised it is their legal duty to notify the Driver and Vehicle Licensing Agency (DVLA) if they have had laser treatment.

- Occasionally, central vision may deteriorate. People with diabetes should understand that this is a possibility. It can be permanent.

- The person with diabetes should have access to a trained health professional to answer any queries prior to laser therapy.

References

Department of Health (2002). *National Service Framework for Diabetes: Delivery Strategy*. London: DoH.

National Services Division NHS Scotland (2006). *Diabetic Retinopathy Screening*. Edinburgh: NHS Scotland.

UK National Screening Committee (2004). *Essential Elements in Developing a Diabetic Retinopathy Screening Programme*. Version 3.21. UK National Screening Committee.

Further reading

Alexander WD (1998). *Diabetic Retinopathy: A Guide for Diabetes Care Teams*. Oxford: Blackwell Science.

Rudnicka AR, Birch J (2000). *Diabetic Eye Disease Identification and Co-management*. Oxford : Butterworth Heinemann.

Taylor R (2000). *Handbook of Retinal Screening in Diabetes*. Chichester: John Wiley & Sons.

14 Foot care and surveillance

Questions this chapter will help you answer

- Do I have systems in place to detect the 'at-risk' foot?

- Are my patients getting an effective foot check to detect complications?

- How do I perform a basic foot check?

- How do I use a monofilament?

- When should I refer to a chiropodist or podiatrist?

- What questions will help me to determine whether someone has painful diabetic neuropathy?

> *Without good organisational links [between specialties], serious delays in treatments can occur.*
>
> Audit Commission (2000)

People with diabetes should be considered to have 'at-risk' feet unless proven otherwise. Diabetes is still the highest cause of lower limb amputation, and much suffering could be prevented by early detection and management. Peripheral vascular disease, in which the large blood vessels to the lower limbs are damaged, and neuropathy causing pain and/or loss of sensation need to be identified early to prevent deterioration (National Institute for Health and Clinical Excellence, 2004):

- 20–40% have neuropathy.

- 20–40% have peripheral vascular disease.

- 5% of people with diabetes may develop a foot ulcer in any year.

- Amputation rates are often around 0.5% per year.

In the fight to prevent, or halt the progression of, these conditions, a holistic approach needs to be adopted. Certainly, glucose, blood pressure and lipid control are essential, but they should be combined with effective education on lifestyle changes in diet, physical activity and smoking cessation. People with diabetes and their carers need to be involved in education and decision-making, and be given the information to enable them to understand the need for possible change.

- A foot check should form part of the annual review, or be instigated more frequently if signs or symptoms are present.

- The health professional conducting the check should possess the knowledge and skills to enable him or her to do checks. Referral to a podiatrist may be preferable.

- A basic foot check includes:

  - 10 g monofilament testing (Figures 14.1 and 14.2). Monofilaments should not be used to test more than 10 patients in one session and should be left for at least 24 hours to 'recover' (buckling strength) between sessions;

  - palpation of foot pulses;

  - examination for corns, calluses, deformity and skin condition.

- Health professionals carrying out basic checks should have a referral policy in place if abnormalities are detected.

- Recording the results is important.

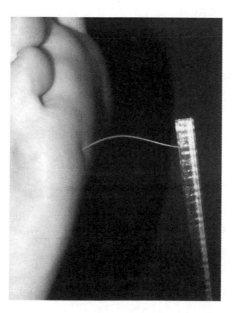

Figure 14.1 Monofilament testing

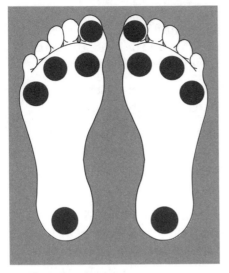

♦ Demonstrate on the patient's hand or arm, so they know what the sensation feels like

♦ Ask the patient to close their eyes and say 'yes' when they feel the filament

♦ Place the tip of the filament perpendicular to the skin and increase the pressure until it bends. Hold for 1–2 seconds

♦ Use the filament on all test sites on the feet

♦ Do not test over callus as sensation will be reduced

♦ The various sites should be tested randomly. Sites to which patients do not respond should be re-tested.

Test sites
Test sites shown are based on the most common sites of foot ulceration. Additional sites may include the dorsum of the foot, especially the 1st toe

Figure 14.2 The monofilament test sites for neuropathy
(With thanks to Blackwater Valley & Hart PCT Podiatry Department)

There are difficulties in education relating to foot care: patients can have difficulties taking messages on board when they cannot feel the damage that is being done. In addition, patients at risk need specifically to be made aware if they have existing neuropathy and ischaemia, and what that means to them.

Foot risk can be classified as:

■ low current risk

■ increased risk

■ high risk

■ ulcerated foot.

Low current risk of foot ulcers

(normal sensation, palpable pulses)

■ Agree a management plan including foot care education with each person. Add this to the patient-held record.

■ Arrange annual recall.

Increased risk of foot ulcers

(neuropathy, absent pulses or other risk factor)

■ Arrange a regular review, 3–6-monthly, by trained and knowledgeable health professionals. Referral to podiatry or a specialist practitioner is desirable.

■ At each review:
 ◆ inspect the person's feet
 ◆ consider the need for vascular assessment
 ◆ evaluate footwear
 ◆ enhance foot care education
 ◆ record the results.

Note: Those who have had a previous foot ulcer, deformity or skin changes should be managed as high risk.

High risk of foot ulcers

(neuropathy or absent pulses plus deformity or skin changes or previous ulcer)

■ Arrange frequent review (1–3-monthly) by the foot protection team or appropriate health professional with skills and knowledge in foot care.

■ Consider a referral to the podiatry service.

■ At each review:
 ◆ inspect the patient's feet;
 ◆ consider the need for vascular assessment;
 ◆ evaluate and ensure the appropriate provision of intensified foot care education;
 ◆ consider specialist footwear and insoles;
 ◆ review skin and nail care.

■ Ensure special arrangements for those people with disabilities or immobility.

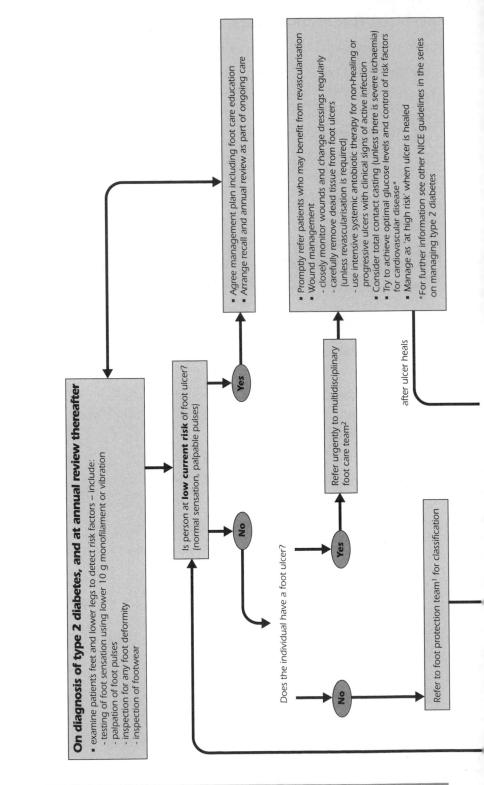

On diagnosis of type 2 diabetes, and at annual review thereafter

- examine patients feet and lower legs to detect risk factors – include:
  - testing of foot sensation using lower 10 g monofilament or vibration
  - palpation of foot pulses
  - inspection for any foot deformity
  - inspection of footwear

Is person at **low current risk** of foot ulcer?
(normal sensation, palpable pulses)

No **Yes**

Does the individual have a foot ulcer?

No **Yes**

Refer to foot protection team[1] for classification

Refer urgently to multidisciplinary foot care team[2]

- Agree management plan including foot care education
- Arrange recall and annual review as part of ongoing care

- Promptly refer patients who may benefit from revascularisation
- Wound management
  - closely monitor wounds and change dressings regularly
  - carefully remove dead tissue from foot ulcers
    (unless revascularisation is required)
  - use intensive systemic antibiotic therapy for non-healing or
    progressive ulcers with clinical signs of active infection
- Consider total contact casting (unless there is severe ischaemia)
- Try to achieve optimal glucose levels and control of risk factors
  for cardiovascular disease*
- Manage as 'at high risk' when ulcer is healed

*For further information see other NICE guidelines in the series
on managing type 2 diabetes

after ulcer heals

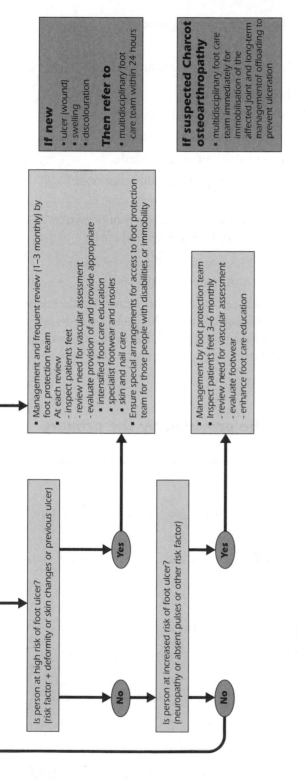

Is person at high risk of foot ulcer?
(risk factor + deformity or skin changes or previous ulcer)

No → **Is person at increased risk of foot ulcer?**
(neuropathy or absent pulses or other risk factor)

Yes →
- Management and frequent review (1–3 monthly) by foot protection team
  - At each review
    - inspect patients feet
    - review need for vascular assessment
    - evaluate provision of and provide appropriate
  - intensified foot care education
  - specialist footwear and insoles
  - skin and nail care
- Ensure special arrangements for access to foot protection team for those people with disabilities or immobility

No

Yes →
- Management by foot protection team
- Inspect patients feet 3–6 monthly
  - review need for vascular assessment
  - evaluate footwear
  - enhance foot care education

If new
- ulcer (wound)
- swelling
- discolouration

Then refer to
- multidisciplinary foot care team within 24 hours

If suspected Charcot osteoarthropathy
- multidisciplinary foot care team immediately for immobilisation of the affected joint and long-term management of offloading to prevent ulceration

Figure 14.3 Algorithm for care provided by the diabetes team
(Reproduced with permission from NICE)

[1] A team with expertise in protecting the foot: typically members of the team include podiatrists, orthotists and footcare specialists
[2] A team of highly trained special podiatrists and orthotists, nurses with training in dressing diabetic foot wounds and diabetologists with expertise in lower limb complications

Care of people with foot care emergencies and foot ulcers

- Refer to the multidisciplinary foot care team within 24 hours.
- Expect that team, as a minimum, to:
  - ◆ investigate and treat vascular insufficiency;
  - ◆ initiate and supervise wound management;
  - ◆ use dressings and debridement as indicated;
  - ◆ use systemic antibiotic therapy for cellulitis or bone infection as indicated;
  - ◆ ensure an effective means of distributing foot pressures, including specialist footwear, orthotics and casts.
- Support the patient to achieve optimal glucose levels and control of risk factors for cardiovascular disease.

Members of the general practice diabetes care team should ensure that all people are receiving assessment and education on foot care at least annually wherever their care is organised. Information from specialist letters should be updated on practice computer systems or templates.

What foot care should be provided by the primary care team?

(Figure 14.3.)

- Identification of people with diabetes who are 'at risk' of foot problems.
- An annual (more often for those 'at risk') examination of both feet.
- An annual examination of shoes.
- Education about foot care and footwear.
- Appropriate and timely referral for chiropody (podiatry) treatment.
- Appropriate and timely referral to a specialist foot clinic (if needed).

How to organise foot care in general practice

- Those with diabetes and their carers should be involved in education and decision-making.

- Arrange recall and annual review as part of ongoing care.

- Healthcare professionals and other personnel involved in the assessment of the at-risk foot should have the necessary knowledge and skills.

- As part of the annual review, trained personnel should examine patients' feet to detect risk factors for ulceration.

- An agreed management plan should be in place and findings recorded in the patient-held record (where available).

- Extra vigilance should be used for people who are older or frail, have had diabetes for a long time, have poor vision, have poor footwear, smoke, are socially deprived or live alone.

- Strategies, for example a district nurse visit or domiciliary podiatry, need to be agreed by members of the primary care diabetes team to address those who cannot attend the practice.

- Structured patient education should be made available to all people with diabetes at the time of initial diagnosis, and then as required on an ongoing basis, based on a formal, regular assessment of need.

- Use different patient education approaches until optimal methods appear to be identified in terms of desired outcomes.

The diabetic foot

The two major complications of diabetes, causing foot ulceration, are (Figure 14.4 and Table 14.1):

- abnormal circulation (micro- and macrovascular disease – ischaemia);

- diabetic neuropathy (autonomic and peripheral; see below).

It is important to recognise that one or other or both of these complications may be present in the same patient, and to be able to recognise the differences between them and the associated factors leading to foot ulceration.

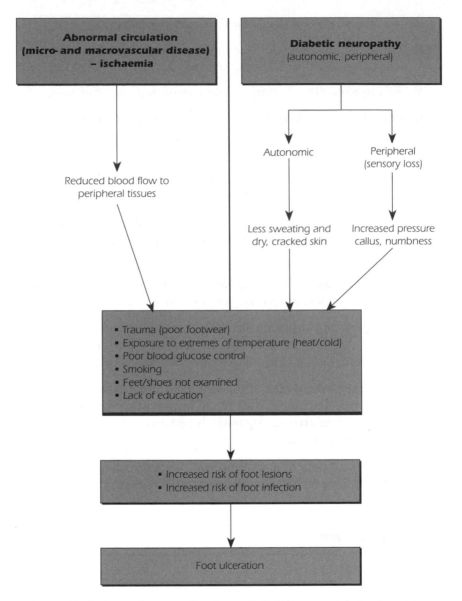

Figure 14.4 The major complications of diabetes causing foot problems

Diabetic neuropathy

Diabetic neuropathy is most often reported as pain and/or loss of feeling (numbness) in the feet, but it may appear in other areas. It can be difficult to identify. Neuropathic pain is caused by a problem in the nervous input to the affected part as opposed to pain coming from the affected part. Traditional therapies that treat the affected area may therefore be

Table 14.1 The ischaemic and the neuropathic foot

The ischaemic foot	The neuropathic foot
History	History
The presence of intermittent claudication (calf pain), present when walking and relieved by rest	Corns, calluses and ulcers are usually painful
Rest pain is a constant severe pain in the toes, foot, calf or even thighs and buttocks when severe	Questioning may reveal that the patient is unaware of lesions or that they are not troublesome
Pain occurs at rest and is aggravated in the sleeping position	Enquire about general sensation (feeling in the legs and feet)
	A lack of feeling or 'pins and needles' or burning may be reported
Examination	Examination
Colour: pale to cyanosed	Colour: normal to pink
Temperature: cold	Temperature: warm
Pulses (dorsalis pedis, posterior tibial): diminished or absent	Pulses (dorsalis pedis, posterior tibial): present or may be full and bounding
Sensation: present	Sensation: diminished or absent
Knee/ankle jerk: present	Knee/ankle jerk: diminished or absent

ineffective as they do not target the nerve root producing the painful sensation.

- Over 30% of people with diabetes will have painful diabetic neuropathy (Amos et al, 1997).

- Neuropathic pain is a chronic condition.

- It is often worse at night.

- Routine questions may help differentiation from pain due to injury, headache, etc. (nociceptive or somatic pain).

- People with diabetes need reassurance that their pain is real and potentially treatable.

There are some simple questions to ask to assess whether the pain is due to neuropathy (Table 14.2).

Table 14.2 Neuropathic pain

Possible question	Possible answer if due to neuropathy
How would you describe your pain?	Pins and needles, pricking, tingling, shooting, sudden, like a hot knife, electric shock
Does the skin appear different in the painful areas?	Red, patchy, rough Hot, burning sensation
Is the painful area more sensitive?	Worse with light touch, pressure, even bed sheets

Treatment of neuropathic pain

- Oral agents:
  - Tricyclic antidepressants, for example amitriptyline.
  - Anticonvulsants, for example pregabalin and gabapentin.
  - Opioids, for example tramadol or fentanyl.
- Topical agents:
  - Cream, for example capsaicin.
- Transcutaneous electrical stimulation:
  - This only works while the machine is operational but may provide relief for short periods.
- Relaxation, physiotherapy and cognitive behavioural pain management:
  - The pain warrants referral to specialist care.

It is important to reassure individuals that their pain is understood and that they are involved in discussion around therapies that will help.

Examination of the feet

Equipment required for a basic check:

- an examination couch or foot stool (second chair);
- a good light source;
- a 10 g monofilament.

For the health professional with the relevant skills and knowledge:

- a patella hammer (to test the knee/ankle jerk);
- a Rydell-Seiffer C64 fixed weight tuning fork (to test perception of vibration).

Note: Doppler ultrasound can be used to measure blood flow, and a biothesiometer can be used to detect diminished vibration perception. These two items of equipment are expensive but should be available through local podiatry specialists. Contact your local service for information and referral policy.

The examination

- Shoes, socks and tights or stockings must be removed.
- The patient should be examined lying on a couch or seated comfortably with both legs and feet raised (on a foot stool or second chair).
- Both feet should be checked for:
    - the condition of the skin (lower legs and feet);
    - dry, flaky skin;
    - cracks or evidence of fungal infection between each toe (athlete's foot);
    - the colour of the skin (lower legs and feet);
    - corns, calluses and other deformities (particularly on pressure-bearing points, such as the metatarsal heads);
    - the condition of the toenails (whether thickened, long or horny);
    - nail-cutting technique and ingrowing toenails;
    - discoloration and abnormal skin lesions;
    - evidence of infection, i.e. pain, lack of pain, numbness, inflammation, cellulitis or exudate (which may be purulent);
    - ensure that both the upper and lower surfaces of the feet and toes (including the heels) are carefully examined.
- All abnormalities/changes should be recorded.
- A doctor or suitably trained member of the primary care team should complete the examination of the feet:
    - The dorsalis pedis and posterior tibial pulses should be palpated.

- If ischaemia is severe, pulses throughout the lower limb should be palpated.

- Changed, diminished or absent pulses should be recorded.

- Sensation-testing with a 10 g monofilament – for comparison, the stimulus should first be applied to the patient's outstretched hand and then repeated on the lower limbs and feet, with the person's eyes closed.

- Testing for motor neuropathy should include examination for weakness or deformities in the toes and feet.

■ Foot ulcers should be examined for inflammation and discharge (and a swab taken for bacterial analysis).

■ Foot problems identified should be recorded and discussed with the patient as appropriate.

Examination of the shoes

Shoes should be examined inside and outside (Figure 14.5) for:

■ evidence of wear and tear generally;

■ the need for repair;

■ evidence of gait change (one shoe more worn than the other);

■ evidence of excessive weight-bearing (heel or sole worn down);

■ evidence of perforation of the soles or heels (by nails, etc.);

■ evidence of abrasive heels (especially with new shoes);

■ evidence of damaging projections inside the shoes (causing pressure);

■ evidence of worn insoles (causing pressure);

■ problems identified with shoes should be recorded and discussed with the patient.

Examination of socks, stockings and tights

Socks, stockings or tights should be examined (Figure 14.6) for:

■ type of material (whether constricting – nylon or elasticated);

■ type of washing powder used (as biological washing powders can be irritant);

Shoes 'fit for walking'

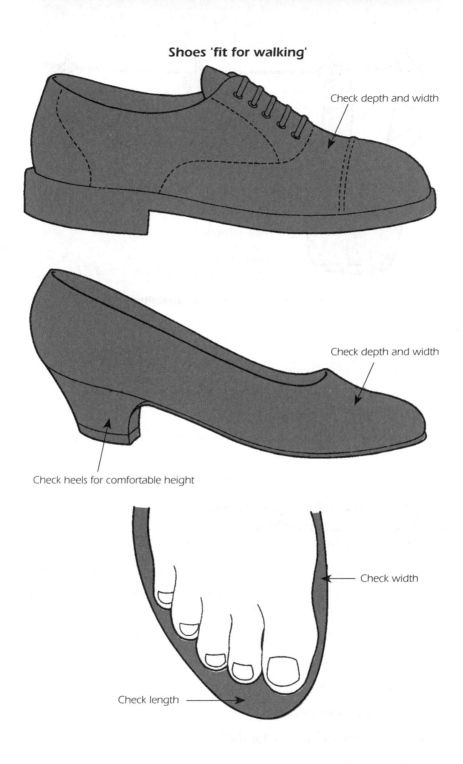

Figure 14.5 Shoes

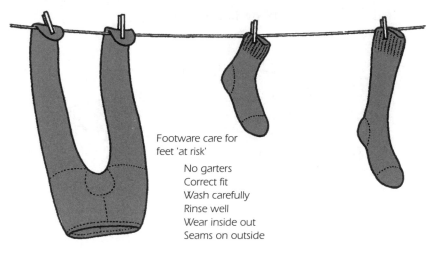

Footware care for
feet 'at risk'

No garters
Correct fit
Wash carefully
Rinse well
Wear inside out
Seams on outside

Figure 14.6 Socks/stockings/tights

- the method of holding up (e.g. garters should not be used);
- the presence and thickness of seams (which can cause traumatic ulcers);
- problems identified should be recorded and discussed with the patient.

Identification of people at risk of diabetic foot problems

People with diabetes who are 'at risk' of foot problems should be identified and recorded on the diabetes register, and/or on the recall system, for more frequent follow-up. Those at risk are those:

- with peripheral vascular disease (ischaemia);
- with neuropathy;
- who are elderly;
- who have poor vision;
- who are unable to care for their own feet;
- living alone;

- with poor mobility/dexterity;
- with foot deformities;
- with a history of foot ulceration;
- who are heavy smokers;
- with poor glycaemic control.

Treatment

Foot care advice

- Advice about foot care should be individually given and reinforced as and when appropriate and at least annually.
- Foot care advice should preferably be provided for the relative or carer, as individuals with diabetes (particularly if they are 'at risk') may be unable to follow the advice themselves.
- Printed information may be available locally or from Diabetes UK (see Appendix 4).
- Information and advice for patients about foot care, shoes and footwear (socks, stockings, tights) are given in Tables 14.3–14.5.

Treatment of diabetic foot ulcers by the primary care team

If foot ulcers are reported to, or detected by, the primary care team, the following procedure should be carried out:

- Both feet should be examined.
- Glycaemic control should be reviewed.
- A wound swab should be taken (if appropriate).
- If infection is present, antibiotics should be prescribed (these may be required long term).
- The foot and lower limb should be rested whenever possible.
- When resting, the foot and lower limb should be elevated (at least to hip level).
- Light, non-adherent dressings should be used.

- Constricting (elastic) bandages should not be used.

- Both feet should be examined regularly.

- If infection persists, the ulcer does not heal or glycaemic control is poor, referral to a diabetes foot clinic (or the specialist diabetes team) should be made. The multidisciplinary foot care team should comprise highly trained specialist podiatrists and orthotists, nurses with training in the dressing of diabetic foot wounds, and diabetologists with expertise in lower limb complications. They should have unhindered access to suites for managing major wounds, urgent inpatient facilities, antibiotic administration, community nursing, microbiology diagnostic and advisory services, orthopaedic/podiatric surgery, vascular surgery, radiology and orthotics.

- Education should be reinforced with the person with diabetes, with particular reference to foot care.

Table 14.3 Patient information: diabetes foot care advice

1 Inspect feet daily (if possible; use a mirror if you cannot reach your feet)

2 Keep feet clean (wash well and dry between the toes)

3 Avoid extremes of temperature – heat/cold

4 Avoid very hot baths (put cold water in first, then add hot water and test with an elbow)

5 Avoid hot fires and radiators

6 Avoid hot water bottles (use an electric heat pad and check its safety annually; alternatively, wear warm bed socks)

7 Report sores and skin damage immediately to your doctor or nurse

8 Cut the nails according to the shape of the toe. If you cannot cut your nails, go to a podiatrist (chiropodist)

9 Do not treat corns or calluses yourself – go to a podiatrist (chiropodist). Do not use surgical blades or corn-paring knives on your feet

10 Keep the skin supple (by using hand cream, olive oil or E45 cream)

11 Wear shoes or slippers at all times

Table 14.4 Patient information: diabetes care shoe advice

1   Feel inside and check the outside of your shoes before putting them on (check for ridges, sharp points and protruding nails)

2   Buy shoes that fit well (depth, width and length; heels not too high – approximately 3–7 cm (1–2 inches)

3   Go to a shoe shop that will measure and fit your shoes correctly

4   Remember that shoes should be fitted individually (as each foot is slightly different in shape and size)

5   If the shape of your foot has altered, you may need specially fitted insoles or shoes (which can be supplied by your chiropodist [podiatrist] or shoe-fitter)

6   Do not wear new shoes for long (no more than 1–2 hours at a time)

7   Newly fitted shoes should be slightly longer than your longest toe when you are standing – your foot lengthens when you walk (and your toes should move freely inside your shoes)

8   Make sure shoes are not too tight (watch out for creases when you walk)

9   Make sure shoes are not too loose (watch out for your feet sliding or heels/toes rubbing)

10 Do not wear rubber boots for too long. Do not wear 'work' boots for too long (change into shoes as soon as you can)

Criteria for referral to a podiatrist (chiropodist)

There is no difference between podiatrists and chiropodists. The term 'podiatrist' was adopted in 1993 to bring us into line with other English-speaking countries. The titles 'podiatrist' and 'chiropodist' are protected in law, and only those registered with the Health Professions Council can legally use them. This replaces the old title of 'state-registered chiropodist'. If assisting people with diabetes to find a chiropodist or podiatrist, ensure that the latter is registered with the Health Professions Council. Further information is available on The Society of Chiropodists and Podiatrists website (see Appendix 4).

Members of the primary care team who have not seen a podiatrist at work should arrange to observe the scope of work they do. It is not all cutting toenails, by any means. Podiatrists undergo extensive training over 3 or 4 years and may specialise in a variety of topics: sport, diabetes, footwear or surgery, for example.

Referral should be made for the following reasons:

- the toenails cannot be cut by the person with diabetes (as a result of visual impairment, etc.);

- the toenails cannot be cut by the relative or carer;

- corns or calluses require treatment;

- insoles or special shoes may be required;

- general foot care or footwear advice is needed;

- urgent chiropodist (podiatrist) treatment is required;

- an assessment is needed;

- regular surveillance is required.

Table 14.5 Patient information:
diabetes care footwear advice (socks, stockings, tights)

---

1 If possible, change socks, stockings or tights daily

2 Wear the correct size

3 Socks should be of natural fibres (wool or cotton) and loose-fitting

4 Do not wear garters

5 Wash in non-irritant detergent (e.g. non-biological washing powder) and rinse well

6 If you have poor circulation or nerve damage, wear socks, stockings or tights inside out (so that the seams are on the outside)

7 Repair damaged socks, stockings and tights or discard them and use new ones

8 If you have varicose veins requiring support stockings, seek medical advice (for the correct type and size of stocking when you obtain your prescription)

Criteria for referral to specialist foot clinic or specialist diabetes team

Referral should be made for the following reasons:

- the presence of a foot ulcer;
- severe ischaemia;
- autonomic or peripheral neuropathy causing sensory loss;
- pain or numbness in the feet or lower limbs;
- a history of foot ulceration;
- foot deformity (which may be caused by neuropathy);
- suspicion of osteomyelitis (an X-ray is required to confirm this);
- a need for 'custom-made' insoles or special shoes;
- for those identified as being 'at risk' who require regular chiropody (podiatry) and surveillance (outside the scope of the primary care team).

References

Amos AF, McCarty DJ, Zimmer P (1997). The rising global burden of diabetes and its complications: estimates and projections to the year 2010. *Diabetic Medicine* **14**: S1–S85.

National Institute for Health and Clinical Excellence (2004). *Management of Type 2 diabetes. Prevention and Management of Foot Problems*. London: NICE.

Further reading

Edmonds ME, Foster AVM (2000). *Managing the Diabetic Foot*. Oxford: Blackwell Science.

Hutchinson A, McIntosh A, Feder G, Home PD, Young R (2000). *Clinical Guidelines for Type 2 Diabetes: Prevention and Management of Foot Problems*. London: Royal College of General Practitioners.

Munro N, Rich N, McIntosh C, Foster A, Edmonds M (2003). Infections in the diabetic foot. *British Journal of Diabetes and Vascular Disease* **3**: 132–136.

15   Aspects of culture relating to diabetes care

Questions this chapter will help you answer

- What cultural differences should I understand when conducting an initial assessment?
- What dietary restrictions occur in particular faiths?
- What advice should I give around festivals and holidays?
- Where can I get further information for my patients?

> *I do not read English or Urdu. Therefore my care information should be in another format, like an audio tape in mother tongue language. There should always be an interpreter available at the clinic.*
>
> Audit Commission (2002)

Culture is defined as a set of learned beliefs, values and behaviours; the way of life shared by the members of a society; the values, traditions, norms, customs and institutions that a group of people, who are unified by race, ethnicity, language, nationality or religion, share. The overarching term of 'ethnic' is used to relate to a group of people with racial, religious or linguistic characteristics in common, and more emphasis is being placed on the needs of British Minority Ethnic groups in relation to the provision of diabetes care.

The purpose of this chapter is to explore the differences that occur and provide some practical advice on ways of adapting diabetes care to suit those differences. What it does not attempt to do is provide a description of the different faiths or racial groups living in the UK. Further information on culture, race and religion can be found in the resources at the end of the chapter.

We all live in a rapidly changing environment – not least the social and demographic make-up of the population. In some circles, this is described as a diverse and vibrant multicultural ethnic mix; in health circles, it presents challenges to our traditional method of providing care.

The National Health Service is under a legal and moral obligation to provide services to all people who need them, regardless of their gender, age or ethnic background. Healthcare professionals, as part of their continuing professional development, need to examine their practice and identify areas in which specific knowledge and skills to meet the demands of caring for a diverse community may be required.

While examining our own practice, knowledge and skills in addressing the needs of all peoples, we may meet challenges within ourselves that must be overcome in order to provide high-quality care. Our levels of understanding about cultures other than our own may vary. Our grasp of different beliefs may be superficial; it may also be highly developed in those with experience of working in areas with a multiethnic population. To cater adequately for minority ethnic groups, we must acknowledge our level of awareness and sensitivity in order to show respect for others.

Diabetes prevalence and complications

The results of the 2001 Home Office Census showed 7.9% of the total UK population to be made up of ethnic minorities from a variety of backgrounds (Figure 15.1). Overall, the census demonstrated a rise in

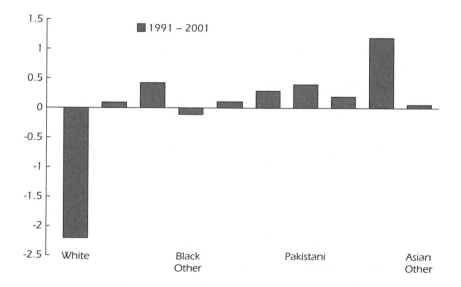

Figure 15.1 Changes in the make-up of the UK population, 1991–2001
(Data from the 2001 Home Office Census)
Note: Some categories are not listed owing to a change in classification between 1991 and 2006

ethnic groups and a decline in the total white population. The ethnic minority populations tend to be concentrated in large urban centres, with nearly half, 45.7%, living in the London region, where they make up 29% of London population.

In 1997, the worldwide incidence of diabetes was 2.1%, with many more cases undiagnosed. It is expected that, by 2010, the incidence will increase by 3%, with 61% of people with diabetes living in Asia (Amos et al, 1997). India has the largest number of people with diabetes (35 million) and the fastest growing prevalence of the condition (Marso, 2003).

Diabetes appears to develop at a relatively younger age in people from a South Asian background, and therefore it is more likely that the prevalence and complications will increase with advancing age and socio-economic status. Type 2 diabetes tends to develop around 5 years sooner in people from African/Caribbean and Asian backgrounds (Greenhalgh, 1997), and the prevalence of the condition is at least five times higher among these communities (Department of Health, 2004). There is also increasing evidence of type 2 diabetes in children, particularly in South Asian populations.

The effect of diabetes in ethnic communities

- Death from coronary artery disease and the incidence of end stage renal failure are higher in the Indo-Asian population.

- African/Caribbean and South Asian men with diabetes have a 40% and 70%, respectively, higher risk of stroke than the general population (Burlace, 2001). The reasons for poor outcomes have been identified as poor glycaemic control and poor knowledge of diabetes in Indo-Asians.

- The prevalence of diabetes in the UK is 3.6%, rising to 20–40% in older people. This is expected to be higher in ethnic groups and is rising rapidly.

There are several points to consider in relation to diabetes:

- Food is important in all cultures. Diabetes management may need to be tailored to suit a variety of lifestyles.
  - ◆ Eating habits vary widely between ethnic groups.
  - ◆ Sweet foods commonly form part of festivities.
  - ◆ Fasting is normal in some cultures.
  - ◆ Religion may form the basis of meal times.

- ◆ Certain substances (e.g. meat or alcohol) may be prohibited.
- ◆ Timing of meals varies within ethnic groups.
- ■ Pork or beef insulin may be unacceptable to some people.
- ■ Herbal medications may be taken alongside prescribed medication.
- ■ Holy days or holidays may influence when a person can attend a clinic.
- ■ Being overweight reflects prosperity and well-being in some communities.
  - ◆ Physical activity may not form part of daily life in some cultures.

Barriers to effective communication

Communication and language

Different languages remain a major barrier to communication. Fortunately, many migrants to the UK are from the old or new commonwealth where English remains the second language in the country of origin. Medicine and law are still practised in English in most of the commonwealth countries. Therefore peoples from these countries are used to having interpreters. Not all people who volunteer to be interpreters for a patient are, however, considered suitable.

Inappropriate interpreters are:

- ■ *children*, as parents may not want the child to know the details of their illness;
- ■ *relatives*, as there may be a stigma attached to diabetes that patients do not want publicised;
- ■ *family friends*, as personal details are unlikely to be discussed fully through a friend.

Appropriate interpreters, however, are:

- ■ *Language line*, a subscription translation service (see Appendix 4);
- ■ *official interpreters*;
- ■ a *health professional* who speaks both languages well;
- ■ *patient advocates*.

Training is now available for local community-based spokespeople to help them play a significant role in ensuring better health for people disadvantaged through a variety of means.

Not everyone speaks English well, so an initial assessment should be made and 'ground rules' agreed for future meetings:

- Is an interpreter needed?

- Who is going to supply the interpreter?

- Where and when can the meeting take place?

- Will family members be present?

- What language should written information be provided in?

- Is written information acceptable; for example can the patient read?

Link workers, patient advocates and telephone translation services are available in many health authorities for use in communicating with those who have little knowledge of English. Enquire at your primary care organisation and through community and social services.

Cultures, customs and manners

Problems can arise when doctors or nurses from one culture are dealing with patients who are from other cultures. It is not possible to describe all the cultures represented in the UK, but some explanation of aspects that could give rise to health hazards is necessary to avoid diagnostic or management traps.

Personal communication

Different people have different normal systems of social communication. It is not possible to provide a diabetes clinic for multiple cultures without understanding some of the issues inherent in personal contact.

The English have a personality profile of 'vision, hearing, touch'. African/Caribbeans, Asians, Chinese, East Europeans and even Americans have a personality profile of 'touch, hearing, vision'.

- Direct eye contact is seen as a positive trait in Caucasian groups yet is a sign of authority in Asian communities.

- Asian school children avert their eyes from their teacher as a sign of respect – health professionals may expect similar treatment.

- Examples of English manners include constant eye contact,

speaking out loud, holding a conversation, standing at ease with a confident smile, listening without speaking and also being at ease with silence. It is the opposite in Eastern cultures. You may notice deferential eye contact and the husband taking control of the conversation for the whole family.

■ Individuals from one culture may be expected to behave in a prescribed fashion but may not fit the expected norm. People may not adopt the norms of the country they are living in and not conform to expectations. It is important at the outset to assess relevant behaviours and beliefs.

Consultation and examination

British patients are only too happy to give their life and family history to the doctor or nurse, but African-Asian patients resist answering this line of questioning and view it with grave suspicion. The word 'I' is never used by African-Asian patients; the words 'please' and 'the' may also not exist in their language. Their politeness is conveyed by gesture.

Many women would prefer to be examined by a woman doctor, and men would be very embarrassed to be examined by a woman doctor. Rectal examinations, enemas or giving suppositories may be taboo, and referral to psychiatrists may have a social stigma attached in some cultures. Many Asian people feel very strongly stigmatised with a diagnosis of diabetes. It is still considered as a contagious disease, and marriage potential may be affected by admitting to a diagnosis of and treatment for diabetes: women may fear that they will not be accepted in marriage.

Herbal medication

Many people with diabetes use various types of traditional/herbal medicines in conjunction with their therapeutic medications. These herbal medicines are mostly vegetables (Karela or gourd – *Memordicca carrantia* – having a proven insulin-like substance). Diabetes UK has issued a warning on the use of Karela, the hypoglycaemic effects of which are well documented. It is used traditionally in Asian cookery and as a traditional medicine to lower blood glucose levels. In practice, however, it is difficult to take enough of the Karela plant to have a significant effect.

Herbal medicines are easily available in this country, and some have hypoglycaemic properties. Also available in this country are some tablets and concentrated juices of these traditional medicines. Most of the tablets have four or five ingredients, some of which are hepatotoxic. With the above in mind, it is important to ask any people with diabetes if they are taking any of the above medications.

Festivals

All festivals share one thing in common: the exchange of sweets/dried fruit or other sweet items. People visit each other and share sweets and rich fried food. Many people with diabetes find it very difficult to refuse these sweetmeats and end up with hyperglycaemia or take extra oral hypoglycaemic agents without informing their doctor/nurse.

Hot and cold foods

In many communities around the world, it is believed that certain foods are 'hot', whereas others are 'cold'. The hot or cold nature of foods bears no relation to the temperature or the spiciness of the dish: it is believed to be an inherent property of the food, supposedly giving rise to physical effects in the body.

Hot foods are supposed to raise the body temperature, excite the emotions and increase activity. Cold foods are believed to impart strength, cool the body and also cause cheerfulness.

A diet containing hot and cold foods is normally consumed, but during certain illnesses and in certain conditions, preference will be given to the nature of the foods. Some foods with their hot and cold properties are listed in Table 15.1.

Betel chewing

Betel is an after-dinner delicacy used by adult South Asians, particularly Bangladeshi and Bengali women, and Malaysians; therefore, it is quite commonly used by people with diabetes. It can have metabolic effects that need to be excluded in consultations.

- Acute effects of betel chewing include exacerbation of asthma, hypotension and tachycardia.

- The effects of anticholinergic drugs may decrease when used in combination with betel nut or its constituent arecoline.

- Use with cholinergic drugs may cause toxicity (salivation, increased tears, incontinence, sweating, diarrhoea, vomiting, fever).

- Betel nut may slow or raise the heart rate, and can alter the effects of drugs that slow the heart, such as beta-blockers, calcium channel blockers and digoxin.

- Betel nut may alter blood sugar levels, so caution is advised when using medications that may also alter blood sugar. Patients taking oral hypoglycaemic agents or using insulin should be monitored closely by a healthcare professional. Medication adjustments may be necessary.

Table 15.1 Examples of the 'hot' and 'cold' foods

Food group	Hot	Cold
Cereals		Wheat, rice
Green leafy vegetables		All
Root vegetables	Carrot, onion	Potatoes
Other vegetables	Capsicum, pepper, aubergine or bringle	Cucumber, beans, cauliflower, marrow, gourd, ladies fingers (okra), etc.
Fruits	Dates, mango, pawpaw or papaya	All other fruits, e.g. apples, oranges, melons, etc.
Animal products	Meats, chicken, mutton, fish, eggs	
Milk products		Milk and cream, curds or yoghurt, buttermilk
Pulses	Lentils	Bangalgram or chickpea, greengram, peas, redgram
Nuts	All types, including ground or peanuts, cashew nuts	
Spices and condiments	Chillies, green and red powder, cinnamon, clove, garlic, ginger, mustard, nutmeg, pepper	Coriander, cumin, cardamom, fennel, tamarind
Oils	Mustard	Butter, coconut oil, ground nut oil
Miscellaneous	Tea, coffee, honey, jaggery or brown sugar	

■ Betel nut may increase the effects of monoamine oxidase inhibitors, angiotensin-converting enzyme inhibitors, phenothiazines, cholesterol-lowering drugs or stimulant drugs.

Smoking

Smoking in some cultures is accepted social practice, yet little is available in a variety of languages to help people quit. Cardiovascular disease, as mentioned above, is higher in some ethnic groups, and smoking multiplies this risk. Various forms of smoking, all of which should be discouraged, are available. Health professionals should discuss smoking cessation with people with diabetes, include it in their education plans and record the results.

Hookah smoking

Healthcare professionals should be aware that this is a common practice and social custom among adult Asian men and women (particularly Muslim and Bangladeshi). The hookah is a smoking apparatus that consists of a flask filled with water, with two tubes attached. One tube is topped by a funnel containing lighted coals, beneath which is a metal lid over a layer of tobacco leaves or paste. The second tube has one end under the water in the flask, the other end being fitted with a mouthpiece. Tobacco vapour filtered through the water is then inhaled through the mouthpiece.

Cigarette and beedi smoking

This is a quite common practice. There are 'cigarette shops' in various parts of the country where beedi can be bought. Beedi is rolled tobacco, with a very high tar content, in a tobacco leaf and is commonly available in the Asian grocery shops as well as these 'cigarette shops'. People of Asian backgrounds commonly go for a walk after the evening meal to these 'cigarette shops', which are more of a social meeting place analogous to pubs in the indigenous culture of Britain.

Alcohol

Alcohol is commonly consumed and abused by many cultures and is prohibited in some religions. It is because of this it can be seem as offensive to question a Muslim on alcohol drinking (see also Chapter 10).

Religions

Figure 15.2 shows the signs of some different religious groups.

Some behaviours are governed by religion. Factors that are relevant to diabetes are discussed here under the following headings:

- Buddhists
- Christian Scientists
- Christians
- Hindus
- Jehovah's Witnesses

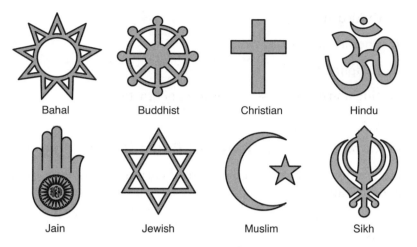

| Bahal | Buddhist | Christian | Hindu |
| Jain | Jewish | Muslim | Sikh |

Figure 15.2 Signs of different religious groups

- Jews
- Muslims
- Sikhs.

It is not possible to provide dates for all festivals/holidays as many are moveable feasts. Multifaith calendars are listed in Further Resources at the end of this chapter.

Buddhists

Buddhists may be strict vegetarians or vegans, but many eat meat. The health professional should discuss this as part of the initial assessment. Smoking and alcohol are sometimes frowned upon also.

Christian Scientists

Drugs, including those for pain relief, and blood products are not acceptable within the teachings of Christian Science, but personal choice may waive this direction. Alternative methods of pain relief should be explored:

- Relaxation techniques: meditation, hypnosis, yoga.
- Music therapy – audiotapes and CDs may be available through the local library.

- Guided imagery.
- Therapeutic touch.
- Acupuncture.

Fasting and dietary restrictions are not practised.

Christians (Catholic, Church of England and others)

There are no restrictions on diet or medication practised within the Christian Church.

Hindus

Three important festivals celebrated by many Hindus:

1 *Holi*: a festival of colour welcoming the arrival of spring with colours (February/March).

2 *Dessehra*: a festival celebrating the death of Demon Ravana (mostly October).

3 *Diwali*: a festival of light, joy and sharing (October/November). It is similar to Christmas. People celebrate the return of Lord Rama after killing the Demon Ravana. It follows the start of the New Year for the trading community.

Hindus (Buddhist and Jains) are mainly vegetarian; cows are sacred to orthodox Hindus and prayed to, so beef is not eaten by Hindus. Sweets are consumed more or less daily, and rich, fried food is consumed at celebrations and festivities. Many women fast for one or two days in a week or on certain festive occasions; men may fast too. They may consume fruits, sweets or milk puddings. Full-cream milk is commonly used for puddings, etc.

- It is common to offer sweets and dried or fresh fruit to God during times of prayer. These are consumed by the family members on a daily basis.

- Hindus have strict religious instructions to do no harm to any living thing, so most of them will be strict vegetarians.

- Some Hindus may not even eat eggs or fish, although most will probably accept dairy products. These tend to be high fat.

- It is important to discuss diet as part of your initial assessment.

- The cow is considered to be a sacred representation of the bounty of the gods. Beef insulin (although little used nowadays) would not be acceptable.

- Some Hindus may fast when they are ill in an attempt to restore health and balance to the body.

- Some Hindus may fast as a religious exercise, to give thanks for a successful recovery. At the end of a period of fasting, a Hindu patient's family may bring them some sweets that have been blessed (prashad).

- Older and especially devout Hindus may also choose to fast during the full moon as a cultural tradition, but most will agree to eat when their health requires them to.

- During times of fasting, Hindus may be encouraged to take hot milk, fruit, tea, salad and yoghurt, but careful monitoring of glycaemic control is essential and medication may need to be altered until the blood glucose level is stable.

Jehovah's Witnesses

- Jehovah's Witnesses prohibit the use of blood and blood products – to the extent of not allowing the storage of blood samples and refusing surgery that is not 'bloodless'. Individuals may interpret the teaching in a more relaxed manner.

- Alcohol is allowed but not drunkenness.

- Smoking is not allowed.

- Dietary restrictions may apply; it is best to discuss this in the initial assessment.

Jews

Various festivals take place in the Jewish calendar, for example:

- *Rosh Hashanah*: the Jewish new year – celebrated with such delicacies as honey cake.

- *Yom Kippur*: the Day of Atonement. This involves fasting (including no drink or even toothbrushing) from sunset to an hour after sunset on the next day. Children under 13, pregnant women and anyone with a health problem are exempt.

- *Sukkot*: harvest festival – celebrated with lots of fruit and vegetables.

- *Chanucah*: an 8-day celebration of the fight against the Greeks in the final century BC, when a small jar of oil kept the everlasting light burning for 8 days. It is traditional to eat foods cooked in oil, for example doughnuts and potato pancakes.

- *Purim*: the festival of Esther – poppy seed cakes are traditionally eaten.

- *Passover*: the celebration of the exodus from Egypt under Moses. This lasts 8 days, and no leavened food must be eaten for the duration (matzos are the unleavened bread consumed).

- *Shavuot*: the festival of weeks (on which Pentecost is based). It is traditional to eat dairy products.

There are many other minor fast days and festivals that are usually kept only by Orthodox Jews. As with the Sabbath, all festivals start (and finish) at sunset.

Food must be kosher:

- Animals must have cloven hooves and chew the cud. Cows, goats and sheep are kosher; horses and pigs are not.

- Fish must have scales and fins. For this reason, shellfish and eels, for example, are not kosher.

- Food must have been butchered and prepared in a kosher way.

- Fruit is always kosher, unless damaged by rot or insects.

Orthodox Jews observe the Sabbath and certain holidays. They will not have tests, investigations or clinic appointments on these days. Some may not even be willing to take medication on these days, but health takes precedence if the condition is life threatening. Insulin may need to be prepared the night before.

Muslims

Muslims are strictly forbidden to drink alcohol. Eating pork is totally prohibited, so porcine insulin is unacceptable to Muslims; human insulin is preferred. Only food that has been declared by Allah as good (Halal) is acceptable to the majority of Muslims.

The Muslim year is divided into 12 lunar months, alternating between 29 and 30 days. Every festival is approximately 10 days earlier than the previous year.

- *Moharram*: an anniversary of the killing of the prophet's grandson Hussein. It is celebrated by Shi'a Muslims.

- *Ramadan*: the birthday of the prophet Mohammed. A strict fast is practised from the first day until day 21, which is called the night of prayer.

- *Eid-ul-Fitr*: A two-and-a-half day festival to mark the end of Ramadan.

- *Eid-ul-Azho*: A 3-day celebration of completion of a pilgrimage to Mecca.

- *Mawild Al-Nabi*: the birthday of the prophet Mohammed (mostly in June).

- *Layat Al-Qadr* (night): day 26 of Ramadan.

Foods that are not permitted include:

- wine and other alcoholic drinks, or anything (including medicine) that contains alcohol;

- blood, bloody meat or any product made with animal blood or blood products;

- pork and all other pork products including fat;

- meat not killed in accordance with strict halal conditions;

- fish without fins or scales (such as shellfish).

Muslims traditionally observe a strict fast during the month of Ramadan. They are not allowed to eat or drink between sunrise and sunset. Muslims who have a chronic condition do not have to fast but may decide to do so (see below).

Ramadan

Ramadan is the holy month for Muslims, falling in the ninth lunar month in the Islamic calendar year. Because the timing of Ramadan is linked to the sighting of the new moon, the timing of this month varies. Ramadan is a period of worship, self-discipline, austerity and charity. During this month, foods and fluids are only allowed at night so fasting extends from dawn to sunset – the exact length of time dependent on geographical location and season. In the summer months in the UK, fasting can last for up to 18 hours a day.

Fasting is obligatory for all healthy adult Muslims. Exemption from fasting is granted to certain people, including children under 12, the sick, the elderly, pregnant and breast-feeding women and travellers.

There are various items that need discussion with the person with diabetes and his or her carers:

- Hypoglycaemia is more likely when people are fasting if they are taking insulin or sulphonylureas (e.g. gliclazide).

- People with diabetes can be exempt from fasting.

- Home monitoring may only be possible during hours of darkness.

- During Ramadan, people with diabetes may not attend clinics as they cannot give blood during this time.

- Friday is the day on which most Muslims attend the Mosque and may not attend a clinic.

- Only two meals are taken daily during Ramadan – sunrise and sunset – and they tend to contain sweet and rich foods.

- People taking sulphonylureas such as gliclazide may need to change the timing of taking their medication and/or may need less medication during periods of fasting.

- People taking metformin and/or glitazones, such as rosiglitazone and pioglitazone, may need to change the timing of their medication but will generally be able to continue their medication.

- Individuals on insulin will need to alter their medication. Referral to a diabetes specialist nurse is recommended unless the care team has the knowledge and skills to manage this complex therapy.

Sikhs

The temple, Gurudhwara (or Gurdwara), serves three free vegetarian meals with chapattis (Langer) every day all year round. These contain high amounts of fibre and starch. Desserts are invariably made of full-cream milk, dry nuts and sugar. Sikhs do not eat beef.

Karah (prasad) is an offering to Guru and served to people visiting the temple. It is made with ghee (clarified butter), dry nuts and full-cream milk. It is worth asking an Asian person with diabetes how much is consumed.

Festivals include the following:

- *Baisakhi-Sikhs*: New Year celebrated with prayers and an exchange of presents.

- *Guru Nanak*: Sikhism was founded by Guru Nanak, and present-day Sikhism is still based on his teachings and those of the nine Sikh Gurus who followed him.

- *Diwali*: celebrated by prayer, an exchange of presents and a distribution of sweets to friends and relatives.

All these festivals are associated with enjoyment and overindulgence in highly saturated carbohydrate sweets, syrups, dairy products and fried foods.

- Alcohol and tobacco are prohibited.

- Different beliefs surround the eating of meat, and the health professional should discuss dietary habits as part of the initial assessment.

- Some Sikhs – mainly older people – fast.

African/Caribbean populations

African/Caribbean people have a high prevalence of diabetes (three to four times higher than in the white population) and poor outcomes from the condition. There is a notable difference in the outcome of diabetes in the African/Caribbean community, with a higher incidence of stroke and of end stage renal failure than in the diabetic community as whole.

As there has not been much research on this group's health beliefs and experiences, there is a lack of specifically focused patient material. Healthcare professionals should try to address the health practices and beliefs of this group, so that they can make informed decisions on how they manage their condition.

Beliefs

The cultural understandings of Caribbean people are important because they can be used to interpret signs of illness and guide the selection of treatments, as well as evaluate the efficacy of these treatments.

There can be vast differences in how Caribbean people understand biomedicine and the functioning of the human body. Many Caribbean people have distinct beliefs about blood, which can lead to fasting and taking laxatives.

Caribbean people often categorise blood as 'good' or 'bad', and this categorisation is more likely among older people and people with diabetes. Most describe 'bad blood' as blood from a sick person – it is viewed as an index of poor health, often as a result of not eating properly. Suggested ways of keeping blood 'good' include healthy eating, exercising and taking laxatives and home remedies such as vinegar, onions, garlic and cod liver oil. Many of these are positive practices, which can be incorporated into a diabetes management plan. There may also be a reluctance, especially among elder members of the community, to have blood tests, because these can be seen as 'harmful'.

Healthcare professionals have often reported their perception that obesity can be viewed in positive terms within the African/Caribbean community, but this does not appear to be the case – having a normal BMI is associated with health and attractiveness. There does seem, however, to be a great unawareness of the link between obesity and the onset of diabetes. It is important to make African/Caribbean patients aware of this link and to encourage them to eat healthily.

Providing diabetes care

New ways of providing information that meets the needs of patients should be available in primary care, such as websites, videos, CDs and multilingual publications (see Further Resources below and Appendix 4).

The Expert Patient Programme empowers people of all cultures to self-care. Find out where your nearest course is run (see Further Resources below).

Men and women may need to be targeted separately for health advice and support. Find out what is available in your local area to support ethnic groups in terms of healthy eating, weight loss and increasing activity.

The education of patients, carers and the general public is paramount to changing attitudes. Ensure that patients have access to up-to-date dietary advice on lower-fat alternatives to ghee, milk and yoghurt, and involve the family in structured education (see Chapter 16).

Good schemes exist involving local community centres, link workers and patient advocates to overcome cultural barriers. Your local primary care organisation, council and/or social services may be able to provide information.

Remember that healthcare beliefs vary widely within ethnic groups, so make a full assessment at your initial meeting. Record important information such as the language(s) spoken, whether written information is appropriate and 'ground rules' (see above) for future reference. Client satisfaction with nursing care is tied to the degree to which expectations are shared and met.

At the initial assessment, discuss normal dietary habits through open questions:

- 'Tell me about what you normally eat.' Remember that this may only elicit information on meals. Snacks may not be considered to be 'food'.

- 'At what times do you normally eat your meals?' Wide variances within and outside ethnic groups are prevalent, and medication may need to be tailored to suit.

- 'What changes to your normal eating plan do you have at holidays or festivals?' Suggest low-fat alternatives and discuss foods with lower sugar contents, such as fresh fruit, for celebrations.

Remember to avoid medical jargon.

Some ethnic communities may not be used to taking long-term medication. A careful explanation of what is expected of the drug, its side effects and the possible length of treatment need to be included in education plans.

Individuals with diabetes should be encouraged to participate in decision-making related their own care. Goals and targets should be agreed with them and preferably entered in the care record by the person themselves for discussion at the next appointment. This encourages active participation in meeting targets.

Where possible, the extended family should also be involved in educational activities. Healthcare professionals provide on average only 4 hours contact with their clients each year – families and those with diabetes themselves provide the vast majority of care. They need the understanding to do that job effectively. Support groups are successful and might be organised within the practice if space allows.

Check understanding by asking individuals and their carers to repeat advice back to you. Remember that nodding agreement may be just a sign of respect – not necessarily understanding. As an example, Andrews and Boyle (2002) have suggested some questions to elicit an understanding of hypertension:

- What do you think caused your high blood pressure?

- What effect do you think it will have on you?

- Some people forget to take their daily pills; does this happen to you?

- What frightens or worries you about high blood pressure?

SUMMARY

■ Health professionals in primary care can do much to increase the knowledge and understanding of the wide variety of cultural communities within the UK.

■ They must, however, first examine their own understanding and seek training and education to enable them to interact effectively with those from backgrounds different from their own.

■ Much research locally may need to be undertaken to ensure that resources are available to provide people with diabetes with appropriate information for their needs.

■ If this is achieved, good rapport will lead to an increased quality of life for those engaged in their own care.

References

Amos AF, McCarty DJ, Zimmer P (1997). The rising global burden of diabetes and its complications: estimates and projections to the year 2010. *Diabetic Medicine* **14**: S1–S85.

Andrews M & Boyle J (2002). *Transcultural Concepts in Nursing Care*, 4th edn. Philadelphia: Lippincott Williams & Wilkins.

Burlace, S. (2001). Reducing stroke risk in ethnic minorities. *Best Practice* 18 July: 14–15.

Department of Health (2004). *Health Survey for England 2004*. London: DoH.

Greenhalgh PM (1997). Diabetes in British South Asians: nature, nurture and culture. *Diabetic Medicine* **14**: 10–18.

Marso SP (ed.) (2003). *The Handbook of Diabetes Mellitus and Cardiovascular Disease*. London: Remidica Publishing.

Further resources

A multifaith calendar is available from Swindon Borough Council giving dates of festivals and holidays. There is a small cost.

The Equality Challenge Unit has online calendars with dates of multifaith festivals. www.ecu.ac.uk.

A multifaith calendar is also available at www.shap.org/calendar.html.

Richard Hourston, podiatrist, has published practical foot care leaflets in 31 languages on his website. These are freely available to print out and photocopy. They do not rely on text alone – pictures are used to illustrate points. www.diabeticfoot.org.uk.

Diabetes UK has many publications (some listed below) in a variety of languages either from its catalogue or available online at www.diabetes.org.uk.

◆ Healthy lifestyle, fasting and diabetes

◆ Hypoglycaemia

◆ Ramadan and diabetes

◆ A guide for African-Caribbean people – your key to better health.

The Expert Patient Programme (www.expertpatients.nhs.uk) has local courses to support patients in understanding how they can look after themselves and communicate effectively with health professions.

Further reading

Patroe L (2001). *An Executive Summary of the Diabetes Development Fund for Black and Minority Ethnic Communities in the North West of England.* London: Diabetes UK.

Pinar R (2002). Management of people with diabetes during Ramadan. *British Journal of Nursing* **11**:1300–1303.

Scott P (2001). Caribbean people's health beliefs about the body and their implications for diabetes management: a South London Study. *Practical Diabetes International* **18**: 94–98.

16 Structured patient education

Questions this chapter will help you answer

- What is meant by structured patient education?
- Is it available to my patients locally?
- How can I engage patients in education and ensure that learning takes place?
- Should I organise group education sessions?

> *My attitude has always been 'it ain't going to beat me' and I believe that the most important care is education in all aspects of the disease ... I have been insulin-dependent for 43 years and can still do 10 press-ups ... it is not all doom and gloom!*
>
> Audit Commission (2000)

In 2003, the National Institute for Health and Clinical Excellence (2003) published guidance on structured education. This defined structured education as:

> a planned and graded programme that is comprehensive in scope, flexible in content, responsive to an individual's clinical and psychological needs, and adaptable to his or her educational and cultural background.

The UK Department of Health announced that all primary care organisations needed to implement this guidance from January 2006. The report identified two programmes that met National Institute for Health and Clinical Excellence standards – Dose Adjustment for Normal Eating (DAFNE) and Diabetes Education and Self Management for Ongoing and Newly Diagnosed (DESMOND) – with others such as X-PERT in development (see below and Appendix 4).

In summary, the guidance suggests the following:

- It is recommended that structured patient education is made available to all people with diabetes at the time of initial diagnosis and then as required on an ongoing basis, based on a formal, regular assessment of need.

- Neither specific methods of providing education nor frequency of sessions were defined proscriptively. Some principles of good practice were, however, made clear:

  - ◆ Educational interventions should reflect established principles of adult learning.

  - ◆ Education should be provided by an appropriately trained multidisciplinary team to groups of people with diabetes, unless group work was considered unsuitable for an individual.

  - ◆ Sessions should be accessible to the broadest range of people, taking into account culture, ethnicity, disability and geographical issues, and could be held either in the community or at a local diabetes centre.

  - ◆ Educational programmes should use a variety of techniques to promote active learning (engaging individuals in the process of learning and relating the content of programmes to personal experience), adapted wherever possible to meet the different needs, personal choices and learning styles of those with diabetes, and should be integrated into routine diabetes care over the longer term.

To provide further guidance, Diabetes UK and the Department of Health (2005) published a report from the Patient Education Working Group. Key criteria for structured education were identified, based on a philosophy that the programme would be evidence based, dynamic and flexible to the needs of the individual, and that users should be involved in its ongoing development.

Key criteria

Key criteria required to deliver this effective teaching and learning system are as follows:

- **A structured curriculum**. The curriculum needs to:

1 have a philosophy of supporting self-management attitudes, beliefs, knowledge and skills for the learner;

2 be person centred, incorporating the assessment of individual learning needs;

3 be reliable, valid, relevant and comprehensive;

4 be theory driven and evidence based;

5 be flexible and able to cope with diversity;

6 be able to use different teaching media;

7 be resource effective and have supporting materials;

8 be recognised as an evolving one based on new evidence and be written down.

■ **Trained educators**. Trained educators need to:

1 have an understanding of education theory appropriate to the age and needs of the programme learners;

2 be competent in the delivery of the education theory of the programme they are offering;

3 be competent in the delivery of the principles and content of the specific programme they are offering.

■ **Be quality assured**. A quality assurance programme needs to be in place. The programme needs to be peer reviewed by independent assessors who assess against agreed criteria:

1 the environment;

2 the structure;

3 the process;

4 the content;

5 the use of materials;

6 whether the programme has actually been delivered;

7 evaluation and outcome information.

■ **Be audited**. The outcomes from the programme need to be audited. The outcomes might include:

1 biomedical parameters;

2 quality of life;

3 satisfaction;

4 patient experience;

5 user involvement;

6 the degree of self-management achieved as a result of the programme.

Structured programmes must:

■ have a structured, written curriculum;

■ have trained educators;

■ be quality assured;

■ be audited.

Box 16.1 DAFNE: Dose Adjustment for Normal Eating – type 1 diabetes

The main principles of the DAFNE course are:

1 skills-based training to teach flexible insulin adjustment to match carbohydrate in a free diet on a meal-by-meal basis;

2 an emphasis on self-management and independence from the diabetes care team;

3 the use of adult education principles to facilitate new learning in a group setting.

Participants attend the course for the full 5 consecutive days in groups of 6–8. In theory, those using twice-daily insulin regimens might benefit, but in practice, participants in DAFNE switch to a multiple injection regimen on the first day of the course to maximise the opportunities for dose adjustment.

The course consists of three main areas:

■ nutrition topics;

■ insulin dose adjustment at meal times and special circumstances (exercise, illness);

■ other topics such as hypoglycaemia, complications, sick day rules and pregnancy.

There is also a course handbook for participants.

Topics to be covered in the programme are more fully explained in Diabetes UK's (2005) recommendations, available online on their website (see Appendix 4):

■ the nature of diabetes;

■ the day-to-day management of diabetes;

■ specific issues;

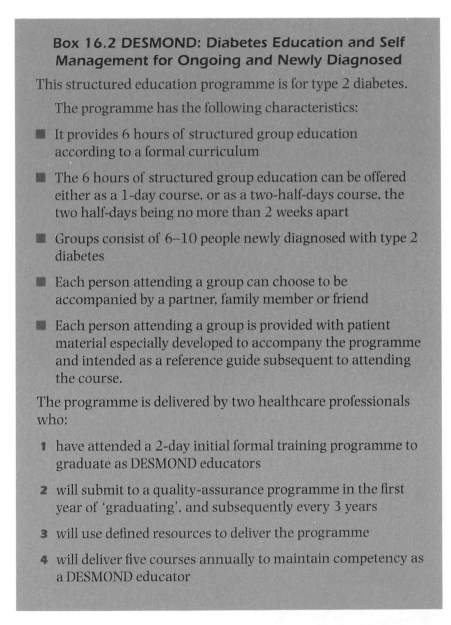

Box 16.2 DESMOND: Diabetes Education and Self Management for Ongoing and Newly Diagnosed

This structured education programme is for type 2 diabetes.

The programme has the following characteristics:

■ It provides 6 hours of structured group education according to a formal curriculum

■ The 6 hours of structured group education can be offered either as a 1-day course, or as a two-half-days course, the two half-days being no more than 2 weeks apart

■ Groups consist of 6–10 people newly diagnosed with type 2 diabetes

■ Each person attending a group can choose to be accompanied by a partner, family member or friend

■ Each person attending a group is provided with patient material especially developed to accompany the programme and intended as a reference guide subsequent to attending the course.

The programme is delivered by two healthcare professionals who:

1 have attended a 2-day initial formal training programme to graduate as DESMOND educators

2 will submit to a quality-assurance programme in the first year of 'graduating', and subsequently every 3 years

3 will use defined resources to deliver the programme

4 will deliver five courses annually to maintain competency as a DESMOND educator

- living with diabetes;
- 'sick day rules'.

Programmes such as DAFNE for people with type 1 diabetes, DESMOND for people with type 2 diabetes and X-PERT have been evaluated (Boxes 16.1–16.3; see Appendix 4 for websites). Programmes relevant to ethnic groups are in development, and other programmes are being refined to meet the standards.

Box 16.3 The diabetes X-PERT programme was designed in conjunction with patients and the local branch of Diabetes UK, Burnley, Lancashire

- A 6-week programme for people with diabetes
- 16 participants (plus carers) at each session
- A 2-day 'Train the Trainers' course
- Patient empowerment and activation
- Subject of a randomised controlled trial
- An Urdu-speaking programme for South Asian participants

Each X-PERT session used visual aids to explore health issues related to diabetes, and each participant received a copy of their own health results with an explanation. The X-PERT programme aimed to increase knowledge, skills and confidence so that individuals were able to make informed decisions regarding their diabetes self-management.

The X-PERT programme has won four national awards:

- The Diabetes UK 2003 Diabetes Education Award (March 2003)
- The National Obesity Forum Weight Management in Diabetes Care Award (October 2003)
- The *Health Service Journal* Patient-Centred Care Award (November 2004)
- The Secretary of State's Excellence in Healthcare Management Award (November 2004)

Living with diabetes

Living with diabetes requires knowledge and experience, built up over time. The level and pace of learning vary greatly between individuals. It is important for healthcare professionals to appreciate the gaps between 'learning', 'understanding' and 'doing', and why such gaps occur.

Reasons for 'learning', 'understanding' and 'doing' gaps

The newly diagnosed person
Considerable shock often accompanies the newly diagnosed person with diabetes. A sense of bereavement is felt, caused by the loss of health and fear of the unknown or of the future. This sense of shock and fear may also be felt by relatives and have a considerable impact on a whole family. It is at this time that a great deal of information may be passed to the person concerned, much of which is unnecessary at this stage and may even be counterproductive and confusing.

Alternatively, the person may consider their diabetes to be 'mild' and be unaware of the importance of self-care and regular review.

- Always assess prior knowledge and understanding in order to tailor education to the individual's needs.

Preconceived ideas
Experiences of diabetes previously learned from family members or friends may have been negative and even horrific, resulting in extreme fear and concern. This may block any constructive discussion at an early stage regarding self-management.

- Ensure people with diabetes understand that each person is different and that what happens to one person need not apply to others.

Fear of living with diabetes
Preconceived ideas may lead to particular concerns of living with diabetes, such as restrictions on eating, drinking and everyday activities. Worries may be expressed regarding employment, driving, travel, holidays and, in younger people, the implications of diabetes on attending college, leaving home, starting work and starting a family. Similarly, preconceived ideas and previous knowledge of diabetes may result in extreme concern (even a morbid fear) of complications, particularly regarding eyes and blindness, feet and amputation.

■ Encourage people with diabetes to express their fears and address them before embarking on the health professionals' priorities.

Culture
Culture and personal health beliefs have a considerable bearing on attitudes to disease and coping with a life-long progressive condition such as diabetes. In certain societies, being overweight in a woman is regarded as beautiful and desirable; in others, the opposite is true. The diagnosis of diabetes in some cultures may place the person concerned into a 'sick role', rendering the concept of living a healthy life with diabetes difficult to grasp. For further details of how to deal with cultural aspects, see Chapter 15.

Mental difficulties
People with learning difficulties, mental illness or disability require particular care in their management. Much of the burden of their diabetes and concerns over its progression will fall on relatives or carers, who require special support.

The ageing process affects the memory as well as the ability to take in information and act on it. As people become older, they may appear to cope quite well with living with diabetes, but they may be reluctant to change certain habits built up over a lifetime.

Literacy and education
Literacy is assumed, both in our own society and in others. An illiterate person should not be deemed stupid; in fact, the reverse may be true. Compensation by the person for illiteracy may be such that the problem is effectively disguised.

Educational levels, particularly with regard to how the body works, should not be taken for granted. A highly intelligent and well-educated person is often assumed to be knowledgeable and coping when, in fact, the diagnosis may be denied or a fear of complications may lead to an obsessional monitoring and control of blood glucose levels ruling the person's life.

■ Health professionals should ensure that people with diabetes can reiterate advice discussed with them to enable learning to take place.

Language
Language is obviously a barrier to communication when English is not the mother tongue. It is important that appropriate translation

methods are used, such as help from health link workers or a telephone translation scheme such as Language Line (available in some health districts; see Appendix 4). Contact with local ethnic minority groups may also generate local interest in diabetes, translating expertise and materials into the appropriate language.

The greatest difficulty with language used by healthcare professionals is the use of medical terminology, which is either not understood or is misunderstood and, in most instances, is inappropriate. Most people are grateful for a simple, non-technical explanation and will enquire further if this is insufficient.

Information-giving

There are six main problems of information-giving as identified by people with diabetes:

1 *Incorrect information* – when facts given about diabetes are wrong. It is much better for the healthcare professional to admit ignorance and offer to find out the correct information.

2 *Inconsistent information* – when several healthcare professionals are involved and different educational messages are received, giving a confusing picture.

3 *Too much information* – when too many messages are given, often at the same time, particularly at or near the time of diagnosis.

4 *Too little information* – when the information supplied or requested is insufficient for the person concerned to find it useful or helpful.

5 *Inappropriate information* – when the information given is not appropriate to the diabetes requirements or the age and lifestyle of the person concerned.

6 *Lack of up-to-date information* – when information is given at diagnosis or when it is specifically requested and no further or new information is offered.

Motivational interviewing

Most people do not like being told what to do; their personal freedom is threatened. As healthcare professionals, we need to avoid the message that 'I am the expert and I'm going to tell you how to run your life'. It is not enough to know what people with diabetes should change in their life in order to keep their diabetes 'under control'. We also need to know how we can help our patients to make the changes that they want to make. One process that can help is called 'motivational interviewing' (Table 16.1).

Motivational interviewing is a particular way to help people recognize and do something about their present or potential problems. It is particularly useful with people who are reluctant to change and ambivalent about changing. It is intended to help resolve ambivalence and to get a person moving along the path to change. For some people, this is all they really need. Once they are unstuck, no longer immobilized by conflicting motivations, they have all the skills and resources they need in order to make lasting change. All they need is a relatively brief motivational boost.

(Miller and Rollnick, 1991)

Table 16.1 Old and new interview models
The old model vs. the new

The patient says	And the health professional replies	
	(Old model)	(New model)
I hate this exercise plan	Why don't you try having a 10-minute walk after dinner every evening with your partner?	What do you hate about it? What would help you do better at it?
I'm too busy to take more exercise	You need to do this to prevent complications	What sort of activity do you enjoy? What would help you incorporate that in your busy life?
I don't think I can quit smoking	Smoking is the leading cause of preventable death	Why do you think that? What has happened in the past when you tried to quit? What worries you most when you think about trying to quit?
I can't lose weight	You'll need to go on insulin if we can't get your sugar levels down. Losing weight might prevent that	What have you tried that has worked? What do you understand about the local schemes available to you?
I haven't been able to test my blood sugar four times a day	It's hard at first, but just keep trying. You really need to keep track of it	What is preventing you from doing that? Do you know what the numbers mean?
I haven't been taking those pills regularly	They are really important. Do keep trying to remember	Tell me about your reasons. Do you know what they are for and how they work?

Reasons why patients don't remember advice

Patients may remember a strikingly small amount of information if it is just told to them.

- Up to 80% of information may be forgotten.

- Almost half may be remembered incorrectly.

- Shorter appointments and busier clinics reinforce this problem.

- People are more likely to remember the first statements they are told but even more likely to remember a decision they have made themselves.

- Pictures and printed matter assist memory.

Home, work and social life

Home, work and social life influence the control and even the progression of diabetes. Unemployment, financial concerns and loneliness may be hidden, but they may be the reason for a change in eating habits, shoes of a poorer quality, disinterest or depression.

Opportunities in careers, employment, sport and other common life experiences may be overshadowed by the stigma of diabetes.

Lifestyle changes

Leaving home for the first time, a change of home or job, retirement or the loss of a partner may cause a major change in attitude and behaviour. Extra support and further education may be needed at these times.

Assessment for diabetes self-management and education

This should take place at annual review and, if appropriate, at every routine review. The assessment (by enquiry) should include:

- demographic information/changes;

- family status/changes;

- employment status/changes;

- medical history/changes;

- lifestyle history/changes;

- diabetes management/changes.

In addition, at diagnosis (or for a person with diabetes who has recently joined the practice), the assessment (by enquiry or observation) should include:

- any family history of diabetes;
- preconceived ideas about diabetes;
- a knowledge of diabetes and its complications;
- the circumstances surrounding the diagnosis;
- the individual's feelings surrounding diagnosis;
- the feelings of the family and/or carers related to diagnosis;
- culture/language;
- physical difficulties;
- mental difficulties;
- literacy/education;
- attitude to diabetes.

Getting the message across

Initially, education about diabetes in the general practice situation is best provided individually after assessment, although it can be helpful for a newly diagnosed person to meet someone who has had the condition for a time and has come to terms with it. In association with the information provided, the practice should be able to offer the following resources (see also Appendix 4):

- Titles of books or a book loan scheme.
- Booklets and leaflets (available from pharmaceutical companies or Diabetes UK).
- The address, telephone number and website address for Diabetes UK.
- The address and telephone number of the local branch of Diabetes UK.
- Where applicable, the address, telephone number and website of the British Heart Foundation.
- Local information regarding diabetes care and associated services (e.g. dietetics, chiropody/podiatry).

- Supportive agencies including those for smoking cessation where applicable.

- Social services.

- Environmental health (for 'sharps' disposal)

As the general population logs into the Internet, people with diabetes and those caring for them can join supportive diabetes networks across the world, as well as accessing the very latest developments in diabetes research and technology. It is important that IT is used sensitively and is not a replacement for the personal touch. It is a tool for the development of understanding and should, whenever possible, be planned into a structured, monitored and evaluated diabetes education programme.

Group diabetes education in the practice

Group education sessions for 8–10 people (more than this may be too inhibiting) can be held around a cup of tea and involve various health professionals, for example dietitians.

A variety of initiatives will be developing across the UK in response to ongoing research. Before embarking on unstructured group education that does not fit into today's ethos, health professionals should liaise with their local specialist team. There may be accredited schemes planned or in place (see information on the DAFNE, DESMOND and X-PERT programmes, above).

Organisation

- Select the group to be invited (e.g. people treated with diet, tablets or insulin).

- Select members of the primary care team to be involved and ensure that they have knowledge and skills in teaching and learning methods.

- Decide the time, length and place of sessions.

- Arrange tea, coffee and snacks.

- Set objectives for the session (to be agreed by the participants).

- Invite participants (with a minimum of 2 weeks' notice; Figure 16.1).

- Design a simple evaluation form for participants to complete after the session (Figure 16.2).

Practice Telephone No.: 222333
The Medical Practice
Woolley End Road
Airedale Edge
SHEFFIELD
South Yorkshire S2 3AB

January 2006

Mrs P Johnson
The Tannery
Black Terrace
SHEFFIELD S1 1XX

Dear Mrs Johnson

Re: Diabetes Care

We are planning to hold a lunchtime session for people with diabetes to discuss:

- Planning meals

- Testing for sugar

- Other topics, as required.

on Wednesday 18 April 2006, at 12.30pm.

The session will finish at 2 pm and a snack lunch will be provided.

You and your husband are warmly invited to attend. If you are unable to come, we would be grateful if you would let us know.

Yours sincerely

Dr A Smith (General Practitioner)   Mrs M Jones (Practice Nurse)

Figure 16.1 Sample letter of invitation for a group diabetes session

Invitations can be given verbally to people attending the diabetes clinic if the group session is planned well ahead (to save the cost of telephone calls and stamps).

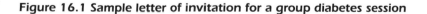

The Medical Practice
Woolley End Road
Airedale Edge
SHEFFIELD
South Yorkshire S2 3AB

Diabetes care – group session

Date:

In order to assess today's session, we would be grateful if you would fill in this form. Thank you.

Please delete the answers that do not apply to you and make your own comments.

1. Are you   A person with diabetes?

                       A relative?

                       A friend?

2. Did you receive sufficient notice to attend today's session?

                                                  YES/NO

3. Meal-planning

    (a) Was the topic covered sufficiently for you?   YES/NO

    (b) Were there aspects of the topic not covered?   YES/NO

    (c) What aspects of this topic would you have like to discuss further? Please write them down:

    _____

    _____

    _____

    _____

    _____

    _____

    _____

    _____

4. Testing for sugar

    (a) Was the topic covered enough for you?   YES/NO

    (b) Were aspects of the topic not covered?   YES/NO

    (c) What aspects of this topic would you have liked
        to discuss further? Please write them down:

    _____

    _____

    _____

    _____

5. What other topics discussed did you find useful
   in the session? Please write them down:

    _____

    _____

    _____

    _____

6. Did you find that today's session helped you to understand
   more about living with diabetes?   YES/NO

7. Would you be interested in attending further
   group sessions relating to diabetes care?   YES/NO

8. Do you have any suggestions for future sessions?
   Please write them down:

    _____

    _____

    _____

    _____

Thank you for filling in this form.

**Figure 16.2 Sample evaluation form for use following a group
diabetes session**

Facilitating the session

This includes the following:

- Preparation of room.
- Greeting participants.
- Domestic arrangements (coats, toilets, etc.).
- Introductions.
- Arrangements for tea, coffee and snacks.
- Stating the aims of the session and discussing these with participants.
- Identifying topics requested by participants.
- Introducing topics.
- Allowing discussion to progress around topics.
- Time-keeping.
- Summarising the session.
- Organising an evaluation form to be completed.
- Arranging follow-up or further session.
- Dealing with any personal problems identified during the session.
- Supervising the departure of participants.
- Clearing up.
- Discussing the evaluation forms and session with other members of the team.
- Recording the education session in the practice and patient records.

'Getting the message across' in diabetes education, whether to individuals or to groups, involves the following:

- Discussing and planning education concerned with the person with diabetes, relative and/or carer.
- Listening.
- Hearing what is being said.
- 'Picking up' hidden worries and difficulties.

- Responding to questions.

- Dealing with urgent problems.

- Asking the right questions in the right way (open questions such as 'Tell me about how you feel . . .' rather than 'Are you well?').

- Being non-judgemental.

- 'Staging' information.

- Providing small pieces of information at one time.

- Obtaining feedback on the information given.

- Summarising the information given.

- Demonstrating practical skills.

- Observing the practical skills learned.

- Being positive, encouraging and supportive.

- Recording the information given and skills learned.

- Discussing and planning further education with the person with diabetes, relative and/or carer.

References

Diabetes UK/Department of Health (2005). *Structured Patient Education in Diabetes. Report from the Patient Education Working Group.* London: DoH.
Diabetes UK (2005) *Recommendations for the Provision of Services in Primary Care for People with Diabetes.* London: Diabetes UK.
Miller WR, Rollnick S (1991) *Motivational Interviewing. Preparing People to Change Addictive Behavior.* New York: Guildford Press.
National Institute for Health and Clinical Excellence (2003). *Guidance on the Use of Patient-education Models for Diabetes.* Health Technology Appraisal No. 60. London: NICE.

Further reading

Deakin TA, Cade JE, Williams R, Greenwood DC (2006). Structured patient education: the diabetes X-PERT programme makes a difference. *Diabetic Medicine* **23**: 944–954.

Personal diabetes records and care plans

(hand-held records, patient-held records)

Questions this chapter will help you answer

- What is the difference between personal diabetes records (hand-held records, patient-held records) and care plans?

- What information should I include in the patient-held record?

- How will the patient benefit from these?

- Where can I get a template to use?

> *I would like more information about the results of the various blood tests and blood pressure test. I feel somewhat in the dark as to how I am progressing; one is given the impression 'all is well'. How well? Is there more I should be doing? What are the latest developments – could they help me?*
>
> Audit Commission (2000)

Personal diabetes records should be used to record investigations and therapy regimens.

Care plans – which should be an integral part of a patient-held record – are an agreed plan of action between an informed person with diabetes and members of the care team.

In 2002, the Department of Health published its National Service Framework for Diabetes Delivery Strategy. It set criteria for meeting the standards set in 2001 and outlined areas for individuals' involvement in their own care. It recognised that those in poorer areas were more likely to suffer the complications of diabetes and suggested local systems be put in place to tackle those most at risk. Two particular areas highlighted for consideration were:

- information and appropriate psychological support and the opportunity to participate in structured (usually group) education to people diagnosed with diabetes after April 2003 (see Chapter 16);
- an agreed care plan, a personal diabetes record and named contact within the local service to all those diagnosed with diabetes after April 2003, along with people with poor blood glucose control (glycated haemoglobin (HbA_{1c}) level greater than 7.5%).

The components of a personal diabetes record (Box 17.1) had been under discussion with Diabetes UK, and this provided formal recognition of a need to involve people with diabetes in their own care.

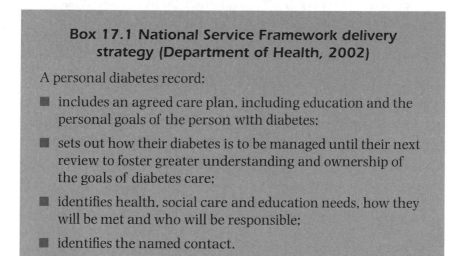

Box 17.1 National Service Framework delivery strategy (Department of Health, 2002)

A personal diabetes record:

- includes an agreed care plan, including education and the personal goals of the person with diabetes;
- sets out how their diabetes is to be managed until their next review to foster greater understanding and ownership of the goals of diabetes care;
- identifies health, social care and education needs, how they will be met and who will be responsible;
- identifies the named contact.

What is a care plan?

The National Service Framework delivery strategy describes a care plan in the following terms (Department of Health, 2002):

- A care plan is at the heart of a partnership approach to care and a central part of effective care management. The process of agreeing a care plan offers people active involvement in deciding, agreeing and owning how their diabetes will be managed. Whilst the overall goal is a genuine partnership, the person with diabetes must feel that they are comfortable with what is proposed and that they do not have to bear more responsibility than they wish.

- PCTs [primary care trusts] should ensure systematic treatment regimens are in place for people with diabetes. Ultimately, at the heart of these will be regular reviews, which will be based on a diabetes record and a care plan developed and agreed jointly between the person with diabetes and a member of the diabetes team.

- People with diabetes may be seen by many different health and social care professionals over the years. Unless services are co-ordinated, this can prove problematic for them and compromise the quality of care. Experience from other care groups has shown the benefit of designating one member of the care team as a named contact for each person with diabetes. This person acts as an initial point of contact, helping the person with diabetes navigate the service and access other members of the multidisciplinary team as appropriate. They may also be the team member who takes the lead in reviewing the diabetes management. The role of the named contact is particularly important at those times when diabetes care is most difficult – for example, at diagnosis, when changing treatment, or during adolescence and the transition to adult services. Good practice shows that they should be identified in discussion with the person with diabetes.

Patient-held records can:

- serve as an aid to structured care (i.e. help to ensure that all people with diabetes get regular checks of their blood glucose control, eyes, feet, blood pressure, etc.);

- help to educate the individual and the health professional in the principles of good diabetes care;

- involve the patient or carer more closely in the management plan;

- facilitate continuity of care when individuals move house, change doctor, go on holiday or need emergency care.

Some information records should contain are:

- contact details for the person with diabetes;

- the individual's medical details;

- explanatory notes;

- treatment;

- instruction for emergencies;
- an education checklist;
- a personal treatment plan;
- regular (3- or 6-monthly) checks;
- annual review checks;
- space for the individual's own notes;
- a glossary of medical terms;
- in some cases, clinical education and published advice relevant to the individual.

Figure 17.1 can be used as a template.

While electronic methods of sharing information are being developed, primary care organisations and networks are working to agree locally acceptable forms of patient-held records. Diabetes UK (2003) have published a template that is reproduced here (Figure 17.1) with permission; an example of a care plan is given in Figure 17.2.

Examples of personal diabetes records and care plans in use were found to be scarce by the Department of Health (2005), few having been evaluated for effectiveness. Both health professionals and people with diabetes appreciated their worth but found difficulty in implementing them. An example provided by the Department of Health is given in Figure 17.2.

References

Department of Health (2002). *National Service Framework for Diabetes: Delivery Strategy*. London: DoH.

Department of Health (2005). *Empowering People with Diabetes. An Exploration of the Role of Personal Diabetes Records and Care Plans*. London: DoH.

Diabetes UK (2003) *Care Recommendation. Patient-held Records*. London: Diabetes UK.

1. Diabetes Record Card

This record card will help you receive the best care for your diabetes, and could provide vital information if you are taken ill. Please complete all the relevant details on this card, or ask the nurse or doctor to do so for you. You should bring it to all your appointments and ask the person who sees you to fill it in.

Name:

Address

Phone Number: (H)   (W)

Date of Birth: NHS Number:

Ethnic Origin: Religion:

Interpreter Phone: Language Spoken:

Emergency Contact Name: Phone Number:

GP Name & Address:

GP Phone: (day)   (out of hours)

Community Pharmacist   Name/Phone:

Diabetes Nurse Name: Phone:

Chiropodist Name: Phone:

Dietitian Name: Phone:

Hospital Diabetes Specialist: Phone:

Hospital Number:

Diabetes UK Careline: 0845 120 2960
(the lines are open Monday to Friday 9am to 5pm)
Diabetes UK website: www.diabetes.org.uk

Figure 17.1 Diabetes record card

2. Medical Details

Diabetes History

Type of diabetes:

Date diagnosed: Weight at diagnosis:

Symptoms at diagnosis:

Family history of diabetes, blood pressure, heart disease, stroke
or high cholesterol etc.:

Initial treatment:

Past Medical History

Note especially any high blood pressure, high cholesterol levels, angina,
heart attack or heart surgery, and stroke or similar event:

3. Explanatory Notes

This is your Personal Diabetes Record, it is your record of important
information about your diabetes care. The information collected in this record
will help to improve communication between yourself and the healthcare
professionals looking after you.

Please take your record with you to all appointments including the following:

- your GP
- the hospital diabetes clinic
- the eye clinic
- your optician
- the diabetes nurse
- the dietitian
- your chiropodist/podiatrist
- the hospital accident and emergency department

4. Medication

Allergies:
....

Date prescribed	Name of medication	Strength	How many and when	What it's for

Insulin Delivery Device:
....

Type of Monitoring: Blood   Urine
....

Monitoring Device and Strips Used:
....

5. Emergencies and Illnesses

Hypoglycaemic attack ('hypo') – This occurs when the blood glucose level is too low, usually when a meal or snack has been missed, too much insulin has been taken or after unaccustomed exercise. It comes on SUDDENLY in a person who was not unwell. The symptoms may include: sweating, shaking, irritability, confusion, and feeling faint. **Action:** TAKE SUGAR OR A SUGARY DRINK IMMEDIATELY (such as glucose tablets, Lucozade or other non-diet drink), stop exercising and follow the short-acting carbohydrate with some long-acting carbohydrate (eg sandwich, milk, a biscuit, or next meal if due).

Hyperglycaemic coma – This occurs when the blood glucose level is very high. It builds up over days or weeks, so the person may have been feeling unwell for a few days. They become drowsy and their breath may smell sweet. **Action:** measure the blood glucose level with strips to confirm that it is high. Call a doctor or an ambulance.

Not sure? If unsure whether it is hypo- or hyperglycaemia, give sugar anyway.

Illness – People with diabetes who are ill and take insulin need more insulin not less, even if they do not feel like eating. NEVER STOP INSULIN TREATMENT. If people with diabetes on insulin cannot drink fluids they need to seek professional medical help. Regular checks of blood glucose and for ketones in the urine during any illness are essential whether on tablet or insulin treatment.

6. Checklist for Education Sessions

Below is a list of topics that you may need to know about. Some are very important; the nurse or doctor should discuss them with you regularly. Some may not be relevant to you. If you are unsure, please ask.

Topic	Dates Discussed		
What is diabetes?			
Diet			
Tablets			
Physical activity			
Insulin & injection technique			
Hyperglycaemia			
Illness			
Blood testing			
Urine testing			
Foot care			
Importance of eye checks			
Smoking			
Alcohol			
Complications			
Driving/insurance			
Travel			
Sexual health			
Planning pregnancy			
Diabetes UK			
Free prescriptions			
Benefits			

7. Diet Plan and Progress Record

This is a plan agreed between the person with diabetes and the health professional giving dietary, physical activity and weight targets and advised frequency of regular check-ups etc.

Dietary Goals:

Comments (with dates):

Physical Activity Plan and Progress Record

Physical Activity Goals:

Comments (with dates):

8. Diabetes Surveillance Record (check-ups)

This may be presented in a fold-out format or as several pages in a booklet; Diabetes UK recommended intervals are shown but should be modified if necessary.

Date	3-monthly	6-monthly	9-monthly	Annual
Review control				
Weight / BMI / waist circumference				
Blood pressure 　Lying or sitting				
Standing				
Foot examination 　General condition				
Pulses				
Sensation				
Urine tests 　Glucose				
Protein				
Microalbuminuria				
Blood tests 　Glucose level				
HbA_{1c}				
Total cholesterol 　HDL 　LDL				
Triglyceride				
Eye examination				
Fundoscopy				
Visual acuity				
Retinal photograph				

Date of next visit: ....

9. Personal Notes and Queries

This section is for you to note anything about your diabetes that you would like to discuss.

_____

_____

_____

_____

_____

_____

_____

_____

_____

_____

_____

_____

_____

_____

_____

_____

_____

_____

_____

_____

What Diabetes Care to Expect

Research has shown that people with diabetes get fewer complications, and may live longer, if they have regular check-ups, even if they do not feel ill in any way. You should agree with your doctor how often these checks should be, but at the very least, you should make sure someone examines the back of your eyes once a year. For more details, see the leaflet, 'What diabetes care to expect' available free from Diabetes UK. To order this leaflet call freephone **0800 585 088**.

10. Terms and Tests

Blood glucose level – the amount of glucose (sugar)in the blood.

Blood pressure (BP) – the pressure level within the arteries, which indicates how hard the heart is working to pump the blood round the body.

Body mass index (BMI) – a measure of how overweight or underweight you are. A BMI above 28 kg/m² means that you are seriously overweight. It is calculated by

BMI = Weight (kg) / Height² (m²).

Cataracts – cloudiness and thickening of the lens of the eye.

Cholesterol – a type of fat in the blood. Too much cholesterol in the blood may increase your risk of developing heart disease.

Foot pulses and sensation – checks made on the blood supply and amount of feeling in the feet.

HbA1 (or HbA1c) – a blood test which indicates the average level of your blood glucose during the past three months. Known also as Glycated Haemoglobin.

HDL – high density lipoprotein, often referred to as good cholesterol, it carries cholesterol away from the arteries. High levels of these can protect people from heart disease and stroke.

Hyperglycaemia – high blood glucose level.

Hypoglycaemia – low blood glucose level.

Hyperlipidemia – another name for high cholesterol or triglyceride levels.

LDL – low density lipoproteins, known as bad cholesterol; too much LDL in the blood can cause it to collect on the artery lining, leading to narrowing and hardening.

Microalbuminuria – a test for very tiny amounts of protein in the urine.

Protein – urine protein is checked (with test strips) to test for damage to the kidneys. Protein is also found when there is an infection in the urine.

Retinopathy – damage to the back of the eye (retina).

Triglyceride (TG) – a type of fat in the blood.

Urea and creatinine – blood tests to check for kidney damage.

Visual acuity – an eye test which involves reading a letter chart.

CARE PLAN			
Named Contact:		Completed By:	Date:

PATIENT ISSUES/CONCERNS

EDUCATIONAL NEEDS

KEY CLINICAL DATA	MY AIM	IDEAL RANGE
Eye Assessment		
Foot Assessment		
Renal Assessment		
HbA1c		
BP		
Cardio-Vascular Risk		
Food Issues		
Physical Activity		
Other conditions/concerns		

AGREED KEY ISSUES

PATIENT'S PRIORITIES (for action by patient or the team)

Figure 17.2 Sample care plans: empowering people with diabetes.
An exploration of the role of personal diabetes records and care plans
(Reproduced from Department of Health, 2005, with permission)
BP, blood pressure; HbA1c, glycated haemoglobin

DATE	PATIENT SELECTED TARGET	ACTIONS TO DO	EVALUATION

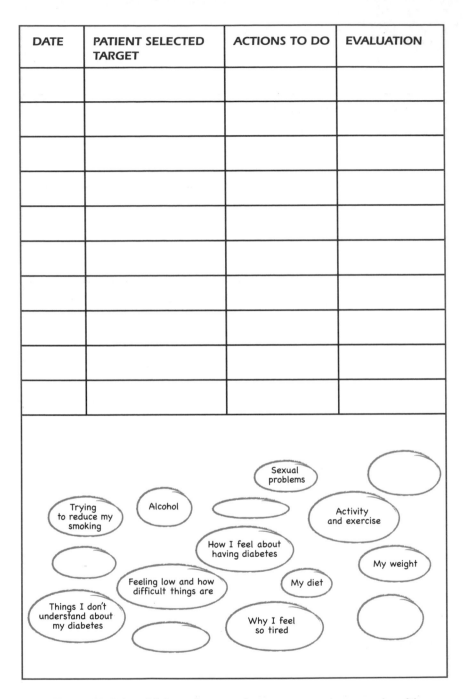

Figure 17.2 (cont'd) **Sample care plans: empowering people with diabetes. An exploration of the role of personal diabetes records and care plans**

(Reproduced from Department of Health, 2005, with permission)

BP, blood pressure; HbA1c, glycated haemoglobin

18 Living with diabetes

Questions this chapter will help you answer

- What should I be including in my education plans?
- What are the rules on driving with diabetes?
- Are there specific issues with women's health and diabetes?
- What should I advise travellers with diabetes?
- What do I do to detect and manage depression?

> *... it is important that [patients'] psychological and educational needs are treated as seriously as their medical needs.*
>
> Audit Commission (2000)

As part of structured education, people with diabetes need to understand the condition. Health professionals need to help them gain the educational tools they need to look after themselves. After all, who provides the majority of patient care? Those with diabetes themselves. They may see a health professional for a total of only a few minutes to a few hours in a year; therefore, it is important to engage them in the learning process. Areas to be discussed with people living with diabetes are included here, with expanded information in the relevant chapters.

After confirmation of diagnosis

Advising and working with people newly diagnosed with diabetes needs to be undertaken with understanding and in a sensitive manner, taking account of their level of understanding, culture and beliefs. They need to be encouraged to share their anxieties and express concerns for their future.

A care plan (see Chapter 17) should be agreed that focuses on continuing support and education, with the person with diabetes taking an active role. The care plan should be a useful document, renegotiated at each stage of the care pathway and containing a past history of goals, investigations and education. Topics for discussion, not all of which need be covered in one session, are listed below, with thanks to Diabetes UK (Diabetes UK, 2005).

Nature of diabetes

- Significance and implications of a diagnosis of diabetes; the impact of diabetes (see Chapter 7).

- Aims and different types of treatment (see Chapter 11).

- Continuation of drug supply – ordering of prescription; is notice required by the practice?

- Relationship between blood glucose level, dietary intake and physical activity (see Chapter 10).

- Short- and long-term consequences of poorly controlled diabetes (see Chapter 24).

- Nature and prevention of long-term complications (see Chapter 24).

- Importance of annual surveillance for complications (see Chapter 8).

Day-to-day management of diabetes

- Importance of a healthy lifestyle, especially physical activity, a balanced diet and not smoking (see Chapter 10).

- Importance of self-management (see Chapter 17).

- Smoking.

- Self-monitoring – glucose monitoring (urine testing being less used nowadays) (see Chapter 12).

- Interpreting the results of self-monitoring and tests of long-term blood glucose control (see Chapter 12).

- Adjusting insulin dosage (for those on insulin) (see Chapter 11).

- Importance of systematically using different injection sites (for those on insulin) (see Chapter 11).

- Storage of insulin; disposal of 'sharps' (see Chapter 11).

- Importance of regular foot care, choice of footwear, foot hygiene and the role of podiatry (see Chapter 14).

- Importance of oral hygiene and regular dental check-ups.

Specific issues

- Care provision (where, how and who?) (see Chapter 8).

- Prescription exemption (if taking hypoglycaemic agents or insulin) (see Chapter 11).

- Educational materials in different formats, for example DVDs, leaflets and websites (see Chapter 16).

- Hypoglycaemia (see Chapter 12).

- Hyperglycaemia (see Chapter 12).

- Alcohol (see Chapter 10).

- Car driving and insurance (see later in this chapter).

- Other illness – 'sick day rules' must be given to all people with diabetes (see Chapter 12).

- Immunisations, such as for influenza or pneumococcal pneumonia, should be offered to all those with diabetes.

- Importance of regular eye examinations – both visual acuity and fundal examination (see Chapter 13).

- Blood glucose monitoring (see Chapter 12).

Other possible topics for follow-up visits

Pre-conception advice (for women of childbearing age) must encompass the importance of excellent control at the time of conception as well as during pregnancy.

- Oral hypoglycaemic agents must be stopped.

Blood pressure

See Chapter 24.

Special occasions, celebrations, eating out

See Chapters 10 and 15.

Annual review

The importance and reasons for the annual care plan should be stressed.

Eye care and screening

See Chapter 13.

Foot and shoe care

See Chapter 14.

Chiropody/podiatry (may be required)

See Chapter 14.

Cervical screening

- This should be offered to women with diabetes.

Breast screening

- Breast screening should be offered to women with diabetes.

Diabetes and depression

Depression may affect at least twice as many people with diabetes than members of the general population. The former also tend to have more recurrences of the condition. This is linked to:

- poor self-care;
- a lack of achievement of metabolic targets;
- a higher incidence of complications including cardiovascular disease and stroke.

Depression may be underdetected in the rushed diabetes clinic and is addressed in the GMS contract, with QOF points being available for detection and management (Table 18:1; for further information, see Chapter 3).

National Institute for Health and Clinical Excellence guidance on depression (2004) advises that depression screening should be undertaken in primary care for high-risk groups, including those with diabetes and heart disease. Two questions were highlighted in assessing mood:

- During the past month, have you often been bothered by feeling down, depressed or hopeless?

- During the past month, have you often been bothered by having little interest or pleasure in doing things?

A 'yes' answer to either question is considered to be a positive test. A 'no' response to both questions makes depression highly unlikely.

Primary care teams should consider asking these questions as part of their care plans, but clear systems need to be agreed on what action to take if depression is diagnosed. A further assessment of other symptoms such as tiredness, guilt, poor concentration, change in sleep pattern and appetite, and suicidal ideation will be required, and only those with the knowledge and skills to manage this condition should undertake this role. Referral to psychologists and/or other health professionals proficient in dealing with depression may be required.

For those with a new diagnosis of depression, tools are available to assess the severity of the condition:

1 the Patient Health Questionnaire (PHQ-9);

2 the Beck Depression Inventory Second Edition (BDI-II);

3 the Hospital Anxiety and Depression Scale (HADS).

It is advisable for a practice to choose one of these three measures and become familiar with its questions and scoring systems.

Table 18.1 Depression in the General Medical Services contract

Indicator	Points	Payment stages
Diagnosis and initial management		
DEP1: The percentage of patients on the diabetes register and/or the CHD register for whom case finding for depression has been undertaken on one occasion during the previous 15 months using two standard screening questions	8	40–90%
DEP2: In those patients with a new diagnosis of depression, recorded between the preceding April to 31 March, the percentage of patients who have had an assessment of severity at the outset of treatment using an assessment tool validated for use in primary care	25	40–90%

CHD, coronary heart disease

The **PHQ-9** (which can be downloaded free from www.depression-primarycare.org) is a nine-question self-report measure of severity that takes approximately 3 minutes to complete. It uses criteria contained in the fourth revision of the *Diagnostic and Statistical Manual of Mental Disorders* (DSM-IV), and scores are categorised as minimal (1–4), mild (5–9), moderate (10–14), moderately severe (15–19) and severe (20–27) depression.

The **BDI-II** (available to purchase) is a 21-item self report instrument that also uses the DSM-IV criteria. It takes approximately 5 minutes to fill in. A total score of 0–13 is considered minimal range, 14–19 is mild, 20–28 is moderate and 29–63 is severe.

The **HADS** (available to purchase) has, despite its name, been validated for use in community and primary care settings. It is self-administered and takes up to 5 minutes to complete. The Anxiety and Depression scales both comprise seven questions rated from a score of 0 to 3 depending on the severity of the problem described in each question. The two subscales can also be aggregated to provide an overall anxiety and depression score. The anxiety and depression scores are categorised as normal (0–7), mild (8–10), moderate (11–14) and severe (15–21).

Family planning advice

- Fertility is not impaired in diabetes, except in the presence of severe renal disease.

- Oral contraception is 99% effective if taken according to instructions. Fewer than 1 woman in 100 will then become pregnant in 1 year.

- Combined oral contraceptives (COCs) should be avoided where possible owing to the possibility of arterial disease. Women should take COCs for the shortest time possible and should:
  - be under 25 years old;
  - have had diabetes for only a short time;
  - be free of complications;
  - be non-smokers;
  - have a body mass index of less than 30;
  - be normotensive.

- Gestational diabetes and a strong family history of diabetes do not contraindicate the use of COCs.

- Barrier methods, the progestogen-only pill, implant and intrauterine systems/devices (IUS/IUDs) are preferable to COCs:
  - ◆ The progestogen-only pill may have adverse metabolic effects. Newer types, for example Cerazette, are preferred. Other contraceptive options may be preferable.
  - ◆ IUS/IUDs need good diabetes control in order to limit the small risk of infection, especially at insertion.
- Ultra-low-dose COCs are permitted in young people with diabetes with a lipid friendly progestogen, e.g. Mercilon or Femodette 20 μg oestrogen.

Pre-conception

- Blood glucose levels should be well controlled 3 months before conception.
- Pre-pregnancy counselling, education and support should be planned.
- Early referral is necessary.

Pregnancy

- Continuing support and surveillance by obstetric and diabetes teams are necessary throughout pregnancy and in the postnatal period.
- Early referral is recommended.
- Dietary adjustments may be required during the establishment of breastfeeding.
- Protection should be provided against rubella during pregnancy.

Hormone replacement therapy

- Hormone replacement therapy can and should be used in women with diabetes (the pros and cons of its effect on coronary heart disease should be discussed with the individual to allow her to make an informed choice).
- Progestogens may have an anti-insulin effect.
- Blood glucose levels should be carefully monitored.
- Insulin doses may need adjustment.

Erectile dysfunction

This is frequently not discussed owing to embarrassment. The person with diabetes needs to know that:

- it is common in men who have had diabetes for some time;
- glycaemic control is important;
- there are several treatments available, including Viagra, and most men can be helped;
- specialist referral for assessment may be necessary.

Children and young people with diabetes

These groups will be referred to specialist care.

- The individuals themselves require special care and management.
- Their parents need support.
- They should be referred appropriately on diagnosis.
- They may have particular problems at certain stages of childhood and development (e.g. change of school, onset of puberty), requiring extra support.
- Diabetes control can deteriorate quickly (especially during an illness). Urgent admission to hospital may be required.
- All immunisations should be offered to children and young people with diabetes.
- As adult life approaches, support and counselling are required to deal with higher education, employment, social pressures, driving and living away from home for the first time.

Employment

People with diabetes must consider their safety, and that of others, if they are taking hypoglycaemic agents or insulin.

The Discrimination Disability Act (1995) says that it is illegal for employers to treat people who have diabetes differently from other employees, but there are some exceptions:

- the armed forces
- the police service

■ the fire service.

There is also a blanket ban on these jobs:

- airline pilot, cabin crew with most airlines and air traffic control;
- train-driving;
- taxi-driving in some areas.

Others jobs to consider carefully are:

- working at heights;
- deep-sea-diving;
- working on oil rigs;
- coal-face work;
- truck- and bus-driving.

Shift work can be accommodated with flexible insulin regimens.

Sport and leisure

- The safety of the person with diabetes and the safety of others (in association with hypoglycaemia) must be considered.
- People on insulin need to understand the effect of exercise on blood glucose level and how to manage blood glucose fluctuations. If they are on insulin, they need to understand the principles of dose adjustment.
- Having an accompanying person is a sensible precaution.
- A few sports apply restrictions to those with diabetes.
- Extra food and/or a reduction in insulin dose may be needed relating to the degree of activity.
- Extra food (if the person is treated with medication) may be needed relating to the degree of activity.
- There is a possibility of delayed hypoglycaemia (after strenuous activity), which may occur many hours later.
- The symptoms, prevention and treatment of hypoglycaemia in association with sport and leisure activities should be understood.

Car-driving

Car-driving licences should be kept up to date through the Driver and Vehicle Licensing Agency (DVLA; see Appendix 4 for the website address).

- Car-driving licences can be held by people with diabetes.

- People with diabetes need to be aware they must inform the DVLA if they are being treated with hypoglycaemic agents or insulin. (It is not necessary to inform the DVLA about treatment with oral agents unless there is a concomitant condition, but it is wise to do so and to keep relevant correspondence.)

- Licences are renewed every 1, 2 or 3 years depending on the person's health, or at the age of 70 years if the person is treated with diet alone or some oral agents. Each application will be assessed by the DVLA.

- Licence renewal forms are sent automatically before the expiry date. There is no fee for renewal.

- Licence renewal is granted after completion of the form by the person with diabetes. (The form must include signed consent for the individual's doctor to be consulted by the DVLA if required.)

- A medical check may be requested by the DVLA.

- The driver must inform his or her driving insurance company of the presence of diabetes. Some insurance companies load the driver's premium; this should be challenged. It is sensible to 'shop around' because the Disability Discrimination Act 1995 has improved this situation.

Driving larger vehicles

- People treated by diet alone or by diet and tablets are normally allowed to hold LGV (previously HGV) and PCV (previously PSV) licences, provided they are otherwise in good health.

- People treated with insulin are not allowed to hold these licences. This has important employment implications. The person with diabetes must understand that he or she must stop driving this type of vehicle and inform the DVLA. The only exception is for the small number of people who had insulin-treated diabetes and were issued with such a licence before April 1991, when the law changed.

- Holders of vocational driving licences must inform the DVLA when they start insulin treatment. There should be a place in their care plan to record this information.

- The decision to follow this advice is the responsibility of the individual concerned. If it is not followed, the licence will be revoked.

- There is, however, a statutory right of appeal (details being sent from the DVLA when the licence is revoked).

- General advice regarding appeals against the withdrawal of car and vocational driving licences can be obtained from Diabetes UK (contact details in Appendix 4).

- People with visual impairment should not drive.

- People who have lost their warning signs of hypoglycaemia should not drive. Support to regain lost warning signs of hypoglycaemia should be available through the specialist team.

- Drivers should know the symptoms, prevention and treatment of hypoglycaemia. Sweets/biscuits should always be available in the vehicle.

- If warning signs of hypoglycaemia occur, the driver should:
  - move as safely as possible to the side of the road;
  - stop the car and remove the keys from the ignition;
  - move to the passenger seat and eat some sweets or biscuits;
  - resume driving only when it is safe to do so;
  - have a substantial starchy snack or meal as soon as possible.

Life assurance

- As with motor insurance, life assurance is calculated according to a person's age and state of health.

- A life assurance policy already held should not be affected by the diagnosis of diabetes. It is not necessary to declare the diabetes.

- If a new policy is taken out, the diabetes must be declared and the policy may be loaded. This can be challenged.

- Advice about sympathetic insurance companies can be obtained from Diabetes UK (details in Appendix 4).

Haslemere Health Centre
Church Lane
Haslemere
Surrey
GU* *BQ

Tel: 01483 ******

Re: ....

....

....

Date: ....

To whom it may concern:

This is to confirm that the above named person has diabetes mellitus requiring regular injections of insulin. He/she is carrying insulin, pen injection devices, needles, a blood glucose meter, lancets, finger pricking device and testing strips. He/she is also carrying food, GlucoGel dextrose gel and Glucagon in case of hypoglycaemia. It is essential that he/she keep these items with him/her in the aircraft cabin in order to manage his/her diabetes safely. Insulin **must not** be put into the hold as it may freeze, which would render it inactive.

Thank you for your understanding in this matter.

Yours sincerely,

Jemima Smith
Diabetes Specialist Nurse in Primary Care

Figure 18.1 Sample letter for use when travelling abroad

Travel and holidays

- Immunisation may be required. Exact details will depend on the country to be visited (available in the practice). Diabetes control may be temporarily affected (by immunisation).

- Travel insurance should include:
  - declaring diabetes (to obtain adequate cover);
  - checking extent of coverage;
  - looking for a premium with a minimum coverage of £250 000;
  - contacting Diabetes UK for further information if required (see Appendix 4).

- Provide leaflets from the practice and/or provide information from the Department of Health website pages on the Travellers' Guide to Health (see Appendix 4).

- Obtain the European Health Insurance Card (EHIC; previously Form E111) from the Post Office or Department of Health website online for medical care in EC countries.

- The following should be considered before travel:
  - identification (card/bracelet);
  - if travelling abroad, a doctor's letter may be helpful when carrying needles, syringes and medications, for example steroids (particularly at customs points; Figure 18.1);
  - travel sickness prevention;
  - antidiarrhoea medication;
  - antimalarial medication (if appropriate);
  - a supply of antibiotics (for long-term travel off the beaten track);
  - simple dressings;
  - sufficient medication or insulin (insulin stored in a cool bag) and carried in the hand luggage (as luggage freezes in the hold). Owing to security measures, insulin and other medication may be stored in a locked cupboard by airline staff. Remember that U100 insulin is not available everywhere;
  - sufficient supplies of syringes and needle-clippers (carried in the hand luggage);
  - monitoring equipment (carried in the hand luggage);

- sunburn protection cream;
- a sun hat;
- water purification tablets (if appropriate);
- appropriate footwear;
- sweets or biscuits for when travelling or for delays at airports.

■ The local specialist team will be able to help with complicated journeys and travel.

■ See Appendix 4 for details on the Foreign and Commonwealth Office, Health Protection Scotland, Travel Health Information and Masta Travel Health, which can provide information.

Dental care

■ Regular dental checks are important.

■ Dental infections may disturb diabetes control.

■ A painful mouth (particularly poorly fitting dentures) may prevent eating and cause a subsequent risk of hypoglycaemia.

■ There is no financial help for people with diabetes relating to dental care.

References

Diabetes UK (2005). *Recommendations for the Provision of Services in Primary Care for People with Diabetes.* Diabetes UK, London.
National Institute for Health and Clinical Excellence (2004). *Depression: Management of Depression in Primary and Secondary Care.* Clinical Guideline No. 23. London: NICE.

Further reading

Walker R, Rodgers J in association with Diabetes UK (2004). *Diabetes. A Practical Guide to Managing your Health.* London: Dorling Kindersley.

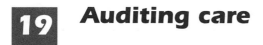

19 Auditing care

Questions this chapter will help you answer

- What is the difference between data-gathering, research and audit?

- Is everyone with diabetes diagnosed and recorded on my practice diabetes register?

- What should I record on specific complications?

- What proportion of those in my practice with diabetes receive the key processes of diabetes care?

- What proportion of people with diabetes achieve treatment targets?

> *... many health authorities were unable to collect data on outcomes of diabetes care.*
>
> Audit Commission (2000)

Audit is an accepted part of patient care. It can lead to improvements for those with diabetes and healthcare professionals alike. To participate, and benefit from, audit, you need to understand the difference between data-gathering for information or research purposes and audit (Table 19.1).

Table 19.1 Difference between research and audit

Research	Audit
Discovers the right thing to do	Determines whether the right thing is being done
A series of 'one-off' projects	A cyclical series of reviews
Collects complex data	Collects routine data
Experiment is rigorously defined	Review of what clinicians actually do
Often possible to generalise the findings	Not possible to generalise from the findings

Definition

Audit is defined as:

> The attempt to improve the quality of medical care by measuring the performance of those providing that care, by considering the performance in relation to desired standards, and by improving on this performance.

- The activity to be audited should represent a problem in the provision of care.

- It should be an area that those involved are keen to improve and, indeed, one in which they perceive that there is a need for change.

The audit cycle (Figure 19.1) follows a set of principles:

1   The team agree a problem or area to be audited.

2   Standards and criteria are set based on local or national guidelines.

3   Data are gathered, on a card index or computer files, and collated.

4   Results are compared with the standards set, and action is planned.

5   Change is implemented.

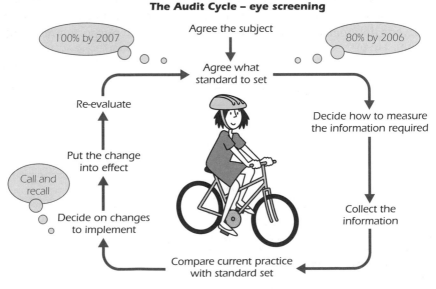

The Audit Cycle – eye screening

Figure 19.1 Example of an audit cycle

6 Re-auditing is undertaken within a given timeframe, for example 1 year.

Audit can prove good practice and patient satisfaction with a service, and boost income through the General Medical Services (GMS) contract (see Chapter 2).

Suitable areas to audit in diabetes might be:

- *structures*: for example, the practice register (does the local practice population compare favourably with other areas with the same demographics?);

- *processes*: for example, recall rates for eye-screening uptake, or whether all people with diabetes are able to get a systematic review;

- *outcomes*: for example, clinical measures outlined in the GMS contract (see Chapter 2).

Continuous data suitable for audit are generally available through general practitioner (GP) computer systems but should not bypass the need for team discussion on what is important to audit.

The Quality Management and Analysis System (see Appendix 4 for website) is a national system that is being developed to support the quality and outcomes framework detailed in the GMS contract.

The National Institute for Health and Clinical Excellence (details in Appendix 4) has recommendations for audit in its many diabetes guidelines.

- Risk of *coronary heart disease* (CHD): greater detail is needed on clinical care for those with diabetes, for example those with a higher CHD risk who have been offered antiplatelet therapy (aspirin), those who have microalbuminuria or proteinuria, and the percentage of patients whose blood pressure is equal to or above 135/75 mmHg.

- *Glycaemic control*: the percentage of patients who have received education about self-monitoring of blood glucose level, lifestyle advice or patient education.

- *Renal*: the percentage of people with type 2 diabetes who have had their albumin:creatinine ratio or albumin concentration measured in the previous 12 months, and the percentage of patients with microalbuminuria or proteinuria who are receiving an angiotensin-converting enzyme inhibitor.

- *Eyes*: for those with severe retinopathy on examination, the percentage of people who receive a specialist opinion within

4 weeks, or for those with new vessels found on examination, the percentage of people who are seen by an ophthalmologist within 1 week.

- *Feet*: the percentage of patients who have a record of an agreed management plan (including patient education) in the previous 15 months, the percentage of patients with recorded diabetes with feet at high risk of ulceration who attend a podiatry service, or the percentage of patients with a new below-ankle (and, separately, those with an above-ankle) amputation in the previous 12 months.

DiabetesE

DiabetesE is a self-assessment service that includes a web-based tool. The service enables primary care organisations (PCOs), specialist diabetes services and primary care practices to systematically and objectively self-assess the management and delivery of diabetes care against the National Service Framework (NSF) Delivery Strategy and Clinical Standards (Department of Health, 2001, 2002). It provides a whole-system view of diabetes care and assists performance improvement on the four key fronts of:

- baseline assessment
- continuous quality improvement
- national benchmarking
- knowledge management.

Self-assessment helps PCOs and individual practices to examine, systematically, whether appropriate mechanisms are in place to plan, deliver and monitor a whole system of diabetes care. Self-assessment can enable the PCOs and practices to analyse their performance, determine whether they are achieving their objectives and support the planning of improvements in the diabetes service. The self-assessment tool will enable PCOs and practices to:

- determine their current achievements and priorities for change;
- measure their progress against themselves and their peers;
- prepare themselves for future Commission for Health Improvement NSF assessments.

The National Diabetes Audit (The Information Centre, 2005) is designed to complement DiabetesE. Information about more than half a million people with diabetes has been collected through the National Diabetes Audit 2004/05. A total of 106 PCOs, 1868 individual GP practices, and many hospital trusts and specialist paediatric units have registered for the audit.

When compared against National Institute for Health and Clinical Excellence guidelines, the results of the audit show:

Glycated haemoglobin (HbA_{1c}):

- 22% of people with diabetes achieved the best HbA_{1c} target range of less than 6.5%;
- 58% of people achieved the target of less than 7.5%.

Blood pressure:

- 24% of people with diabetes achieved the blood pressure target of less than or equal to 135/75 mmHg;
- 88% of people achieved the target of less than 160/100 mmHg.

Cholesterol:

- 68% of people achieved the target of less than 5 mmol/l;
- 10% more men achieved the cholesterol target than women. A possible explanation for this may be the greater screening for and prevalence of CHD among men and a resulting increased use of statins.

Key findings

A number of important findings including significant variations in services have been identified from the 2004/05 data:

- Around 81% of people predicted to have diabetes are recorded as doing so.
- Significant differences exist in the complication rates of myocardial infarction, cardiac failure, renal failure and major amputations among people with diabetes.
- Only 61% of people with diabetes have eye-screening recorded.
- 58% of people with diabetes reached a target level of 7.5% HbA_{1c}.

Key recommendations

It is recommended that diabetes networks, clinicians and PCOs should:

1 Continue the improvements in diagnosing and recording people with diabetes and aim to ensure that at least 90% of the predicted number are identified and registered.

2 Strive to improve the accuracy and completeness of recording diabetes type in order to better understand the population of people with diabetes and their needs.

3 Also improve the accuracy and recording of ethnicity in order to better understand the population of people with diabetes and evaluate their needs.

4 Use detailed local knowledge to:

◆ identify and investigate reasons for significantly high complications rates where they occur. The NDA Analysis toolkit, PIANO (available from The Information Centre; see Appendix 4), contains the relevant statistical process charts;

◆ share understanding of the factors contributing to the achievement of significantly low complications rates. Again, PIANO contains the relevant statistical process charts.

5 Review rates of carrying out and recording key processes of care and aim to make further improvements to aspire to achieve the benchmarks as set by the upper quartiles seen in the audit (Table 19.2). Local services should aim to complete the gaps in undertaking the key care processes, particularly where they are poorly filled. The upper quartiles in the audit should be considered as a minimum to be achieved, and continued improvement should be based on this. Where services are clearly lagging, local organisations should examine the specific reasons for this.

6 Consider the provision of services for people in the younger age bands (under 16 years) and aim to maximise the rates of carrying out the key processes of diabetic care in order to minimise complications. Consideration must also be given to provision of services for the 16–24-years age bands in order to ensure ease of transition of care into adulthood.

7 Aspire to achieve the upper quartile rates for each of the treatment targets (Table 19.3).

Table 19.2 Care process rates

Care process	Minimum rate to achieve
Blood pressure	93%
Smoking status	87%
Creatinine	88%
Cholesterol	87%
HbA$_{1c}$ (glycated haemoglobin)	85%
Body mass index	85%
Eye examination	66%
Foot examination	68%
Urinary albumin level	58%
All care processes	34%

Again, the upper quartiles in the audit should be considered as a minimum to be achieved, and continued improvement should be based on this. Where local services are achieving the upper quartile targets, they should show year-on-year improvement in order to meet National Institute for Health and Clinical Excellence guidelines and implementation of the NSF for diabetes.

Table 19.3 Treatment targets: minimum rate to achieve

	Treatment targets	Minimum rate to achieve
HbA1c (glycated haemoglobin)	<6.5%	26%
	≤7.5%	62%
Cholesterol	<5 mmol/litre	72%
Blood pressure	≤135/75 mml lg	26%
	<160/100 mmHg	90%

References

Department of Health (2001). *National Service Framework for Diabetes: Standards*. London: DoH.

Department of Health (2002). *National Service Framework for Diabetes: Delivery Strategy*. London: DoH.

The Information Centre (2005). *National Diabetes Audit. Key Findings About the Quality of Care for People with Diabetes in England, Incorportaing Registration from Wales*. Leeds: HSIC.

Further reading

Audit Commission (2000). *Testing Times: A Review of Diabetes Services in England and Wales*. London: Audit Commission.

Khunti K, Baker R (2002). The effect of audit on the quality of diabetes care in primary care. *Journal of Clinical Excellence* 4: 3–8.

Part III

About diabetes

Diabetes mellitus: a history of the condition

Questions this chapter will help you answer

- What are the different classifications of diabetes accepted today?

- Who classified them?

- When was insulin first used?

- When were oral medications introduced?

- How has medical technology advanced care of people with diabetes?

Diabetes is a wonderful affection, not very frequent among men, being a melting down of the flesh and limbs into urine . . . life is short, disgusting and painful, thirst unquenchable, death inevitable.

Aretaeus the Cappadocian (AD 2)

Thankfully, times have changed!

Classification and types

Diabetes mellitus is a complex metabolic disease characterised by high blood glucose concentrations. It is associated with impaired insulin production and/or action, resulting in the body's inability to utilise nutrients properly. It is believed that various genetic and environmental or lifestyle factors influence the cause and prognosis of the condition. Important differences in the frequency of diabetes and its complications have been reported between countries, ethnic and cultural groups.

It has never been easy to classify and diagnose diabetes mellitus because its very heterogeneity and characteristics have rendered most attempts at subdivision not entirely accurate and unable to reflect its underlying nature. There were anomalies in the earliest classification by age of onset (juvenile-onset diabetes, maturity-onset diabetes) and then a replacement of these names by identified pathogenic mechanisms (type 1 diabetes, type 2 diabetes, impaired glucose tolerance, impaired fasting glucose). New diagnostic criteria set by the World Health Organization were ratified in 2000 (see Chapter 7).

At the present time, the major clinical classes of glucose intolerance include type 1 and type 2 diabetes mellitus, malnutrition-related diabetes mellitus, impaired glucose tolerance (IGT), impaired fasting glycaemia (IFG) and gestational diabetes (which includes gestational IGT and gestational diabetes mellitus). The terms and definitions used to describe and diagnose diabetes were unified and adopted in 1979/80, being updated in 1985, reflecting the tenth revision of the International Classification of Diseases and Health-related Problems (ICD-10). New terms were introduced by the World Health Organization in 1999.

History

Diabetes has been known and recognised for many thousands of years as a disease characterised by weakness, thirst and frequency of micturition. Aretaeus, a contemporary of Galen, noted that the Greek word for a siphon had been given to diabetes because 'the fluid does not remain in the body, but uses the body as a ladder, whereby to leave it!'

Early treatments are described in the Ebers Papyrus, written around 1500 BC, found in a grave in Thebes in Egypt in 1862. The treatment – 'to drive away the passing of too much urine' – described a medicine including a mixture of bones, wheat grains, fresh fruits, green lead, earth and water. These ingredients the user was to 'let stand moist, strain it, take it for 4 days'.

In more modern times, the sweet taste of urine passed by people with this disease was noted by Willis in the late 17th century, and Matthew Dobson of Liverpool demonstrated that the sweet taste was caused by sugar. The Latin word for honeysweet – 'mellitus' – was added to distinguish the disease from diabetes insipidus, a pituitary disorder, in which a large volume of sugar-free urine is passed.

In 1815, the French chemist Chevraul showed that the sugar in diabetic urine was glucose. The association between diabetes and the pancreas was not recognised until much later. Paul Langerhans described the pancreatic islet cells in the mid-19th century, and in 1889, Mering and Minkowski produced fatal diabetes by removing the pancreas in animals.

The real breakthrough came in 1921–22, when insulin was discovered in Toronto by Frederick Banting and Charles Best:

> Those who watched the first starved, sometimes comatose diabetics receive insulin and return to life saw one of the genuine miracles of modern medicine. They were present at the closest approach to the resurrection of the body that our secular society can achieve and at the discovery of what has become the elixir of life for millions of human beings around the world.

So wrote Michael Bliss, the Canadian historian, in his definitive work on the discovery of insulin (Bliss, 1982). Further research, however, revealed the complex physiology involved in the aetiology of the disease and in the development of complications. It was recognised that there were a number of different forms of diabetes. The discovery of insulin marked the therapeutic period. It confirmed the concept of a deficiency of insulin action as the basic abnormality in diabetes, and gave rise to the differentiation between type 1 diabetes mellitus and non-type 1 diabetes mellitus.

Pharmaceutical research and development relating to type 1 diabetes has concentrated on developing 'purer' and more effective forms of insulin and new methods of delivery by 'pens' and 'pumps'. Recombinant technology developed during the 1980s dramatically changed the availability and use of insulin. Animal insulin was no longer the sole source of the hormone. Insulin could now be produced in unlimited quantities at a purity close to that of 'human' insulin. This technology enabled the genetic blueprint of porcine insulin to be altered to produce an alternative insulin, close to that of the human species.

Oral hypoglycaemic agents were first introduced in Germany in 1955 and have been extensively developed. There are four main groups: the sulphonylureas, the biguanides, thiazolidinediones and postprandial glucose regulators (see Chapter 11). The sulphonylureas act mainly by stimulating the release of insulin from the beta-cells in the pancreas. The action of the biguanide group is less clear but is believed to increase the peripheral uptake of glucose. The thiazolidinediones reduce blood glucose and insulin levels by reducing insulin resistance. Postprandial glucose regulators have a mode of action similar to that of sulphonylureas but with a faster onset and shorter duration.

Diet is the 'cornerstone' of treatment. An interesting observation on the effect of food on the incidence and progression of diabetes was made by the French physician Bouchardat in 1875, during the Prussian siege of Paris. The siege was prolonged and, as food supplies ran out, forcing the population to eat cats and dogs, he noticed the absence of new cases in his practice and an improvement in the condition of those already diagnosed. Similar observations were made in the two World Wars when national death rates for diabetes fell noticeably.

Dietary recommendations have changed from a restricted carbohydrate intake to a regimen low in fat and high in unrefined carbohydrates and dietary fibre. For the overweight, a reduction in energy intake remains the most important aim. Carbohydrate should make up about 50–55% of the energy intake, preferably from foods naturally high in dietary fibre (Nutrition Subcommittee of the Diabetes Care Advisory Committee of Diabetes UK, 2003). Up to 25 g of added sucrose per day may be allowed, provided it is part of a diet low in fat and high in fibre.

Dietary advice for the treatment of diabetes is aimed not only at the control of blood glucose, but also at the prevention of cardiovascular disease. In general, it is the same advice as that offered to the general population.

The discovery of insulin by Banting and Best highlighted and accelerated the quest for understanding the condition. As more has become known, the search for the causes of diabetes has moved towards further study of the immune system and the role of infection and the genetic implications already identified.

References

Bliss, M. (1982). *The Discovery of Insulin*, pp 304. London, UK: Macmillan Press.

Nutrition Subcommittee of the Diabetes Care Advisory Committee of Diabetes UK (2003). The implementation of nutritional advice for people with diabetes. *Diabetic Medicine* **20**: 786–807.

World Health Organization (1999). *Definition, Diagnosis and Classification of Diabetes Mellitus and its Complications*. Geneva: WHO.

Further reading

Williams G, Pickup J (2004). *Handbook of Diabetes*. Oxford: Blackwell Publishing.

21 Type 1 diabetes mellitus

Questions this chapter will help you answer

- What are the symptoms of type 1 diabetes?

- What causes it?

- Who gets type 1 diabetes?

- Is there a place for the management of type 1 diabetes within primary care?

> *When in hospital for eight days, it was not until the third or fourth day I was given my insulin injection before food . . . Listen to those who need insulin injection(s). They know what insulin they need and when.*
>
> Audit Commission (2000)

Formerly termed 'acute diabetes' or 'juvenile-onset diabetes', this type commonly occurs in childhood, in adolescence and on into adult life.

Symptoms generally develop suddenly. There is:

- profound weight loss

- excessive thirst

- polyuria

- lethargy

- abdominal pain.

Insulin is needed for life. Should insulin treatment not be available, ketoacidosis, coma and death are inevitable. The onset is sudden (within days or weeks).

People with type 1 diabetes are often managed within specialist care unless staff have additional knowledge and skills in this area. It is not within the scope of this book to advise on specific regimens – local advice should be sought and a good working relationship encouraged with specialist colleagues (see Chapter 11).

Diagnosis

Diagnosis is usually straightforward, based on the presenting symptoms and raised blood glucose levels (see Chapter 7). After diagnosis, insulin therapy is started, together with appropriate family support and structured education about living with diabetes in all its aspects. Discussion about modifying food intake and activity in relation to the person's life is staged alongside the stabilisation process. A careful multidisciplinary approach with empathy and consistent, correct advice is vital in fostering a healthy 'life with insulin' and in the reduction of acute and long-term complications.

Two acute complications (hypoglycaemia and hyperglycaemia) occur in relation to insulin therapy and are associated with the extremes of blood glucose levels (see Chapter 12).

Pregnancy

The self-regulation of blood glucose is particularly important during pregnancy, when strict blood glucose control is vital even before conception. Pre-pregnancy counselling and blood glucose levels between 4 and 7 mmol/l are recommended to avoid fetal abnormality or death. Thirty years ago, about one quarter of pregnancies in women with diabetes ended in fetal death. Now almost all are successful. This improvement is the result of major developments in obstetric, diabetic and paediatric care. Major congenital abnormalities, however, still occur more frequently than in non-diabetic pregnancies.

The causes of type 1 diabetes

Factors involved in the causation of type 1 diabetes are complex. Not only are genetic factors involved, but also environmental factors, demonstrated by changes in the islet cells and destruction of the beta-cells, either directly or by triggering an autoimmune response. Possible environmental agents suggested are infective conditions (perhaps occurring some years before) as well as physical, chemical and psychological factors.

The prevalence of type 1 diabetes varies considerably in different countries, based on estimates, varying levels of ascertainment and the population age structure. The prevalence appears to be higher further from the Equator, in particular in Scandinavia, and lower than average in Japan.

Seasonal variations in incidence are also of interest as they are consistent and occur all over the world. Higher incidence rates are reported during the autumn and winter months than over the spring and summer periods. Seasonal variations are thought to be associated with the presence of infective agents such as viruses. These may trigger the onset of the disease in susceptible people, in particular young people, in whom the incidence is age related and peaks around the ages of 5 and 12 years, coinciding with changes in school environments and the onset of puberty.

SUMMARY

- The prevalence of type 1 diabetes is about one tenth that of type 2 diabetes in Western communities.

- Clinical onset most commonly occurs during childhood, particularly around the time of puberty.

- The condition also appears in early and later adulthood.

- Consider the possibility of type 1 diabetes in the older person, especially if he or she is slim.

- There is a higher incidence in autumn and winter and an increasing gradient in incidence from southern to northern latitudes.

- People need structured care and education throughout their life to enable them to achieve continuing good health.

- Children with type 1 diabetes and their families need specialist support and education.

Further reading

Hanas R (3rd edn, 2006). *Type 1 Diabetes in Children, Adolescents and Young Adults. How to Become an Expert on Your Own Diabetes.* London: Class Health.

National Institute for Health and Clinical Excellence (2004). *Type 1 Diabetes: Diagnosis and Management of Type 1 Diabetes in Children, Young People and Adults.* London: NICE.

Confidential Enquiry into Maternal and Child Health (2004). *Pregnancy in Women with Type 1 and Type 2 Diabetes. CEMACH Report 2002–2003.* London: CEMACH.

Type 2 diabetes mellitus

Questions this chapter will help you answer

- What percentage of my diabetes patients are likely to have type 2 diabetes?

- What causes it?

- How does it differ from type 1 diabetes?

- What education on lifestyle should I engage in with people with type 2 diabetes?

- Which groups are more likely to be affected?

> *I did not realise how serious diabetes was at first. Perhaps I might have taken it more seriously if I knew then what I know now.*
>
> Audit Commission (2002)

The International Diabetes Federation has published the following facts and figures:

- About 40–50% of people with impaired glucose tolerance will develop type 2 diabetes (accompanied by an increased risk of cardiovascular disease and microvascular complications) within 10 years.

- Until the mid-1980s, type 2 diabetes was considered to be a disease of the middle-aged and elderly, developed after years of poor diet and lack of exercise. These same causes have led to a rise in the disease in children and adolescents as young as 5 years of age.

- Diabetes increased by one third during the 1990s owing to the prevalence of obesity and an ageing population.

- Type 2 diabetes is the most common type of diabetes and accounts for 90–95% of all people with diabetes.

- At least 50% of all people with diabetes are unaware of their condition. In some countries, this figure may rise to 80%.

- Cardiovascular complications associated with type 2 diabetes (e.g. increased atherosclerosis) begin to develop well before type 2 diabetes is diagnosed. By that time, macrovascular damage may already be well advanced.

- Between 70% and 80% of people with diabetes die of cardiovascular disease.

- People with diabetes can have a heart attack without even realising it.

- People with type 2 diabetes have the same risk of heart attack as people without diabetes who have already had a heart attack.

Several ethnic groups (South Asians, African/Caribbeans, Pima Indians) have a greater genetic predisposition to type 2 diabetes than do Caucasians. In the absence of effective interventions, the prevalence of type 2 diabetes in all populations is likely to rise due to increased longevity, an increased number of elderly people and increases in the rates of obesity, lack of regular physical exercise and inappropriate diet.

Efforts to prevent obesity through diet alone have been generally unsuccessful (House of Commons, 2004). Physical activity, however, appears to have an important role in the prevention of type 2 diabetes through its association with reduced body weight and through independent effects on insulin resistance and glucose tolerance. Further research is needed to assess the magnitude of the benefits of activity and to determine the most effective programmes for reducing the incidence of type 2 diabetes. To date, research has failed to demonstrate an association between type 2 diabetes and specific genetic markers even though it is a familial disease.

Both sexes are affected in type 2 diabetes, although in some communities a male preponderance is shown, for example in India and in Asian Indians in the UK. In other communities, females make up most of those with the disease. In populations in which type 2 diabetes is common, it may be encountered in adolescence and among young adults under the age of 25. This form of diabetes, which has a familial distribution compatible with a dominant mode of inheritance, is sometimes referred to as maturity-onset diabetes of the young.

Diagnosis

The diagnosis of type 2 diabetes is less clear cut than that of type 1 (Table 22.1). Previously termed 'mild' by some, it is now obvious that this is a misnomer. **There is no such thing as mild diabetes.** The onset is insidious and may be revealed only at routine screening. Symptoms of lethargy, thirst and polyuria are the most common but may proceed unnoticed until an episode of stress or an infection precipitates the severity of symptoms, forcing the individual to seek help. The diagnosis will be established by raised blood glucose levels (see Chapter 7).

Table 22.1 Differences between type 1 and type 2 diabetes

	Type 1 diabetes	Type 2 diabetes
Proportion (%)	10–20	80–90
Usual age of onset (years)	<40	>40
Speed of onset	Rapid	Gradual
Likelihood of ketosis	High	Low
Complications at presentation	No	Yes, frequently, especially risk factors for coronary heart disease, e.g. hypertension, dyslipidaemia, obesity
Treatment	Diet and insulin	Diet alone, diet and tablets, or diet and tablets and insulin, or insulin alone
Likelihood of hypoglycaemia	More	Less, but dangerous in elderly people
Precipitated by obesity	No	Yes
Majority of care provision	Specialist	Primary care team

A diagnosis of type 2 diabetes has serious implications for life, employment and family interactions. It must be confirmed by laboratory blood tests (see Chapter 7) and sympathetically discussed with individuals and their carers. The person with diabetes should be at the centre of decision-making around lifestyle and treatment changes agreed.

Treatment

Treatment for people with type 2 diabetes is aimed at alleviating symptoms, reducing blood glucose levels and, where possible, preventing complications. Should the individual be overweight, the first line of treatment consists of dietary and activity modification within the limits of what the person can achieve, and education to reduce weight. If successful, this may lead to a reduction in blood glucose levels and symptomatic relief.

Should this line of treatment be unsuccessful, oral hypoglycaemic agents may be required. The choice and progression of medication is discussed in Chapter 11. Should tablets – remembering that triple therapy may be required – fail to achieve the desired result, insulin therapy may be indicated. The normal-weight or underweight person unable to obtain symptom relief and/or a reduction in blood glucose levels with dietary modification and hypoglycaemic agents will usually require insulin sooner rather than later.

Extreme caution is required when treating elderly people with oral hypoglycaemic agents (sulphonylureas and insulin therapy) in order to avoid the complication of hypoglycaemia. People with type 2 diabetes may require insulin in the short term in times of illness or during surgical intervention. A fear of hypoglycaemic attacks and weight gain may increase reluctance on behalf of patients and health professionals to consider insulin therapy at an early stage. The evidence is, however, now there to prove the efficacy of initiating insulin in type 2 diabetes (UK Prospective Diabetes Study Group, 1998).

The livelihood of people with diabetes must also be considered. People holding particular types of driving licences such as Large Goods Vehicle (LGV) and Passenger-Carrying Vehicle (PCV) will lose these should insulin therapy be instituted. A most difficult problem to be solved occurs when insulin is used in the treatment of symptomless people with type 2 diabetes, in whom weight gain progresses with no improvement in blood glucose level.

References

House of Commons (2004). *Health, Third Report. Obesity.* London: House of Commons Publications.
www.publications.parliament.uk/pa/cm200304/cmselect/cmhealth/23/2302.htm.
UK Prospective Diabetes Study Group (1998). Intensive blood-glucose control with sulphonylureas or insulin compared with conventional treatment and risk of complications in patients with type 2 diabetes (UKPDS 33). *Lancet* **352**: 837–853.

Further reading

Amos AF, McCarty DJ, Zimmer P (1997). The rising global burden of diabetes and its complications: estimates and projections to the year 2010. *Diabetic Medicine* **14**: S1–S85.

Diabetes UK (2000). *New Diagnostic Criteria for Diabetes: Summary of Changes. Factsheet.* London: Diabetes UK.

Rudermann M, Apelian AZ, Schneider SM (1990). Exercise in therapy and prevention of type II diabetes: implications for blacks. *Diabetes Care* **13** (Suppl. 4): 1163–1168.

Turner RC, Millns H, Neil H, Stratton I, Manley S, Matthews E, Holman R (1998). UKPDS study group. Risk factors for coronary artery disease in non-insulin dependent diabetes mellitus (UKPDS 23). *British Medical Journal* **316**: 823–828.

UK Prospective Diabetes Study Group (1998). Tight blood pressure control and risk of macrovascular and microvascular complications in type 2 diabetes (UKPDS 38). *British Medical Journal* **317**: 703–713.

World Health Organization (1999). *Definition, Diagnosis and Classification of Diabetes Mellitus and its Complications.* Geneva: WHO.

Other categories of diabetes

(as defined by the World Health Organization)

Questions this chapter will help you answer

■ What is impaired glucose tolerance?

■ How does it differ from impaired fasting glycaemia?

■ How do I diagnose gestational diabetes?

> *... few professionals in the field doubt that effective*
> *prevention, management and early detection of*
> *problems is cost-effective in the long run.*
>
> Audit Commission (2002)

The International Diabetes Federation reviewed impaired glucose tolerance (IGT) and impaired fasting glycaemia (IFG) and found IGT to be more prevalent in most populations. It is possible to have both, and the Federation found that around half of people with IFG also had IGT, whereas around a third with IGT also had IFG.

Both IFG and IGT are associated with a substantially increased risk of developing diabetes and cardiovascular disease, the highest risk being in people with combined IFG and IGT. Screening measures are being evaluated, but people with IGT and IFG should be engaged in education to help them prevent the sequelae of diabetes and cardiovascular disease.

Impaired glucose tolerance (Unwin et al, 2002)

Previously, the term 'borderline' diabetes had been used to distinguish between people whose glucose tolerance was 'impaired', i.e. did not meet the diagnostic criteria for diabetes, and people who clearly do have diabetes. The IGT category removed the label of 'diabetes' because this level of glucose intolerance is not associated with the development of microvascular complications. It is, however, strongly associated with macrovascular complications and future diabetes.

IGT:

- results from raised hepatic glucose output and a defect in early insulin secretion ;

- is slightly more common among women;

- progresses into older age.

Lifestyle changes can be highly effective in preventing or delaying the onset of diabetes: weight loss (where indicated), increasing activity levels and eating a healthy diet all contribute.

Impaired fasting glycaemia

IFG:

- is typically due to peripheral insulin resistance;

- is much more common in men;

- tends to plateau in middle age.

Gestational diabetes mellitus

The National Institute for Health and Clinical Excellence (NICE) advises that routine screening for gestational diabetes (diabetes diagnosed during pregnancy) is not supported by clinical evidence and is not recommended. It is, however, essential for nurses to have a high degree of suspicion in at-risk groups such as:

- the obese;

- those with a strong family history of diabetes;

- women of Asian or African/Caribbean origin;

- women with a history of large babies;

- older women with a first baby.

The glucose tolerance test is regarded as the gold standard for the diagnosis of gestational diabetes mellitus where screening has proved positive. There is, however, still inconsistency in diagnostic levels (Table 23.1). Owing to the low renal threshold that exists in pregnancy,

Table 23.1 Sample diagnostic criteria employed for gestational diabetes mellitus after a 75 g glucose load
(data from National Institute for Health and Clinical Excellence, 2002)

	American Diabetic Association (mmol/l)	Scottish Intercollegiate Guidelines Network (mmol/l)	World Health Organization (mmol/l)
Fasting	5.3	5.5	7.0
1 hour	10.0	Not given	Not given
2 hour	8.6	9.0	11.1

urine testing is of little value. Overt diabetes is missed, and only a few of those with IGT are identified. A full oral glucose tolerance test is impractical for screening the antenatal population, although it is the only definitive test for the diagnosis of gestational diabetes.

Women whose glucose tolerance returns to normal after delivery are at higher risk of developing type 2 diabetes later in life. It is possible to reduce this risk by attention to diet and physical activity. Regular screening should be advocated to identify those at risk.

Diagnosis

Criteria for diagnosis are based on the current World Health Organization recommendations for the diagnosis of gestational diabetes. Diagnosis should be made if the fasting venous plasma glucose level is greater than 7.0 mmol/l, or the fasting venous plasma glucose is less than 7.0 mmol/l but with a venous plasma glucose level 2 hours after a 75 g glucose load of greater than 7.8 mmol/l. This is tighter than the levels indicated by NICE.

Diabetes UK endorses the use of the World Health Organization definition to allow for comparative studies. However, since glucose tolerance changes with the duration of pregnancy, the gestation at which the diagnosis was made should be recorded and, if this is in the third trimester, the clinician should be cautious about the clinical implications of IGT.

Postpartum

Insulin can usually be stopped immediately postpartum. Breast-feeding should, as always, be encouraged in women with gestational diabetes.

Women with gestational diabetes should have the opportunity to be seen by the multidisciplinary team. They should be advised:

- of the increased risk of developing type 1 or type 2 diabetes;
- that the onset of type 2 diabetes can be reduced by maintaining physical activity and avoiding obesity;
- of the increased risk of gestational diabetes in subsequent pregnancies;
- of the need to ensure that dietary recommendations are being followed prior to conception in future pregnancies;
- of the availability of well-woman clinics to help them to maintain a good weight and general health.

It is important that women at risk of developing gestational diabetes are identified because the condition is associated with an increased incidence of perinatal morbidity and the development of diabetes by the mother in later life.

Antenatal care should include the following assessments:

- Previous gestational diabetes or IGT or IFG
- Family history of diabetes
- Maternal obesity (>120% ideal body weight)
- Previous delivery of a large baby
- Previous unexplained still birth
- Previous obstetric and/or perinatal complications
- Recurrent urinary tract infections or candidiasis.

Management

- Management must be by a multidisciplinary obstetrics and diabetes team.
- Tight blood glucose control is paramount for the health of both mother and baby.
- Any oral hypoglycaemic agents taken by a woman with type 2 diabetes should be stopped.

- Insulin may be indicated; this should be discussed between the patient and the specialist team.

Around 40% of women with gestational diabetes will develop type 2 diabetes within 20 years. An awareness of this is important in the avoidance of long-term complications of diabetes.

References

Unwin N, Shaw J, Zimmet P, Alberti KG (2002). Impaired glucose tolerance and impaired fasting glycaemia: the current status on definition and intervention. *Diabetic Medicine* **19**: 708–723.

Further reading

Diabetes UK (2005). *Recommendations for the Management of Pregnant Women with Diabetes (including Gestational Diabetes)*. London: Diabetes UK.

24 Complications of diabetes

Questions this chapter will help you answer

- What differences are there between microvascular and macrovascular complications?

- When are statins recommended?

- What do I do to help prevent complications in people with diabetes?

- What guidelines are available?

- Do I understand insulin resistance?

> *There is [good] evidence in the field of diabetes about what works and a growing recognition of the serious nature of the disease.*
>
> Audit Commission (2000)

Many of the complications of diabetes have been mentioned in previous chapters. This reflects the seriousness of the condition. Many factors have been identified that may lead to the onset, or worsening, of complications. Some are more linked to microvascular complications, others are more implicated in macrovascular, and several apply to both (Table 24.1).

The journal *Heart* published 10-year risk charts for people with diabetes (Wood et al, 1988), but the Joint British Societies' hypertension guidelines suggest that all people with diabetes should be treated as 'coronary equivalents' (Williams et al, 2004) and their risk considered as high, thus dispensing with the risk charts. This is now accepted by the Joint British Societies (2005) report.

The main risk factors for developing macrovascular complications of diabetes are:

- hyperglycaemia

- hypertension

- increasing age

- duration of diabetes
- smoking
- genetic factors
- raised cholesterol and triglyceride levels.

The long-term complications of type 1 diabetes – those of nephropathy, retinopathy, autonomic and peripheral neuropathy – are rarely seen before 5–7 years' duration of the condition.

In type 2 diabetes, however, components of the metabolic syndrome (hyperglycaemia, dyslipidaemia, hypertension, obesity) may have been present for many years before diabetes is diagnosed, and many individuals will have one or more 'complications' of diabetes at diagnosis. The question now is whether the metabolic syndrome leads to cardiovascular disease (CVD) and diabetes rather than type 2 diabetes leading to the complication of CVD.

Type 2 diabetes is progressive, and complications tend to be more prevalent and become more serious with time. Unknown factors allow some people with type 2 diabetes to be free of complications many years after diagnosis. Genetic markers of susceptibility have not been identified.

Table 24.1 Major complications of diabetes

Macrovascular	Cardiovascular disease	Heart attack and stroke Angina
	Peripheral vascular disease	The 'at-risk' foot
Microvascular	Renal disease	Diabetic nephropathy
	Eye disease	Background retinopathy Maculopathy Proliferative retinopathy
	Neuropathy – autonomic and peripheral	Gastrointestinal disturbances Erectile dysfunction Sensation disturbances Visual disturbance

Macrovascular complications

These are coronary heart disease, stroke and peripheral vascular disease.

Coronary heart disease and diabetes mellitus

Key modifiable risk factors for the development of CVD are:

- smoking
- hypertension
- high cholesterol levels
- poor glycaemic control
- an inactive lifestyle
- obesity
- increased alcohol consumption.

Facts (Rayner et al, 2001)

- About 33 000 deaths in the UK each year are attributable to diabetes – about one in seven of all deaths. At least a half of these deaths are from CVD.
- People with diabetes are said to be 'coronary equivalents'; they have a similar risk of a heart attack to someone without diabetes who has already had one.
- About a quarter of people with newly diagnosed diabetes already have CVD.
- In the UK, about 3% of years of life lost in disability are due to diabetes.
- In the UK, 5% of all days spent in hospital are the result of diabetes. About 60% of these days are caused by CVD.
- About 46% of men and 32% of women are overweight or obese in the UK. About two-thirds of cases of diabetes could be prevented if no one was overweight.

In the battle against CVD, it is essential to take a holistic approach. Many factors are worthy of consideration:

- lifestyle issues, such as obesity, activity levels, dietary factors and smoking;

- blood pressure levels;

- lipids: low-density lipoprotein (LDL), high-density lipoprotein (HDL) and triglycerides;

- aspirin therapy.

The *National Service Framework for Coronary Heart Disease: Modern Standards and Service Models* (Department of Health, 2000) includes the following recommendations as one of its 12 standards:

> preventing CHD in high-risk patients in primary care: GPs and primary health care teams should identify all people at significant risk of cardiovascular disease but who have not yet developed symptoms, and offer them appropriate advice and treatment to reduce their risk.

Treating those who have had a myocardial infarction with insulin has been shown to improve prognosis, particularly in those not already receiving insulin (Malmberg et al, 1995). A second study failed to replicate this, but many specialist centres have adopted this regimen.

Statin therapy in diabetes

The National Institute for Health and Clinical Excellence (2002a) published guidance on lipid control. This advised:

- At diagnosis assess full lipid profile (total cholesterol, LDL, HDL and triglycerides), fasting if possible.

- If levels are normal, with values for total cholesterol of less than 5.0 mmol/l (or LDL less than 3.0 mmol/l) and triglycerides below 2.3 mmol/l:
  - review annually;
  - no therapy being required.

- If values are raised, with a total cholesterol concentration of 5.0 mmol/l or higher (or LDL 3.0 mmol/l or higher) or triglycerides 2.3 mmol/l or above:
  - check alcohol intake and provide advice;
  - check thyroid function to exclude hypothyroidism;
  - check liver function to exclude liver disease;
  - check serum creatinine and proteinuria to exclude renal disease;

- agree targets with the patient for glucose control – aiming for a glycated haemoglobin (HbA$_{1c}$) level of around 6.5% (see Chapter 8);
- work with individuals on possible lifestyle changes in terms of diet, activity, smoking and weight loss;
- consider therapy (Table 24.2).

Note that more recent guidelines suggest that all people with type 2 diabetes should be treated as being of high risk for coronary events as they are 'coronary equivalents' (Williams et al, 2004), and tighter levels are advised by the Joint British Societies (2005) (see Table 8.1).

Table 24.2 Recommendations for the pharmacological management of adverse blood lipid profiles in people with type 2 diabetes

(National Institute for Health and Clinical Excellence, 2002a, reproduced with permission)

Blood lipid profile at start of therapy	10-year coronary event risk	Recommendations
1. TC ≥5.0 mmol/litre (or LDL-C ≥3.0 mmol/litre or TG ≥2.3 mmol/litre and <10 mmol/litre)	Lower (no history of CVD and 10-year coronary event risk ≤15%)	▪ Discuss CHD risk with the patient, and consider whether treatment is appropriate at the time when type 2 diabetes is diagnosed. ▪ Consider offering drug therapy at higher levels of cholesterol or triglyceride. ▪ Following a decision to start treatment: – offer a statin, – assess the effect of statin therapy within 3 months and titrate the dose if required, – monitor the effect of therapy annually. ▪ If a decision is made **not** to start pharmacological therapy, monitor lipid profile and cardiovascular risk annually, to consider the need for therapy.
2. TC ≥5.0 mmol/litre (or LDL-C ≥3.0 mmol/litre or TG ≥2.3 mmol/litre and <10 mmol/litre)	Higher: 10-year coronary event risk >15% but no history of CVD	Primary prevention ▪ Offer a statin, ▪ Assess the effect of statin therapy within 3 months and titrate the dose if required. ▪ Monitor the effect of therapy annually.

Table 24.2 (continued))

Blood lipid profile at start of therapy	10-year coronary event risk	Recommendations
3. TC ≥5.0 mmol/litre (or LDL-C ≥3.0 mmol/litre or TG ≥2.3 mmol/litre and <10 mmol/litre)	Higher: manifest CVD	Secondary prevention • Offer a statin. • Assess the effect of statin therapy. • Assess the effect of statin therapy within 3 months and titrate the dose if required. • Consider adding a fibrate after 6 months if triglyceride remains ≥2.3 mmol/litre. • Ensure there is no evidence of drug interaction between the proposed choices of fibrate and statin preparation.* • Monitor the effect of therapy annually.
4. TC <5.0 mmol/litre (or LDL-C <3.0 mmol/litre and TG ≥2.3 mmol/litre and ≥10 mmol/litre)	Higher: manifest CVD	Secondary prevention • Offer a statin or a fibrate. • Assess the effect of statin therapy within 3 months and titrate the dose if required. • Monitor the effect of therapy annually.
5. Fasting TG ≥10 mmol/litre	Higher or lower	• Offer fibrate therapy and consider referral to a diabetes or lipid clinic.

CHD, coronary heart disease; CVD, cardiovascular disease; LDL-C, low-density lipoprotein; TC, total cholesterol; TG, triglycerides

*Use of a statin and fibrate together increases the likelihood of adverse effects (especially rhabdomyolysis) and should be used with caution (see the British National Formulary)

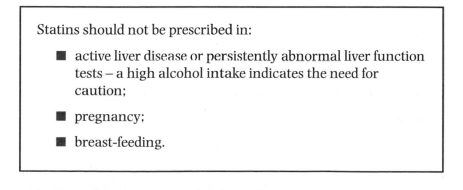

Statins should not be prescribed in:

■ active liver disease or persistently abnormal liver function tests – a high alcohol intake indicates the need for caution;

■ pregnancy;

■ breast-feeding.

Aspirin treatment in diabetes

Diabetes UK (2001) is now recommending that people with diabetes in the groups below should be offered low-dose (75 mg) aspirin treatment or should obtain it for themselves. Anyone considering starting aspirin treatment should initially discuss this with a member of the diabetes care team, a doctor, nurse, pharmacist or podiatrist, taking this information with them.

Aspirin treatment should definitely be considered for anyone over the age of 30 years who is at risk because of:

■ other accepted conditions such as angina, previous heart attack, stroke, transient ischaemic attacks (mini-strokes), atrial fibrillation (a type of irregular heart beat) and peripheral vascular disease;

■ dyslipidaemia; high LDL, low HDL and high triglyceride levels;

■ a diagnosis of raised blood pressure (over 140/80 mmHg): individuals will benefit provided their blood pressure is controlled to less than 150/90 mmHg;

■ microalbuminuria or albuminuria (protein in the urine);

■ a family history of coronary heart disease;

■ smoking;

■ overweight (a body mass index over 25);

■ being from an Indo-Asian background;

■ diabetic retinopathy (eye disease).

Exceptions to this would be those who cannot tolerate aspirin, such as those with known peptic ulceration or those who fall into an unusually high-risk group, for example if there is:

■ aspirin allergy;

■ a bleeding tendency;

■ anticoagulation therapy;

■ a past history of gastrointestinal bleeding;

■ the concurrent use of drugs to prevent gastrointestinal bleeding;

■ active liver disease;

■ a history of aspirin-induced asthma.

The more risk factors, the more likely it is that aspirin treatment will be beneficial. The dosage recommended is at least 75 mg aspirin daily.

Stroke

The same risks that lead to CVD may lead to stroke (see above).

Facts

- People with diabetes are 2–3 times more likely to suffer from a stroke.

- Stroke is responsible for about 15% of deaths in people with type 2 diabetes.

The education and empowerment of people with diabetes to help them alter their lifestyle to prevent stroke is key to improving their health:

- Work with patients to engage them in meeting agreed targets for blood pressure and lipid and glucose levels.

- Agree a management plan to reduce weight (where necessary), maintain good activity levels (appropriate to the person) and help the individual to stop smoking.

Peripheral vascular disease

The 'at-risk' foot may be affected by neuropathy and peripheral vascular disease (see Chapter 14).

Microvascular complications

The kidneys, eyes and peripheral nerves are most affected by diabetes. They may be affected to a different extent, one being severely affected while another is not damaged at all. Complications are caused by thickening of the basement membrane in the kidney, retina, nerves, skin, muscle and adipose tissue.

Diabetic nephropathy (renal disease)

Box 24.1 provides a summary of diabetic nephropathy.

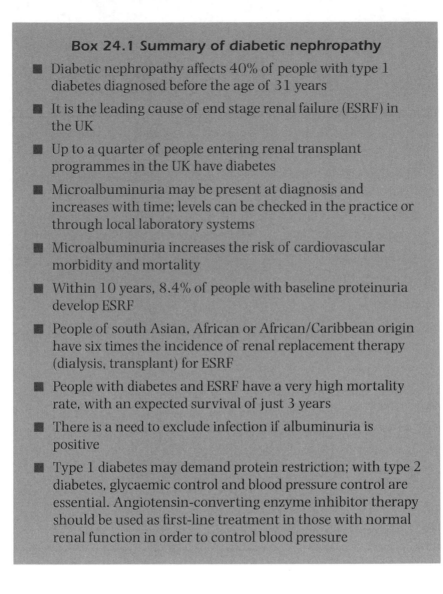

Box 24.1 Summary of diabetic nephropathy

■ Diabetic nephropathy affects 40% of people with type 1 diabetes diagnosed before the age of 31 years

■ It is the leading cause of end stage renal failure (ESRF) in the UK

■ Up to a quarter of people entering renal transplant programmes in the UK have diabetes

■ Microalbuminuria may be present at diagnosis and increases with time; levels can be checked in the practice or through local laboratory systems

■ Microalbuminuria increases the risk of cardiovascular morbidity and mortality

■ Within 10 years, 8.4% of people with baseline proteinuria develop ESRF

■ People of south Asian, African or African/Caribbean origin have six times the incidence of renal replacement therapy (dialysis, transplant) for ESRF

■ People with diabetes and ESRF have a very high mortality rate, with an expected survival of just 3 years

■ There is a need to exclude infection if albuminuria is positive

■ Type 1 diabetes may demand protein restriction; with type 2 diabetes, glycaemic control and blood pressure control are essential. Angiotensin-converting enzyme inhibitor therapy should be used as first-line treatment in those with normal renal function in order to control blood pressure

Facts

■ Diabetic nephropathy is recognised as a major cause of morbidity and mortality in people with type 1 diabetes, affecting some 40% of patients who develop the disease before the age of 31 years.

■ Diabetic nephropathy is the leading cause of end stage renal failure (ESRF) in the UK. Between 15% and 25% of people entering renal transplant programmes in the UK have diabetes. Most of these have type 2 rather than type 1 diabetes.

- At diagnosis:
  - 12–25% (according to various studies) of people with type 2 diabetes already have microalbuminuria;
  - 1.9% of people with type 2 diabetes have frank proteinuria.
- For people with type 2 diabetes:
  - most estimates suggest that around 25% of people with type 2 diabetes have microalbuminuria;
  - most estimates suggest around 15% of people with type 2 diabetes have proteinuria.
- 15% of those with no trace of microalbuminuria will develop it within 5 years, and 5% will develop proteinuria.
- Among people with established diabetes and microalbuminuria, approximately 20% develop proteinuria, 30% revert to normoalbuminuria and 50% remain microalbuminuric after 10 years.
- Once microalbuminuria has developed, there is a considerable increase in the risk of cardiovascular morbidity and mortality. Microalbuminuria, clinical proteinuria and ESRF are progressively stronger risk factors for cardiovascular mortality in people with diabetes.
- Clinical proteinuria is a strong risk factor for ESRF. Within 10 years, 8.4% of people with baseline proteinuria develop ESRF.
- Cardiovascular risk is increased in those with type 2 diabetes with microalbuminuria (2–4-fold increase) and proteinuria (5–8-fold increase), compared with people who have normoalbuminuria.
- People of south Asian, African or African/Caribbean origin have six times the incidence of renal replacement therapy (dialysis, transplant) for ESRF.
- People with diabetes and ESRF have a very high mortality rate, with an expected survival of 3 years.

Diabetic renal disease is defined (National Institute for Health and Clinical Excellence, 2002b) as the presence of raised urine albumin levels and/or raised serum creatinine in the absence of other renal disease. It can further be described as:

- *Microalbuminuria* (incipient nephropathy), defined by a rise in urinary albumin loss to between 30 and 300 mg per day, or a

urinary albumin:creatinine ratio greater than or equal to
2.5 mg/mmol (men) or 3.5 mg/mmol (women), or a urinary
albumin concentration of 20 mg/l or more.

■ *Proteinuria or macroalbuminuria* (overt nephropathy), defined by
a raised urinary albumin excretion greater than 300 mg per
day, or a urinary albumin:creatinine ratio of greater than or
equal to 30 mg/mmol, or a urinary albumin concentration of
200 mg/l or more (Scottish Intercollegiate Guidelines Network,
2001; McIntosh et al, 2002).

Microalbuminuria is the earliest sign of diabetic nephropathy and
predicts increased total mortality, cardiovascular morbidity and mortality, and ESRF.

Box 24.2 What test to use for microalbuminuria

1 The usual method of screening for microalbuminuria is the
urinary albumin:creatinine ratio (ACR), preferably determined
on a sample taken first thing in the morning. This should be
done when the type 2 diabetes is diagnosed and at least
annually thereafter. Local facilities will determine whether
this is done using a laboratory method or near-patient
testing (Micral test II).

2 If the ACR = 2.5 mg/mmol (men) or = 3.5 mg/mmol
(women), repeat the test on two further occasions
(preferably within 1 month). Two positive tests out of three
confirm the diagnosis.

■ **If urinary albumin levels are raised and there is any degree
of diabetic retinopathy, a diagnosis of diabetic renal disease
is likely.** If there is no retinopathy, investigate the possibility
of an alternative, non-diabetic cause of renal disease.

■ Measure the serum creatinine level once a year.

■ The serum creatinine may occasionally be raised without
any detectable presence of albumin in the urine. If there is
no evidence of albuminuria or microvascular disease (e.g.
diabetic retinopathy), consider other causes of renal disease.

■ **Note: if the urine is positive for protein, exclude infection
before undertaking any further investigations.**

There are various tests to identify microalbuminuria (Box 24.2; data from McIntosh et al, 2002).

Table 24.3 provides definitions of lower- and higher-risk albumin excretion.

Table 24.3 Definition of lower-risk and higher-risk albumin excretion
(data from National Institute for Health and Clinical Excellence, 2002b)

Level of risk	Level of albuminuria
Lower risk	Normoalbuminuria: urinary albumin:creatinine ratio <2.5 mg/mmol (men) or <3.5 mg/mmol (women), or urinary albumin concentration <20 mg/l
Higher risk	Microalbuminuria: urinary albumin:creatinine ratio ≥2.5 mg/mmol (men) or ≥3.5 mg/mmol (women), or urinary albumin concentration ≥20 mg/l **or** Proteinuria: urinary albumin:creatinine ratio ≥30 mg/mmol or urinary albumin concentration ≥200 mg/l

Care of people with diabetes to detect and manage renal risk

- Instigate call and recall for microalbuminuria screening. If proteinuria is present, exclude infection before undertaking further investigation.

- Agree goals and targets with patients on lifestyle changes and the management of risk factors such as hypertension, dyslipidaemia, obesity and activity level.

- Assess risk factors and review these at least annually:
  - ◆ If the individual has type 1 diabetes, he or she may need protein restriction. Refer urgently to the dietetic team.
  - ◆ If low-risk type 2 diabetes is present, aim for tight glycaemic control (HbA$_{1c}$ level of 6.5–7.5%) and blood pressure control (<140/80 mmHg) tailored to the individual.
  - ◆ If the diabetes is high-risk type 2, ensure that eye-screening has taken place and record the results; aim for tight blood glucose control (HbA$_{1c}$ 6.5–7.5%) and blood pressure control (<130/75 mmHg) but tailored to the individual. Cardiovascular risk factors should be tackled aggressively. Treat with an angiotensin-converting enzyme (ACE) inhibitor if there are no contraindications (see below).

- Check the albumin:creatinine ratio at least annually and more if the individual is at risk:
  - ◆ Take an early morning specimen.
  - ◆ If this is positive, test twice more, preferably within 1 month.
- Check renal function at least annually.
- The estimated glomerular filtration rate (eGFR) is used to measure kidney function. It is calculated by the laboratory from creatinine in the blood.
  - ◆ A normal eGFR is about 100 ml/min in young adults, so the eGFR is sometimes referred to as the percentage of normal kidney function, as the number is the same.
  - ◆ Some young adults with normal kidneys will have an eGFR as low as 75 ml/min, and this falls by about 1 ml/min per year as people get older, so many healthy people aged 75 will have an eGFR of 50–60 ml/min.
  - ◆ Most laboratories now report eGFR alongside their measurements of blood creatinine levels, and this is the most reliable way to obtain an eGFR result.

Chronic kidney disease

Chronic kidney disease is extremely common, yet the vast majority of individuals affected by it will never require dialysis, although they are at high risk of cardiovascular disease. Because of this, they should receive aggressive management of their risk factors, particularly raised blood pressure.

The stages of chronic kidney disease, along with their estimated prevalence, are as shown in Table 24.4.

Starting ACE inhibitor therapy in people with type 2 diabetes
ACE inhibitor therapy should be used with caution in those with:

- peripheral vascular disease or renovascular disease;
- a raised serum creatinine level.

For all people with type 2 diabetes, measure the serum creatinine and electrolytes 1 week after:

- initiating ACE inhibitor therapy;
- each increase in dose.

Table 24.4 Chronic kidney disease (CKD)

Stage	GFR (ml/min)	Description	Population prevalence (%)
1	>90[1]	Kidney damage with normal or ↑GFR	3.3
2	60–89[1]	Kidney damage with mild ↓GFR	3.0
3	30–59	Moderate ↓GFR	4.3
4	15–29	Severe ↓GFR	0.2
5	<15	Kidney failure	0.2

[1]For a diagnosis of CKD to be made with an eGFR >60 ml/min (ie stage 1 or 2 CKD), other markers of kidney damage, either in terms of imaging or urinalysis (for example polycystic kidneys or microalbuminuria) are required

eGFR, estimated glomerular filtration rate

Guidelines developed by Dr Hugh Gallagher and colleagues (South Thames Renal Unit at St Helier Hospital, Surrey) and available online (see Useful websites in Appendix 4)

Eye disease (diabetic retinopathy)

See Chapter 13.

Diabetic neuropathy

(See also Chapter 14.)

Box 24.3 gives a summary of diabetic neuropathy.

Diabetic neuropathy can be divided into autonomic and peripheral pathology.

The symptoms of diabetic neuropathy may initially be mild, but, without effective treatment, they tend to progress. Symptoms depend on the area affected. There may be:

■ numbness, pain or tingling in the feet or legs (see also Chapter 14 on foot care);

■ weakness in the muscles of the feet;

■ double vision or drooping eyelids;

■ weakness and atrophy of the thigh muscles;

■ problems with the digestive tract;

■ erectile dysfunction;

■ gastrointestinal problems that, when severe, can be debilitating.

> ## Box 24.3 Summary of diabetic neuropathy
>
> - The neuropathy can be autonomic or peripheral
> - It can cause:
>   - numbness, pain or tingling in the feet or legs
>   - double vision or drooping eyelids
>   - weakness and atrophy of the thigh muscles
>   - problems with the digestive tract
>   - erectile dysfunction
>   - gastrointestinal problems that, when severe, can be debilitating
> - Autonomic neuropathy may cause:
>   - postural hypotension
>   - severe diarrhoea
>   - impotence
> - Peripheral neuropathy affects the feet and legs
> - People with diabetes should have at least annual foot checks:
>   - Education on foot care may prevent ulcers or even amputation
>   - Referral policies to podiatry specialists or foot clinics should be in place

Autonomic neuropathy

Many people with diabetes have some abnormality of autonomic function. Insidious in onset, its presence may be undetected until late in its natural history. Dysfunction may be present in the cardiovascular system (causing postural hypotension), the alimentary tract (causing uncontrollable diarrhoea), the respiratory control system and the system for thermoregulation. Genitourinary disturbances are also distressing, one of the major problems being that of impotence. New therapies are proving effective in this area (see below).

Erectile dysfunction (impotence)

Erectile dysfunction is common among men with diabetes, and the longer they have had diabetes the more likely it is to occur. More than half of all men aged over 60 with diabetes may suffer from erectile dysfunction. Unfortunately, many people find sexual health a difficult topic to discuss and may not associate it with their diabetes.

The cause may be physical or psychological. Potential causes are:

■ tiredness;

■ stress;

■ a high alcohol intake;

■ complications (neuropathy or vascular) of the diabetes itself;

■ some medications;

■ previous bladder, bowel or prostate surgery;

■ trauma.

If a man wakes with an erection but finds it difficult to achieve erection when he wants to have sex, it is more likely to be a psychological problem. It is important to stress that this is quite common and to reassure the individual, and his partner, that modern treatments are available.

Treatments available include:

■ oral agents, for agents sildenafil (Viagra), tadalafil (Cialis) and vardenafil (Levitra);

■ vacuum pumps;

■ intercavernosal injections such as alprostadil (Caverject, Viridal Duo);

■ urethral applications, for example e.g alprostadil (MUSE).

Referral to specialist care or a general practitioner with a special interest may be necessary, and this area of therapy should not be undertaken without specific training and experience.

More information can be found in the current edition of the *British National Formulary*, Basu and Ryder (2004), Diabetes UK's leaflet on *Sex and Diabetes – a Guide to Erection Problems*, and the Sexual Dysfunction Association (previously the Impotence Association; see Appendix 4 for contact details).

Peripheral neuropathy

Again, many people with diabetes have neuropathy affecting the peripheral nerves, mainly those of the feet and legs. It has been suggested that more hospital beds in Britain are occupied by patients who have diabetes and lower limb and foot problems than by all those with the other complications of diabetes combined.

The two main features are neuropathy and ischaemia, often present together. Identifying those at risk of foot ulceration and providing preventive education are the most important aspects of the care of the neuropathic foot in a person with diabetes, as well as in preventing prolonged hospital admission and amputation (see Chapter 14).

Association with other conditions

Metabolic syndrome

Metabolic syndrome (also known as syndrome X or Reaven's syndrome; see also Chapter 7) may be present before the diagnosis of type 2 diabetes and is associated with:

- hypertension
- central obesity
- dyslipidaemia
- hyperglycaemia.

Polycystic ovary syndrome may also be involved.

At the heart of this syndrome lies insulin resistance (Figure 24.1). Obesity, especially central obesity, is strongly implicated in insulin resistance.

Insulin resistance

- Insulin resistance is one of the fundamental defects in type 2 diabetes.
- Insulin resistance is an early feature of the development of many cases of type 2 diabetes.
- Receptor sites on the cells do not allow insulin to convert glucose in the blood for storage; therefore, blood glucose levels increase.
- There are subsequent increases in insulin output to try to rectify the problem.
- Insulin-resistant patients may become hyperinsulinaemic.
- Continued insulin resistance leads to the eventual exhaustion

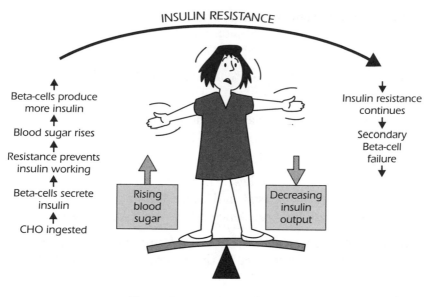

Figure 24.1 Insulin resistance
CHO, carbohydrate

of the beta-cells. This results in a failure to produce adequate insulin and a further increase in blood glucose.

■ In type 2 diabetes, insulin resistance is characterised by impaired (insulin-stimulated) glucose uptake by the fat, liver and skeletal muscle, and overproduction of glucose by the liver.

■ Insulin resistance is central to the development of cardio-vascular risk factors, which are clustered together in the metabolic syndrome described earlier.

■ Regular activity improves oxygen consumption and reduces insulin resistance, even in elderly people.

■ The problems caused by insulin resistance can be reduced by lifestyle changes.

■ Thiazolidinediones (also called PPAR-gamma agonists or glitazones) are drugs that target insulin resistance. They improve glycaemic control by improving insulin sensitivity at key sites of insulin resistance, namely the fat, liver and skeletal muscle.

Hypertension: treatment plans

Facts

- With type 1 diabetes, 30% of people eventually develop hypertension.

- In those with type 1 diabetes and hypertension, hypertension develops after several years and is usually associated with nephropathy.

- In type 2 diabetes, studies do not agree on the prevalence rate as there is no consensus on the level for the diagnosis of hypertension, but prevalence is likely to be at least 50%.

- The UK Prospective Diabetes Study found that good control in type 2 diabetes instigated by the general practitioner produced a:
  - 37% reduction in microvascular end points (nephropathy and advanced retinopathy);
  - 32% reduction in deaths related to diabetes;
  - 24% reduction in diabetes-related end points.

There is increasing evidence that aggressive treatment of raised blood pressure reduces the incidence of vascular complications in diabetes.

- Consider treatment to achieve a systolic blood pressure of less than 140 mmHg or a diastolic blood pressure of less than 80 mmHg:
  - Treat older people with equal enthusiasm, because they are more likely to derive early benefits.
  - Do not treat on the basis of one hypertensive reading; three readings over 2 months is advocated.
  - Discuss lifestyle factors with the individual before prescribing medication. Address shortfalls in activity and diet where appropriate.

Therapy for hypertension

In 2006, the National Institute for Health and Clinical Excellence and the British Hypertension Society updated recommendations for treating people newly diagnosed with hypertension. Based on evidence, beta-blockers were no longer advocated as first-line therapy (Figure 24.2).

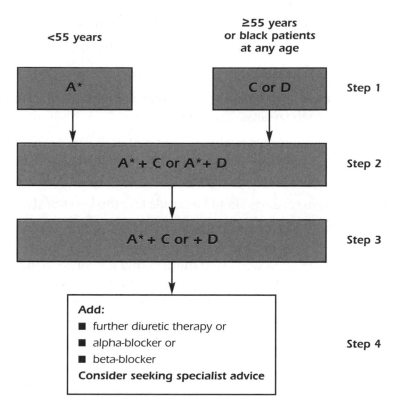

<55 years

**≥55 years
or black patients
at any age**

| A* | | C or D | Step 1 |

A* + C or A*+ D — Step 2

A* + C or + D — Step 3

Add:
- further diuretic therapy or
- alpha-blocker or
- beta-blocker

Consider seeking specialist advice

Step 4

Figure 24.2
Algorithm for the treatment of newly diagnosed hypertension
A = ACE inhibitor (* or ARB if ACEi-intolerant); C = calcium-channel blocker;
D = thiazide-type diuretic. Beta-blockers are not a preferred initial therapy for
hypertension but are an alternative to A in patients <55 years in whom A is not
tolerated, or contraindicated (includes women of child-bearing potential). Black
patients are only those of African or Caribbean descent. In the absence of evidence,
all other patients should be treated according to the algorithm as non-black.
ACEi, angiotensin-converting enzyme inhibitor; ARB, angiotensin receptor blocker
(From National Institute of Health and Clinical Excellence/British Hypertension
Society, 2006)

Blood pressure measurement

It may seem patronising to outline how to take a blood pressure measurement, but a study researching doctors' and nurses' techniques for measuring blood pressure demonstrated they were as bad – or as good – as each other. Digital devices validated by the British Hypertension Society will give true readings, which health professionals may not like as the figures cannot be inadvertently massaged downwards.

- The person should be seated, with arm supported at the level of the heart.

- Remove any tight clothing from the individual.

- A full bladder can increase blood pressure levels.

- If the arm circumference exceeds 33 cm, use a large cuff.

- Deflate the cuff at 2 mmHg per second and measure the blood pressure to the nearest 2 mmHg.

- Record the diastolic pressure at the point of disappearance of the sounds (phase V); if this cannot be identified, use the point at which muffling of the sounds occurs (phase IV).

- At least two readings should be made and the lower of the two readings used.

- There is usually no significant difference in blood pressure between the arms, and using the arm that is nearest to the observer is reasonable. If there is a consistent difference between the two arms, use the arm with the higher blood pressure for routine monitoring (but remember that a difference in blood pressure between the two arms may indicate coarctation of the aorta).

- Check the standing blood pressure in someone with diabetes to exclude postural hypotension, as cardiovascular autonomic neuropathy can cause falsely low or high readings.

All blood pressure machines, whether sphygmomanometers or digital devices, should be quality controlled to ensure accuracy. The British Hypertension Society can provide advice for health professionals, and the Blood Pressure Association information for members of the public (see Appendix 4 for details).

Ambulatory blood pressure monitoring
Ambulatory blood pressure monitors (24-hour blood pressure monitors) also are becoming more reliable and are useful in identifying 'white-coat' hypertension – the rise in blood pressure when a person is approached by a health professional. The average difference between clinic and daytime mean ambulatory blood pressures is approximately 12/7 mmHg.

Drugs used to treat hypertension
(Joint British Societies, 2005; Williams et al, 2004)
The British Hypertension Society recognises that ACE inhibitors are the first-line therapy in diabetic hypertension, not only for their renoprotective properties, but also to reduce cardiovascular risk. The Society

further recognises that two or more drugs may be necessary to achieve the tight goals set.

People with diabetes should be involved in the choice of medication:

- They may not take it if they do not realise its importance; once a day regimes are generally more successful than multiple doses across the day.

- Individuals may not realise that the side effects of one therapy may not occur with another:
  - ◆ Warning signs of hypoglycaemia can be lost with beta-blockers (which may have an impact on driving); also, asthma may worsen and ankle oedema occur.
  - ◆ Thiazides may increase blood glucose levels and contribute to erectile dysfunction.
  - ◆ ACE inhibitors may cause a dry cough so angiotensin inhibitors (angiotensin receptor blockers, or ARBs) may be better.
  - ◆ Calcium channel blockers can cause flushing, headache and oedema.

- Sources of information should be provided as there is too much information to be taken in during a short consultation.

References

Department of Health (2000). *National Service Frameworks. Coronary Heart Disease. Modern Standards and Service Models.* London: DoH.

Diabetes UK (2001). *Aspirin Treatment in Diabetes.* London: Diabetes UK.

House of Commons (2004) *Health, Third Report. Obesity.* London: House of Commons Publications.

Joint British Societies (2005). Guidelines on prevention of cardiovascular disease in clinical practice. *Heart* **91**: 1–52.

McIntosh A, Hutchinson A, Marshall S et al (2002) *Clinical Guidelines and Evidence Review for Type 2 Diabetes – Diabetic Renal Disease: Prevention and Early Management.* Sheffield: ScHARR, University of Sheffield.

Malmberg K, Ryden L, Hamsten A, Herlitz J, Waldenstrom A, Wedel H, Welin L (1995). Randomized trial of insulin-glucose infusion followed by subcutaneous insulin treatment in diabetic patients with acute myocardial infarction (DIGAMI study): effects on mortality at 1 year. *Journal of the American College of Cardiology* **26**: 56–65.

National Institute for Health and Clinical Excellence (2002a). *Management of Type 2 Diabetes. Management of Blood Pressure and Blood Lipids.* Inherited Guideline H. London: NICE.

National Institute for Health and Clinical Excellence/British Hypertension Society (2006). *Hypertension: Management of Hypertension in Adults in Primary Care*. London: NICE.

National Institute for Health and Clinical Excellence (2002b). *Management of Type 2 Diabetes. Renal Disease – Prevention and Early Management*. Inherited Guideline F. London: NICE.

Rayner M, Petersen S, Buckle C, Press V (2001). *Coronary Heart Disease Statistics. Diabetes Supplement*. London: British Heart Foundation.

Scottish Intercollegiate Guidelines Network (2001). *Management of Diabetes*. Report No. 55. Edinburgh: SIGN.

Williams B, Poulter NR, Brown MJ et al (2004). Guidelines for management of hypertension: report of the fourth working party of the British Hypertension Society. 2004 – BHS IV. *Journal of Human Hypertension* **18**: 139–185.

Wood D, Durrington P, Poulter N, McInnes G, Rees A, Wray R (1998). Joint British recommendations on prevention of coronary heart disease in clinical practice. *Heart* **80** (Suppl. II.): S1–S29.

Further reading

Adler AI, Stratton IM, Neil HAW et al (2000). Association of systolic blood pressure with macrovascular and microvascular complications of type 2 diabetes: prospective observational study (UKPDS 36). *British Medical Journal* **321**: 412–419.

Amos AF, McCarty DJ, Zimmer P (1997). The rising global burden of diabetes and its complications: estimates and projections to the year 2010. *Diabetic Medicine* **14**: S1–S85.

Basu A, Ryder R (2004). New treatment options for erectile dysfunction in patients with diabetes mellitus. *Drugs* **64**: 2667–2688.

Chambers R, Stead J, Wakley G (2001). *Diabetes Matters in Primary Care*. Oxford: Radcliffe Medical Press.

Department of Health (2001). *National Service Framework for Coronary Heart Disease: Modern Standards and Service Models*. London: DoH.

Edmonds M, Foster A (2005). *Managing the Diabetic Foot*. London: Blackwell Publishing.

Hansson L et al. (1998). The Hypertension Optimal Treatment (HOT) Study: 24 month data on blood pressure and tolerability. *Lancet* **351**: 1755–1612.

King's Fund (1996). *Counting the Cost of Type 2 Diabetes*. London: King's Fund/British Diabetic Association.

Malmberg K, for the DIGAMI Study Group (1997). Prospective randomised study of intensive insulin treatment on long term survival after acute myocardial infarction in patients with diabetes mellitus. *British Medical Journal* **314**: 1512–1515.

Munro N, Rich N, McIntosh C, Foster A, Edmonds M (2003). Infections in the diabetic foot. *British Journal of Diabetes and Vascular Disease* **3**: 132–136.

National Institute for Health and Clinical Excellence (2002). *Management of Type 2 Diabetes: Retinopathy – Screening and Early Management.* Inherited Guideline E. London: NICE.

National Institute for Health and Clinical Excellence (2002). *Management of Type 2 Diabetes. Management of Blood Glucose.* Inherited Guideline G. London: NICE.

National Institute for Health and Clinical Excellence (2004). *Management of Type 2 Diabetes. Prevention and Management of Foot Problems.* London: NICE.

Stratton IM, Adler AI, Andrew H et al (2000). Association of glycaemia with macrovascular and microvascular complications of type 2 diabetes (UKPDS 35): prospective observational study. *British Medical Journal* **321**: 405–412.

UK Prospective Diabetes Study Group (1998). Intensive blood glucose control with sulphonylureas or insulin compared with conventional treatment and risk of complications in patients with type 2 diabetes (UKPDS 33). *Lancet* **352**: 837–853.

UK Prospective Diabetes Study Group (1998). Effect of intensive blood-glucose control with metformin on complications in overweight patients with type 2 diabetes (UKPDS 34). *Lancet* **352**: 854–865.

UK Prospective Diabetes Study Group (1998). Tight blood pressure control and risk of macrovascular and microvascular complications in type 2 diabetes (UKPDS 38). *British Medical Journal* **317**: 701–713.

UK Prospective Diabetes Study Group (1998). Efficacy of atenolol and captopril in reducing risk of macrovascular and microvascular complications in type 2 diabetes (UKPDS 39). *British Medical Journal* **317**: 713–720.

UK Prospective Diabetes Study Group (1999). Quality of life in type 2 diabetic patients is affected by complications but not by intensive policies to improve blood glucose or blood pressure control (UKPDS 37). *Diabetes Care* **22**: 1125–1136.

Watkins PI (2003). *ABC of Diabetes*, 5th edn. London: BMJ Publishing Group.

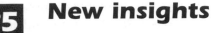

25 New insights

Questions this chapter will help you answer

- Is there evidence that diabetes can be prevented?

- Which studies demonstrate the ability to prevent complications?

- What lessons can I learn from research to inform my practice?

There is continuing new evidence and insight into the management of diabetes. Some recent relevant studies or pieces of research are summarised below.

New research is emerging all the time and can be accessed through the National Diabetes Support Team or the National Electronic Library for Health websites (see Appendix 4).

Prevention of type 2 diabetes mellitus by changes in lifestyle among subjects with impaired glucose tolerance

This study investigated whether improving lifestyle factors, weight, diet and physical exercise could delay the onset of diabetes in people already at risk through impaired glucose tolerance.

- The risk of diabetes was reduced by 58% in the intervention group.

- The reduction in the incidence of diabetes was directly associated with changes in lifestyle.

Conclusions: Progression to type 2 diabetes can be prevented by changes in the lifestyle of high-risk subjects.

Tuomilehto J, Lindstrom MS, Eriksson JG et al (2001). Prevention of type 2 diabetes mellitus by changes in lifestyle among subjects with impaired glucose tolerance. *New England Journal of Medicine* **344**: 1343–1350.

DCCT: The effect of intensive treatment of diabetes on the development and progression of long-term complications in insulin-dependent diabetes mellitus

The landmark DCCT (Diabetes Control and Complications Trial Research Group) study from the USA provided the answer to the argument of whether good glycaemic control halted or even prevented complications in people with diabetes. It only considered type 1 patients on insulin and until UK Prospective Diabetes Study (UKPDS), it was assumed likely that the results applied to type 2 diabetes as well. The UKPDS (see below) furthered that research in type 2 diabetes.

The DCCT found that intensive insulin therapy:

- reduced the risk of developing retinopathy by 76% in those without pre-existing retinopathy;

- slowed the progression of retinopathy by 54% and reduced the progression to severe retinopathy by 47% in those with pre-existing retinopathy;

- reduced microalbuminuria by 39%;

- reduced albuminuria by 54%;

- reduced neuropathy by 60%.

Conclusions: Intensive therapy effectively delays the onset and slows the progression of diabetic retinopathy, nephropathy and neuropathy in individuals with type 1 diabetes. There was an increased risk of hypoglycaemic attacks.

The Diabetes Control and Complications Trial Research Group (1993). The effect of intensive treatment of diabetes on the development and progression of long-term complications in insulin-dependent diabetes mellitus. *New England Journal of Medicine* **329**: 977–986.

UK Prospective Diabetes Study

This is such an important study that all aspects are highlighted here. It was the largest clinical study of diabetes ever conducted and had an impact worldwide.

- It studied the effect of the intensive therapeutic management of type 2 diabetes in reducing long-term complications.

- It demonstrated that long-term complications were reduced with intensive therapy.
- It found that a reduction in glycated haemoglobin (HbA_{1c}) of 1% was associated with a greatly reduced rate of complications.
- It demonstrated that type 2 diabetes is a serious and progressive disease and never 'mild'.
- It found that up to 50% of people with type 2 diabetes had evidence of long-term complications on diagnosis, emphasising the need for the early detection and screening of those in high-risk groups.
- The key treatment targets, reducing long-term complications in the study, related to tight blood pressure and intensive blood glucose control.
- Two papers (numbers 35 and 36) showed the close relationship between complications and the control of blood glucose and blood pressure.

There were several arms to the study.

UKPDS 33: Intensive blood glucose control with sulphonylureas or insulin compared with conventional treatment and risk of complications in patients with type 2 diabetes

Over 10 years, the HbA_{1c} was 7.0% (range 6.2–8.2%) in the intensively treated group compared with 7.9% (range 6.9–8.8%) in the conventional group – an 11% reduction.

- The risk of complications was reduced by:
  - 12% for any diabetes-related end point;
  - 10% for any diabetes-related death;
  - 6% for all-cause mortality.

Interpretation: Intensive blood glucose control with either sulphonylureas or insulin substantially decreases the risk of microvascular complications, but not macrovascular disease, in those with type 2 diabetes.

UK Prospective Diabetes Study Group (1998). Intensive blood glucose control with sulphonylureas or insulin compared with conventional treatment and risk of complications in patients with type 2 diabetes (UKPDS 33). *Lancet* **352**: 837–853.

UKPDS 34: Effect of intensive blood glucose control with metformin on complications in overweight patients with type 2 diabetes

■ Patients allocated metformin, compared with the conventionally treated group, had risk reductions of:

◆ 32% for any diabetes-related end point;

◆ 42% for diabetes-related death;

◆ 36% for all-cause mortality.

■ Metformin showed a greater effect than glibenclamide or insulin for any diabetes-related end point.

Interpretation: Because intensive glucose control with metformin appears to decrease the risk of diabetes-related end points in overweight diabetic individuals, and is associated with less weight gain and fewer hypoglycaemic attacks than are insulin and the sulphonylureas, it may be the first-line pharmacological therapy of choice in these people.

UK Prospective Diabetes Study Group (1998). Effect of intensive blood-glucose control with metformin on complications in overweight patients with type 2 diabetes (UKPDS 34). *Lancet* **352**: 854–865.

UKPDS 35: Association of glycaemia with macrovascular and microvascular complications of type 2 diabetes

■ Each 1% reduction in updated mean HbA_{1c} level was associated with reductions in risk of:

◆ 21% for any end point related to diabetes;

◆ 21% for deaths related to diabetes;

◆ 14% for myocardial infarction;

◆ 37% for microvascular complications.

Conclusion: In individuals with type 2 diabetes, the risk of diabetic complications was strongly associated with previous hyperglycaemia. Any reduction in HbA_{1c} is likely to reduce the risk of complications, the lowest risk being in those with HbA_{1c} values in the normal range (<6.0%).

Stratton IM, Adler AI, Neil HAW et al (2000). Association of glycaemia with macrovascular and microvascular complications of type 2 diabetes (UKPDS 35): prospective observational study. *British Medical Journal* **321**: 405–412.

UKPDS 36: Association of systolic blood pressure with the macrovascular and microvascular complications of type 2 diabetes

■ Each 10 mmHg decrease in updated mean systolic blood pressure was associated with reductions in risk of:
- ◆ 12% for any complication related to diabetes;
- ◆ 15% for deaths related to diabetes;
- ◆ 11% for myocardial infarction;
- ◆ 13% for microvascular complications.

Conclusion: In those with type 2 diabetes, the risk of diabetic complications was strongly associated with raised blood pressure. Any reduction in blood pressure is likely to reduce the risk of complications, the lowest risk being in those with a systolic blood pressure of less than 120 mmHg.

Adler AI, Stratton IM, Neil HAW et al (2000). Association of systolic blood pressure with macrovascular and microvascular complications of type 2 diabetes: prospective observational study (UKPDS 36). *British Medical Journal* **321**: 412–419.

UKPDS 38: Tight blood pressure control and risk of macrovascular and microvascular complications in type 2 diabetes

Mean blood pressure during follow-up was significantly reduced in the group assigned to tight blood pressure control (144/82 mmHg) compared with the group assigned to less tight control (154/87 mmHg).

■ Reductions in risk in the group assigned to tight control compared with that assigned to less tight control were:
- ◆ 24% in diabetes-related end points;
- ◆ 32% in deaths related to diabetes;
- ◆ 44% in strokes;
- ◆ 37% in microvascular end points (predominantly owing to a reduced risk of retinal photocoagulation).

Conclusion: Tight blood pressure control in patients with hypertension and type 2 diabetes achieves a clinically important reduction in the risk of deaths related to diabetes, complications related to diabetes, progression of diabetic retinopathy, and deterioration in visual acuity.

UK Prospective Diabetes Study Group (1998). Tight blood pressure control and risk of macrovascular and microvascular complications in type 2 diabetes (UKPDS 38). *British Medical Journal* 317: 703–713.

Primary Care Diabetes – a National Survey

A national survey in England and Wales aimed to describe:

- the extent and organisation of general practice diabetes care;

- primary care perceptions of support by secondary care;

- cooperation with secondary care;

- the educational experience in diabetes of doctors and nurses in primary care.

The enquiry confirmed that, over the past decade, the focus of diabetes care has shifted and most is now provided in general practice. There are significant geographical variations in the delivery of primary diabetes care and significant differences in the type and amount of training undertaken by those involved in diabetes management.

One in five practices in England and Wales was surveyed. The response to the survey was 70%.

- The median number of individuals with diabetes per practice was 110.

- Of all patients, 75% with diabetes are described as having most or all of their diabetes care in general practice.

- Of all practices, 68% had a special interest in diabetes.

- Of all practices, 96% had diabetes registers.

- Of all practices, 87% used their registers for call and recall.

- Of all practices, 77% had fully computerised registers.

Pierce M, Agarwal G, Ridout D (2000). A survey of diabetes care in general practice in England and Wales. *British Journal of General Practice* 50: 542–545.

Multifactorial intervention and cardiovascular disease in patients with type 2 diabetes

This study demonstrated that targeting multiple risk factors in patients with type 2 diabetes and microalbuminuria reduces the risk of cardiovascular and microvascular events by about 50%.

> Gaede P, Vedel P, Larsen N, Jensen GV, Parving HH, Pedersen O (2000). Multifactorial intervention and cardiovascular disease in patients with type 2 diabetes. *New England Journal of Medicine* **348**: 383–393.

A review of diabetes self-management interventions in disadvantaged populations

The authors reviewed methods of encouraging education for diabetes self-management in ethnic and disadvantaged groups. They recognised barriers to learning associated with language, transport and limited financial resources, and suggested that community education that involved people locally was most effective. Peer support programmes, such as the Expert Patient programme, and new ways of working to suit local populations need to be developed to ensure that disadvantaged people are involved in diabetes education.

> Eakin EG, Bull SS, Glasgow RE, Mason M (2002). Reaching those most in need: a review of diabetes self-management interventions in disadvantaged populations. *Diabetes/Metabolism Research and Reviews* **18**: 26–35.

The Hypertension Optimal Treatment study

The Hypertension Optimal Treatment (HOT) study was a very large study (18 790 subjects) to investigate the optimum target diastolic blood pressure. A subgroup of these hypertensive individuals (1501 patients) also had diabetes.

- In patients with diabetes, a diastolic blood pressure of 80 mmHg led to a reduction of severe cardiovascular events by 51%, compared with a diastolic blood pressure of 90 mmHg.

- The reduction in morbidity was accompanied by a parallel improvement in well-being.

- UKPDS data (paper 36) showed that patients with a normal systolic blood pressure (130 mmHg) had a lower risk of coronary heart disease.

- Thus, the target blood pressure for people with diabetes is 130/80 mmHg.

Hansson L, Zanchetti A, Carruthers SG et al (1998). The Hypertension Optimal Treatment (HOT) study: 24 month data on blood pressure and tolerability. *Lancet* **351**: 1755–1612.

The DECODE Study Group

This study investigated glucose tolerance and mortality, and was a comparison of World Health Organization (WHO) and American Diabetic Association (ADA) diagnostic criteria.

- The ADA proposed that diabetes be defined by a fasting plasma glucose of 7.0 mmol/l alone and did not recommend the use of an oral glucose tolerance test.

- WHO recommended that an oral glucose tolerance test should be used only if the blood glucose concentration was in the uncertain range of 5.5–11.1 mmol/l. For the diagnosis of diabetes mellitus, the WHO recommend the same fasting concentration as the ADA, as well as a 2-hour glucose concentration of at least 11.1 mmol/l.

- A high degree of disagreement in the fasting and 2-hour classifications has been seen between the two recommendations in European populations.

- DECODE assessed mortality associated with the ADA fasting glucose criteria compared with the WHO 2-hour post-challenge glucose criteria.

- Data from 13 prospective European cohort studies were examined, including those for 18 048 men and 7316 women aged 30 years or older. Mean follow-up was 7.3 years.

Key findings

■ Compared with people who had a normal fasting glucose level (<6.1 mmol/l), those with diabetes newly diagnosed using the ADA fasting criteria (>7.0 mmol/l) had hazard ratios for death of 1.81 (men) and 1.79 (women).

■ For impaired fasting glycaemia (6.1–6.9 mmol/l), the hazard ratios were 1.21 and 1.08.

■ For the WHO criteria (>11.1 mmol/l), the hazard ratios for newly diagnosed diabetes were 2.02 in men and 2.77 in women.

■ For impaired fasting glycaemia (7.8–11.1 mmol/l), the ratios were 1.51 and 1.60.

■ Within each fasting glucose classification, mortality increased with increasing 2-hour glucose concentration.

■ For the 2-hour glucose classifications of impaired glucose tolerance and diabetes, there was no trend for increasing fasting glucose concentrations.

Significance

■ An increase in 2-hour glucose level resulted in a significant increase in mortality, independent of fasting glucose.

■ Fasting blood glucose concentration is not as satisfactory as 2-hour blood glucose values for predicting mortality.

DECODE Study Group (1999). Glucose tolerance and mortality: comparison of WHO and American Diabetes Association diagnostic criteria. The DECODE study group. European Diabetes Epidemiology Group. Diabetes Epidemiology: Collaborative analysis of Diagnostic criteria in Europe *Lancet* **354**: 617–621.

Collaborative Atorvastatin Diabetes Study

The Collaborative Atorvastatin Diabetes Study (CARDS) was a multi-centre, randomised, placebo-controlled trial to determine hard outcomes of treatment with atorvastatin 10 mg compared with placebo in individuals with type 2 diabetes and at least one additional cardiovascular risk factor. In total, 2838 high-risk patients were followed for 4 years.

CARDS supported the findings of the Heart Protection Study that it is cardiovascular risk and not necessarily an elevated low-density lipoprotein (LDL) level that predicts a beneficial outcome in individuals taking statins. Similar beneficial outcomes were seen regardless of initial LDL and high-density lipoprotein (HDL) levels. Statin treatment (atorvastatin 10 mg a day) in high-risk individuals with type 2 diabetes and at least one additional risk factor significantly reduced their risk of cardiovascular and stroke events even when the initial LDL concentration was already 3 mmol/l or less.

Colhoun HM, Betteridge DJ, Durrington PN et al (2004). Primary prevention of cardiovascular disease with atorvastatin in type 2 diabetes in the Collaborative Atorvastatin Diabetes Study (CARDS). *Lancet* **364**: 685–696.

Anglo-Scandinavian Cardiac Outcomes Trial

The Anglo-Scandinavian Cardiac Outcomes Trial (ASCOT) included more than 19 000 men and women with high blood pressure who were at a moderate risk of strokes and heart attacks. To control their blood pressure, they received either the newer drugs – a calcium antagonist, amlodipine, and the angiotensin-converting enzyme inhibitor perindopril – or a traditional combination of a beta-blocker, atenolol and a diuretic. In addition, 10 000 individuals were also treated with the cholesterol-lowering drug atorvastatin or a placebo. This is the only major European study to-date to have combined these two treatment strategies.

The final results of ASCOT showed that the combination of newer blood pressure-lowering drugs reduced the risk of stroke by about 25%, coronaries by 15%, cardiovascular deaths by 25% and new cases of diabetes by 30% compared with the standard treatment.

The addition of the cholesterol-lowering drug atorvastatin reduced still further the remaining risk irrespective of the patient's original cholesterol level. Indeed, the ASCOT subjects only had average or below-average levels of cholesterol at the outset of the study.

Dahlöf B, Sever PS, Poulter NR et al, for the ASCOT Investigators (2005). Prevention of cardiovascular events with an antihypertensive regimen of amlodipine adding perindopril as required versus atenolol adding bendroflumethiazide as required, in the Anglo-Scandinavian Cardiac Outcomes Trial – Blood Pressure Lowering Arm (ASCOT-BPLA): a multicentre randomised controlled trial. *Lancet* **366**: 895–906.

Poulter NR, Wedel H, Dahlöf B et al, for the ASCOT Investigators (2005). Role of blood pressure and other variables in the differential cardiovascular event rates noted in the Anglo-Scandinavian Cardiac Outcomes Trial – Blood Pressure Lowering Arm (ASCOT-BPLA). *Lancet* **366**: 907–913.

Sever PS, Dahlof B, Poulter NR et al, for the ASCOT Investigators (2004). Prevention of coronary and stroke events with atorvastatin in hypertensive patients who have average or lower-than-average cholesterol concentrations, in the Anglo-Scandinavian Cardiac Outcomes Trial – Lipid Lowering Arm (ASCOT-LLA): a multicentre randomised controlled trial. *Drugs* **64** (Suppl. 2): 43–60.

Heart Protection Study

The study involved 5963 people with diabetes
   The main findings were as follows:

- Statins reduced the risk of myocardial infarction and stroke by at least a third.

- Substantial reductions in the incidence of major events were shown in women, older people, people with diabetes and co-existing heart disease, and those with a total cholesterol level below 5 mmol/l or LDL cholesterol below 3 mmol/l.

- About 5 years of statin treatment typically prevented these major vascular events in:
  - ◆ 100 of every 1000 people who had previously had a heart attack;
  - ◆ 80 of every 1000 people with angina or some other evidence of coronary heart disease;

- ◆ 70 of every 1000 patients who had previously had a stroke;
- ◆ 70 of every 1000 patients with occlusive disease in the leg or other arteries;
- ◆ 70 of every 1000 people with diabetes.

■ In addition, continued treatment with a statin prevented further major vascular events and deaths in those people who had already had one heart attack or stroke.

■ The benefits of treatment increased throughout the 5-year study treatment period, so more prolonged use of a statin would be expected to produce even bigger benefits.

■ The benefits of statins were additional to those of other treatments used to prevent heart attacks or strokes, such as aspirin and blood pressure-lowering drugs.

■ The trial provided uniquely reliable evidence on the safety of the regimen of 40 mg simvastatin daily that was used. There was no support for previous concerns about the possible adverse effects of lowering cholesterol on particular non-vascular causes of death, on cancers or on strokes due to bleeding.

Implications: Based on WHO estimates of the number of people with coronary heart disease, stroke and diabetes, it can be estimated that the results are relevant to the treatment of some hundreds of millions of people worldwide. If an extra 10 million high-risk people were to start statin treatment, this would save about 50 000 lives each year and would prevent a similar number from suffering non-fatal heart attacks or strokes.

Medical Research Council/British Heart Foundation (2003). Heart Protection Study of cholesterol-lowering with simvastatin in 5963 individuals with diabetes: a randomised placebo-controlled trial. Heart Protection Study Collaborative Group. *Lancet* **361**: 2005–2016.

Appendices

Appendices

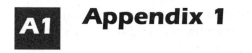

Appendix 1

What diabetes care to expect (2006)

(Diabetes UK; reproduced with permission)

What you should expect from the National Health Service (NHS)

You should receive all health services without discrimination because of age, lifestyle, gender, ethnicity, class, religion, disability, sexuality or your ability to pay.

The NHS should:

- Treat you with respect and dignity.
- Tell you how to contact your diabetes care team.
- Treat you with skill and care, and regularly review your clinical needs.
- Answer any questions about the quality of the services you are getting.
- Provide an interpreting service if English is not your first language, or if you have a sensory impairment or learning difficulties.
- Provide information about local health services and how to contact them.
- Keep you up to date about your diabetes, its care and treatment (and give you access to a second opinion subject to the agreement of your own GP [general practitioner] or consultant).

What care you should expect from your diabetes care team

To achieve the best possible diabetes care, you need to work together with healthcare professionals as equal members of your diabetes care team. It is essential that you understand your diabetes as well as possible so that you are an effective member of this team.

You need to discuss with your consultant or GP the roles and responsibilities of those providing your diabetes care and to identify the key members of your own diabetes care team.

Members in your diabetes care team

- yourself

- consultant physician/diabetologist

- GP

- diabetes specialist nurse (DSN)

- practice nurse

- dietitian

- optometrist/ophthalmologist

- podiatrist/chiropodist

- psychologist

- medical specialists

- pharmacist.

You may see some members of your diabetes care team more often than others.

When you have just been diagnosed, your diabetes care team should:

- Give you a full medical examination.

- Work with you to make a programme of care which suits you and includes diabetes management goals (see the annual review check list below).

- Arrange for you to talk with a diabetes specialist nurse (or practice nurse) who will explain what diabetes is and discuss your individual treatment and the equipment you will need to use.

- Arrange for you to talk with a state registered dietitian, who will want to know what you usually eat, and will give you advice on how to fit your usual diet in with your diabetes – a follow-up meeting should be arranged for more detailed advice.

- Tell you about your diabetes and the beneficial effects of a healthy diet, exercise and good diabetes control.

- Discuss the effects of diabetes on your job, driving, insurance, prescription charges, and if you are a driver, whether you need to inform the DVLA [Driver and Vehicle Licensing Agency] and your insurance company.

- Provide you with regular and appropriate information and education, on food and foot care for example.

- Give you information about Diabetes UK services and details of your local Diabetes UK voluntary group.

Once your diabetes is reasonably controlled, you should:

- Have access to your diabetes care team at least once a year – in this session, take the opportunity to discuss how your diabetes affects you as well as your diabetes control.

- Be able to contact any member of your diabetes care team for specialist advice, in person or by phone.

- Have further education sessions when you are ready for them.

- Have a formal medical annual review once a year with a doctor experienced in diabetes.

On a regular basis, your diabetes care team should:

- Provide continuity of care, ideally from the same doctors and nurses. If this is not possible, the doctors or nurses who you are seeing should be fully aware of your medical history and background.

- Work with you to continually review your programme of care, including your diabetes management goals.

- Let you share in decisions about your treatment or care.

- Let you manage your own diabetes in hospital after discussion with your doctor, if you are well enough to do so and that is what you wish.

- Organise pre and post pregnancy advice, together with an obstetric hospital team, if you are planning to become or already are pregnant.

- Encourage a carer to visit with you, to keep them up to date on diabetes to be able to make informed judgements about diabetes care.

- Encourage the support of friends, partners and/or relatives.

- Provide you with educational sessions and appointments if you wish.

- Give you advice on the effects of diabetes and its treatments when you are ill or taking other medication.

PLUS
If you are treated by insulin injections you should:

- Have frequent visits showing you how to inject, look after your insulin and syringes and dispose of sharps (needles). Also how to test your blood glucose and test for ketones and be informed what the results mean and what to do about them.

- Be given supplies of, or a prescription for the medication and equipment you need.

- Discuss hypoglycaemia (hypos): when and why they may happen and how to deal with them.

If you are treated by tablets you should:

- Be given instruction on blood or urine testing and have explained what the results mean and what to do about them.

- Be given supplies of, or a prescription for, the medication and equipment you need.

- Discuss hypoglycaemia (hypos): when and why they may happen and how to deal with them.

If you are treated by diet alone you should:

- Be given instruction on blood or urine testing and have explained what the results mean and what to do about them.

- Be given supplies of equipment you may need.

It is your responsibility:

- to take as much control of your diabetes on a day-to-day basis as you can. The more you know about your own diabetes, the easier this will become

- to learn about and practise self-care which should include dietary education, exercise and monitoring blood glucose levels

- to examine your feet regularly or have someone check them

- to know how to manage your diabetes and when to ask for help if you are ill, eg chest infection, flu or diarrhoea and vomiting

- to know when, where and how to contact your diabetes care team

- to build the diabetes advice discussed with you into your daily life

- to talk regularly with your diabetes care team and ask questions

- to make a list of points to raise at appointments, if you find it helpful

- to attend your scheduled appointments and inform the diabetes care team if you are unable to do so.

What you should do if you have a complaint

It is important to put your complaint in writing, but also to discuss it with those providing you with your care (eg GP or hospital staff). Each general practice and hospital should have internal procedures to deal with complaints in the first instance.

If this does not solve the problem, you should contact the complaints officer at your health authority or hospital and request that the complaint be considered by an independent review panel (usually a non-executive director of the hospital or health authority concerned) who will be advised by an independent person.

If you are still dissatisfied after these procedures, ask for the Health Service Ombudsman to investigate [see Appendix 4].

Annual review checklist

It is important to remember that your annual review is to enable you to lead a normal and healthy life. It must be about what you want and need as well as what healthcare professionals recommend.

The following should be checked at least once a year.

Laboratory tests and investigations

- Blood glucose control: an HbA1c [glycated haemoglobin] blood test will measure your long-term blood glucose control. The range to aim for should be 7 per cent or below.

- Kidney function: urine and blood tests to check for protein will show that your kidneys are working correctly. There should not be any protein in your urine.

- Blood fats (lipids, cholesterol and triglyceride levels): a blood test that measures your blood fat levels. A total cholesterol of 5.0 mmol/l or less and a fasting triglyceride of 2.0 mmol/l are accepted as national target ranges.*

Please note all normal and good ranges will vary from person to person – it is meant to be a guide so you know what to aim towards. If you have any questions, ask your diabetes care team.

Physical examinations

- Weight is often calculated as a Body Mass Index (BMI) which expresses adult weight in relation to height. From this you will be advised if you need to lose weight to better control your diabetes. Your GP will record your BMI in your notes.

- Legs and feet should be examined to check your skin, circulation and nerve supply. If necessary, you should be referred to a state registered chiropodist/podiatrist.

- Blood pressure should be taken. You should aim for your blood pressure to be at or less than 140/80. If it is at higher levels discuss this with your doctor to discuss why your blood pressure may be high. Keeping your blood pressure down has been proven to be beneficial for people with diabetes (UKPDS research trial).

- Eyes should be examined regularly through a 'fundoscopy' review where your pupils are dilated to enable your optometrist/ophthalmologist to detect any early changes at the back of the eye (retinopathy). Photographs may be taken to record the appearance at the back of your eyes.

- If you're on insulin, your injection sites should be examined.

Lifestyle issues

The review should also provide enough time to discuss:

- Your general well-being; how you are coping with your diabetes at home, work, school or college.

- Your current treatment.

- Your diabetes control, including your home monitoring results.

- Any problems you may be having.

It should include discussion about smoking, alcohol consumption, stress, sexual problems, physical activity and healthy eating issues. You should feel free to raise any or all of these issues with your diabetes care team.

Appendix 2

Groups working in diabetes in primary care

Primary Care Diabetes Society (www.pcdsociety.org)

Healthcare professionals in primary care need a forum for debate, an organisation to promote discussion and awareness of the modern management of diabetes and its complications – to act as a professional voice in the new healthcare environment. This group aims to represent all those involved with diabetes primary care, not only general practitioners (GPs) and practice nurses, but also the 'lost tribe' of GPwSIs (GPs with a special interest) and clinical assistants.

Constitution and aims

1 To promote the awareness of, and interest in, diabetes within primary care.

2 To encourage evidence-based practice in relation to diabetes care by the primary care team, including the implementation of appropriate standards.

3 To promote research and development related to providing good quality diabetes care in the primary care setting.

4 To act as a resource for the provision of high-quality integrated care information about diabetes for the primary care team.

5 To promote the integration of diabetes care amongst all healthcare professionals.

6 To contribute actively to discussion on diabetes issues at national level.

6 To embrace the aims of the Primary Care Diabetes Europe Group, of which PCDS is an active member.

Diabetes and Primary Care journal is the official publication for the society.

Diabetes UK

(See Appendix 4 for details.)

The Diabetes Industry Group
(www.diabetesindustrygroup.com)

The Diabetes Industry Group (DIG) was formed in 1996 to launch Primary Care Diabetes UK, in association with the British Diabetic Association (now Diabetes UK).

DIG assists in raising the profile of diabetes and related disorders. Acting as a non-profit organisation, it aims to enhance diabetes education and make it accessible to the widest number of people. DIG's most recent strategy has been to work in close association with the Department of Health, Diabetes UK and Strategic Health Authorities on the implementation of the National Service Framework for Diabetes. Its main objective is to serve the diabetes community and generate a positive image of the industry, notwithstanding the realities of commercial activity.

Scottish Diabetes Industry Group

The Scottish Diabetes Industry Group was set up in the spring of 2002 under the auspices of the Association of the British Pharmaceutical Industry, Scotland, as a direct response to requests from the Scottish Diabetes Framework Working Group for assistance in implementing the Framework.

Diabetes Research and Wellness Foundation
(www.drwf.org.uk)

Mission statement

The Diabetes Research and Wellness Foundation (DRWF) was established to assist in the relief of persons with diabetes and to raise awareness about diabetes and its associated complications.

DRWF's main objective is 'staying well until a cure is found' and in furtherance of this aim, provides support to those with diabetes by way of a 'Diabetes Wellness Network'.

The Wellness Network was founded because people with diabetes have to make decisions about their general health as well as their diabetes. The Network aims to help people with diabetes deal with these problems, whilst bearing in mind their diabetic condition.

The *Diabetes Wellness News*, the monthly publication, works towards educating, informing and reminding of the best and healthiest choices to make. It is a digest of magazines, newspapers, books and scientific journals – bringing you first class articles from respected diabetes and other healthcare professionals.

With the generous support of many donors, DRWF have been able to fund vital research projects at many leading institutions in the UK. Applications for funds are assessed by the DRWF Research Advisory Board, who are a panel of multi-disciplinary clinicians and scientists. This ensures that funds are distributed to the most viable and current projects, which are most likely to find the cause or cures for diabetes and alleviate its possible complications.

Patient UK (www.patient.co.uk)

Patient UK supplies:

- 699 leaflets on health and disease, some of which have been translated. Most GPs in the UK use these same leaflets to print out for patients and carers during consultations.
- Details of 2001 patient support/self help groups and similar organisations.
- 810 leaflets providing comprehensive information about medicines and online pharmacy.
- Advice on leading a healthy lifestyle, health promotion and preventing illness.
- Explanations and information about tests and investigations commonly performed.
- A directory of UK websites on disease, health news, events, equipment, helplines, benefits, NHS information, carers' issues, dictionaries, women's health, evidence based medicine, etc.
- Health related books.
- Patient Experience – real experiences of medical conditions.
- Find a GP, specialist, hospital, dentist, therapist, counsellor, etc.

Insulin Dependent Diabetes Trust (www.iddtinternational.org)

This is a charity based in the UK that listens to people with diabetes and their carers and supports their needs. The Trust describes itself as follows:

The Insulin Dependent Diabetes Trust (IDDT) is a registered charity and was formed in 1994. We are concerned with listening to the needs of people who live with diabetes, understanding those needs and doing our utmost to offer help and support. We not only want to help those who actually have diabetes but also their carers – the husbands, wives, partners and parents, indeed, all of us who 'live with diabetes'. We recognise that when one person in a family has diabetes, all other family members are affected to a greater or lesser extent and they all have views and needs which may be different from the person with diabetes, but nevertheless are important.

The Trust was set up to look at some of the day to day difficulties of living with diabetes, the worries, fears and concerns that perhaps we don't talk about at the hospital clinic – the ones that many of us experience and understand because we actually live with diabetes. As a charity, IDDT has a Board of Trustees and all our Trustees either have diabetes or have family members with diabetes. So we all know first hand that while diabetes doesn't rule our lives, it is an important part of them. It needs care and attention, it can be a nuisance and it is not without its problems!

Appendix 3

Recommendations for the provision of services in primary care for people with diabetes

This extract is taken from the above document published by Diabetes UK (2005), with permission.

The purpose of this document is to provide guidance to health professionals working in primary care on the organisation and delivery of services for people with diabetes. The emphasis is primarily on the organisation of diabetes care, rather than on the clinical management of individuals with diabetes. Detailed guidelines for the clinical management of diabetes have been produced by the National Institute for Health and Clinical Excellence (NICE), the Scottish Intercollegiate Guidelines Network (SIGN) and the Clinical Resource Efficiency Support Team in Northern Ireland (CREST).

Aims of diabetes care

The overall aim of diabetes care is to enable people with diabetes to achieve a quality of life and life expectancy similar to that of the general population.

Ensuring equitable access to high quality diabetes prevention and care is also a vital attribute of a good diabetes service – this includes ensuring equitable access for vulnerable groups, such as those living in institutional care and those experiencing social deprivation, as well as for black and minority ethnic groups.

The overall prevalence of Type 2 diabetes in the population can be reduced by preventing obesity in the general population and promoting a healthy diet and physical activity. Individuals at increased risk of developing Type 2 diabetes can reduce their risk if they are supported to change their lifestyle by eating a balanced diet, losing weight and increasing their physical activity levels. Multi-agency action is therefore required to reduce the numbers of people who are physically inactive, overweight and obese, by promoting a balanced diet and physical activity across the population. In order to have the greatest impact, action must start in childhood. Action is also needed to help those who are already overweight or obese to lose weight, and people who are physically inactive to increase their levels of physical activity. Primary care professionals have a key role to play in preventing, or at least delaying, Type 2 diabetes by identifying people at increased risk of developing diabetes and supporting them to reduce this risk.

It is now generally accepted that early diagnosis and treatment of people with Type 2 diabetes can also help reduce their likelihood of developing long-term complications and the costs associated with diabetes. Although population-wide screening for diabetes is not considered to be cost effective, it is recommended that screening of those at increased risk of developing diabetes should become a routine part of diabetes services.

The maintenance of near normal blood glucose levels is crucial to the prevention of the microvascular complications of diabetes – diabetic retinopathy, diabetic renal disease and diabetic neuropathy – as well as to the alleviation of the symptoms of diabetes and the avoidance of the acute metabolic crises (hypoglycaemia and ketoacidosis). Regular surveillance for and reduction of cardiovascular risk factors is equally important – this will include, where indicated, the provision of smoking cessation advice, healthy weight management, the promotion of physical activity and the treatment of dyslipidaemia and hypertension.

The active involvement of people with diabetes in the provision of their own care is the cornerstone of good diabetes care. This requires the provision of effective, ongoing education and support, which is matched to the individual's ability and capacity to learn and recognises the importance of the individual's lifestyle, culture and religion. People with diabetes should also be empowered to obtain the maximum benefit from healthcare services so that, as far as possible, they are able to participate in activities open to those who do not have diabetes.

The early detection and treatment of many of the long-term complications of diabetes can reduce morbidity and healthcare costs. In diabetic retinopathy, for example, the early detection of sight threatening retinal disease followed by laser treatment can prevent blindness. Similarly, structured foot care assessment can prevent foot ulcers and amputations. Planned follow-up with effective surveillance for complications is therefore essential.

National standards for the provision of diabetes care have been published in all four nations of the UK. In August 2001, Scotland published their Scottish Diabetes Framework. In December 2001, the Department of Health published the first part of the National Service Framework for Diabetes. This document set out twelve standards for the provision of diabetes prevention and care. These standards have since been adopted by the Assembly for Wales. A national framework for the provision of diabetes care has also been agreed in Northern Ireland. Further information about these frameworks is available on the following websites:

England: www.dh.gov.uk

Wales: www.wales.nhs.uk

Scotland: www.show.scot.nhs.uk

Northern Ireland: www.crestni.org.uk

Provision of diabetes care

Diabetes UK has produced a leaflet for people with diabetes entitled *What diabetes care to expect*. The leaflet, which is available from Diabetes UK (freephone 0800 585 088), explains what treatment and advice people with diabetes should expect from their healthcare team. The leaflet stresses the importance of individuals understanding their diabetes so that they are enabled to manage their own diabetes and become effective members of the healthcare team. Increasingly, people with diabetes will therefore expect to receive the level of care specified in the leaflet, wherever their diabetes care is being provided.

Diabetes care should be person-centred and should aim to empower individuals to manage their own diabetes. Professionals providing diabetes care should support individuals to manage their own diabetes and help them to adopt and maintain a healthy lifestyle. They should actively encourage partnership in decision-making, thereby enabling people with diabetes to have choice, voice and control over what happens to them at each step of their care. A care plan, negotiated and agreed with each individual, set out in an appropriate format and language for the individual, and reviewed as part of the care planning process, is key to the achievement of this aim. Where appropriate, parents and carers should also be fully engaged in this process.

In order to support and encourage self-care and self-management, all healthcare staff should:

- treat individuals with respect and dignity

- ensure that people with diabetes know how to contact members of the team providing their diabetes care and ideally should have a named person who is their main contact

- provide high quality care and regularly review their clinical and psychological needs

- answer any questions about the quality of services received

- provide interpreting services if English is not the person's first language and seek appropriate services for those with sensory impairment or learning disability

- provide information and structured education about diabetes management and local health related services

- remain up to date about diabetes and its care and treatment, in order to keep people with diabetes up to date about their condition

- facilitate access to a second opinion where required (subject to the agreement of the person's GP [general practitioner] or consultant)

- give information about Diabetes UK services and details of local support groups – information is available on the Diabetes UK website (www.diabetes.org.uk).

The responsibilities of the person with diabetes are to:

- take as much control of their diabetes on a day-to-day basis as possible – the more the person knows about his or her own diabetes, the easier this will become

- learn about and practice self-care, which should include dietary management, exercise, taking medication as prescribed, the monitoring of blood glucose levels by blood or urine

- testing and knowing what action to take – decisions about self-care should be made as a result of informed choice

- examine their feet regularly or have someone else check them

- know how to manage their diabetes and when to seek help if they are ill – for example, if they develop a chest infection, flu, diarrhoea or vomiting

- build into their daily life the diabetes advice discussed with their care team

- talk regularly with members of their diabetes care team

- ask questions during consultations, using a list if they find this helpful

- attend scheduled appointments and inform the healthcare team if they are unable to attend.

Skills required to provide care for people with diabetes in primary care

The care of people with diabetes within the primary care setting should be provided by a multidisciplinary team, including, as a minimum, the GP and practice nurse, supported by administrative staff. Other members of the primary healthcare team, including registered dietitians, podiatrists, district nurses, midwives, health visitors and school nurses and counsellors, also have an important role to play in the provision of diabetes care.

Experience suggests that a nurse, usually the practice nurse, is essential to the successful provision of diabetes care within the primary care setting. The GP should also be actively involved, particularly in the optimisation of blood glucose and lipid control, the management of hypertension and the identification and management of diabetic complications.

Key elements of effective diabetes care:

- practice-based registers of people at increased risk of developing diabetes to facilitate the regular testing of and provision of lifestyle advice to people at risk of developing diabetes

- practice-based registers of people with diagnosed diabetes to facilitate the regular call and recall for review of all people with diabetes, which are shared between primary and secondary care

- practice guidelines for the prevention and management of diabetes

- clear patient centred individualised care plans agreed with each person with diabetes that are tailored to meet the needs of the individual and, where appropriate, their carers

- personal diabetes records that can be shared with and accessed by all the health professionals involved in providing care to an individual – as well as the person with diabetes

- a local diabetes policy that includes suggested criteria for referring people with diabetes to specialist diabetes services

- an agreed named contact to help guide the person with diabetes through the healthcare system

Pharmacists are increasingly becoming active members of the primary healthcare team. The new pharmaceutical services contract includes familiar essential services, such as dispensing, signposting and sharps disposal. However, an increasing number of pharmacists are likely to offer additional and enhanced services, which could include full clinical medicines review, diabetes and CHD [coronary heart disease] screening, smoking cessation and care home services. For further information on the role of the pharmacist in diabetes care, see the joint Royal Pharmaceutical Society of Great Britain/Diabetes UK guidance documents at www.rpsgb.org.uk.

The primary healthcare team should be supported by additional personnel, including consultant diabetologists, diabetes specialist nurses, as well as by the provision of a retinal screening programme.

Members of the primary healthcare team involved in the provision of diabetes care need to be trained in:

- **communication** – including the ability to communicate with other members of the primary healthcare team, specialist care colleagues and colleagues working in other agencies, as well as with people with diabetes and their carers. Staff should also be skilled in behavioural change counselling and have the skills necessary to motivate change and to negotiate and agree goals

- **the provision of education, information and support** – including the ability to impart the necessary knowledge, motivation and self-care skills to enable people with diabetes to take responsibility for their own healthcare, and an understanding of the emotional and social problems likely to be faced by people with diabetes

- **diagnosis and examination** – including the identification of the complications of diabetes

- **clinical management** – including the management of diabetes and its complications, associated conditions, cardiovascular risk factors and care planning skills

- **record keeping and administration** – including the maintenance of personal diabetes records, a diabetes register and a call/recall system.

Sufficient time should be allocated and funding provided to enable all members of the primary health care team to attend relevant recognised courses on the management of diabetes. Continuing education and training are essential.

Planning mechanisms across the nations

Since the publication of the national diabetes frameworks, the organisations responsible at local level for commissioning healthcare have been establishing mechanisms to coordinate the effective planning of local diabetes services. The result has been a new emphasis on the development of local diabetes networks to shape policy and practice and enable the provision of high quality, integrated local diabetes services across multiple providers and communities.

Emphasis has been placed upon user involvement in all aspects of diabetes service planning and local planning mechanisms should offer people with diabetes opportunities to get involved in improving the quality of local diabetes services.

In England, responsibility for ensuring local health service provision lies with primary care trusts (PCTs). The National Service Framework for Diabetes: Delivery Strategy recommends an integrated approach to the planning of local diabetes services. This includes:

- a focus on the development of managed diabetes networks

- the reshaping and strengthening of the role of advisory groups as the link between the diabetes networks and PCTs, with accountability for decision-making

- the appointment of diabetes champions and network managers in each PCT.

In Wales, responsibility for local health service provision lies with local health boards, which have the same boundaries as local authorities. The National Service Framework for Diabetes in Wales: Delivery Strategy recommends an integrated approach to local planning, drawing on the Welsh national health strategy Improving Health in Wales. This includes:

- developing the role of local diabetes service advisory groups (LDSAGs) as the mechanism for NSF implementation – or, where LDSAGs do not currently exist, setting up new multistakeholder groups
- the creation of separate user reference groups of people with diabetes, one to relate to each LDSAG.

In Scotland, responsibility for local health service provision lies with regional NHS [National Health Service] boards. The Scottish Diabetes Framework sets out local planning arrangements. These include:

- the identification of local clinical leaders to champion the provision of integrated diabetes services
- the appointment of local 'diabetes coordinators' to improve communication among local diabetes stakeholders, especially between primary and secondary care professionals
- the retention (or creation) of local diabetes service advisory groups with a stronger role in driving change in diabetes services at regional level
- the establishment of managed clinical networks in all regions.

In Northern Ireland, responsibility for local health services and local social services lies with health and social care boards. The Diabetes UK/CREST report on diabetes outlines the importance of lead consultants and GPs working closely together to ensure full integration of diabetes services between primary and secondary care. The report recommends the identification of regional project managers to lead the initiatives on integrated care, eye screening and diabetes registers and information. The report also outlines the following standards for integrated diabetes care:

- there should be agreed guidelines (including indications for referral to hospital) for primary and secondary care
- services should be coordinated between primary and secondary care

- all people with diabetes should have an annual review with a structured format

- the annual review is for screening, prevention and treatment of complications

- management goals are agreed between the person with diabetes and the diabetes team at the annual review

- people with diabetes should be able to contact the diabetes team at any time for advice either in person or by phone

- education and information is an integral part of diabetes care

- people with diabetes can choose to manage their own care in hospital if they are well enough to do so

- all service providers receive regular education and updating on developments in diabetes care.

Diabetes UK

All those concerned with diabetes should be encouraged to join Diabetes UK, including:

- patients, their relatives and friends

- healthcare professionals and managers

Membership benefits for people with diabetes and their carers include:

- six issues a year of our members' magazine, *Balance*, packed with news and information

- Diabetes UK Careline for confidential support and information

- a wide range of booklets packed with information about managing diabetes, eating healthily, reducing the risk of complications and more

- a chance to share experiences with others at over 400 Diabetes UK voluntary groups across the country

- Diabetes UK Services' insurance and financial products designed to meet the needs of people with diabetes

- the opportunity to help yourself and others with diabetes in the UK.

Membership benefits for the healthcare professional include:

- *Diabetes Update* our quarterly magazine for healthcare professionals, keeping you informed of diabetes care and research developments

- *Balance*, our bi-monthly patient focused magazine giving practical advice on living with diabetes

- regular mailings to keep you updated about Diabetes UK activities relevant to healthcare professionals

- *Diabetic Medicine*, our monthly journal publishing reviews and original articles in the fields of diabetes research and practice, available at a substantial discount

- discounted delegate fees for Diabetes UK professional conferences (including the Annual Professional Conference)

- travel grant support for presenting authors at all diabetes-related conferences in Europe

- 25 per cent discount on our information publications.

Contact details can be found in Appendix 4.

Appendix 4

Resources for the provision of diabetes care

- Education
- Books for people with diabetes
- Books for the primary care team
- Reports/papers
- Websites
- Diabetes UK publications
- Journals
- Companies
- Diabetes-focused organisations for professionals
- Patient support organisations

Education

Warwick Diabetes Care
Warwick Diabetes Care
Farmhouse Building, Gibbet Hill Campus, University of Warwick,
Coventry CV4 7AL
Tel: 02476 572958
Fax: 02476 573959
Email: diabetes@warwick.ac.uk
Website: www.diabetescare.warwick.ac.uk

Warwick Diabetes Care provides education and training in diabetes care
to healthcare professionals, from workshops and short courses to part-
time and full-time Masters programmes. Over 5000 doctors, nurses and
other community-based healthcare professionals have undertaken the
certificate in diabetes care (CIDC) since it was launched, and their provision of different delivery methods, in particular distance delivery, has
allowed the course to be delivered in over a third of primary care trusts.

The number of healthcare professionals applying to study continues to grow, reflecting national recognition that it is the premier qualification of its type. A brief introduction to each course is given below.

Masters in Diabetes
The Masters in Diabetes provides a programme dedicated to diabetes for those wishing to specialise. It aims to give hospital doctors, specialist nurses and other health professionals involved in the care of people with diabetes the necessary knowledge and skills to provide high-quality care.

MSc in Health Sciences (Diabetes)
The course has been designed for health professionals who wish to develop a special interest in diabetes care but would also like to take some modules on other topics. This makes it possible for the area of special interest to be reflected in the degree title while allowing the flexibility for work in a wide range of other areas (including medical education, health services management or public health) to count towards the degree.

Masters modules/short courses
Any module from the Masters programmes can be taken as a freestanding short course or as part of a complete part-time Masters programme. Modules are worth 20 Credit Accumulation and Transfer Scheme (CATS) credits.

Certificate in Diabetes Care (Level 2)
The CIDC course is the UK's leading foundation course in diabetes care. It provides healthcare professionals with the practical knowledge and skills necessary to provide an effective and efficient service for people with diabetes.

Postgraduate Certificate in Diabetes Care for Dietitians
This Postgraduate Certificate has been specially developed to give dietitians involved in the care of people with diabetes mellitus the knowledge to further their professional expertise in this specialist area. By addressing the higher educational needs of dietitians, this Postgraduate Certificate will increase knowledge and understanding of the therapeutic role of nutritional management in the provision of diabetes care.

Short courses
Advanced Leaders Programme: this programme trains healthcare professionals with established expertise in diabetes to facilitate and teach the

University of Warwick assessed and accredited CIDC course in their local district. It is a 2-day residential programme held in a purpose-built conference centre with excellent facilities at the University of Warwick.

Intensive Management in Type 2 Diabetes: this course is designed to provide advanced skills to enable the effective management of people with type 2 diabetes, including initiating insulin. A Warwick Diabetes Care accredited trainer will facilitate the course for general practitioner (GP) and nurse teams in their own locality.

Workshops in Diabetes Care: Warwick Diabetes Care has designed a broad portfolio of 1-day diabetes care workshops that can be used flexibly to meet the diverse educational needs associated with diabetes. These can be used to build bespoke programmes to meet individual or organisational needs by choosing relevant topics from the workshop menu.

Primary Care Training Centre (Distance Learning)

Primary Care Training Centre
Crow Trees, 27 Town Lane, Idle, Bradford, West Yorkshire BD10 8NT
Tel: 01274 617617
Fax: 01274 621621
Email: admin@primarycaretraining.co.uk
Website: www.primarycaretraining.co.uk

Diabetes Management in Primary Care

This course, worth 2 CATS credits (Level 2) is suitable for health professionals who hold a relevant qualification in healthcare, for example registered nurses, doctors, registered dietitians, registered podiatrists and pharmacists. As the course is related to clinical practice, applicants are expected to be working with patients who have diabetes.

The content involves practical guidance given for total management within primary care. A multifactorial approach is advocated for insulin resistance and diabetes. The subject is covered in a logical manner from diagnosis through treatment (including insulin and insulin conversion) to monitoring for and the management of complications. Coursework enhances this with every item relevant to improving patient care. Learning continues at the workshops.

In Balance Healthcare UK

Skills-based, quality-assured learning programmes on many aspects of diabetes care.
Website: www.ibhuk.com.

Practical, useful and interesting books for people with diabetes

Bilous RW (2000). *Understanding Diabetes*. London: Family Doctor Publications.

Blair L, McGough N (2005). *Quick Cooking for Diabetes*. London: Pyramid

Cutting D, Maddocks P, Clarke M (2004). *Stop that Heart Attack!* London: Class Publishing.

Day J (2001). *Living with Diabetes: The Diabetes UK Guide for Those Treated with Diet and Tablets*. Chichester: John Wiley & Sons.

Diabetes UK, Bowling A (2001). *The Everyday Diabetic Cookbook*. London: Grub Street.

Estridge B (1996). *Diabetes and Your Teenager*. London: Thorsons.

Fox C, Kilvert A (2007) *Type 1 Diabetes* and *Type 2 Diabetes: Answers at your fingertips*. Both Class Publishing: London.

Hart JT, Fahey T, Savage W (1999). *High Blood Pressure at Your Fingertips*. London: Class Publishing

Hanas R (2006). *Type 1 Diabetes in Children, Adolescents and Young Adults. How to Become an Expert on Your Own Diabetes*, 3rd edn. London: Class Health.

Hillson R (2002). *Diabetes: The Complete Guide*. London: Vermilion.

Jackson G (2004). *Heart Health at Your Fingertips*. London: Class Publishing.

Jarvis S, Rubins A (2003). *Diabetes for Dummies*. Chichester: John Wiley & Sons.

Lewycka M (1999). *Caring for Someone with Diabetes*. London: Age Concern

Walker R, Rodgers J (2004). *Diabetes: A Practical Guide to Managing Your Health*. London: Dorling Kindersley

Walker R, Rodgers J (2006). *Type 2 Diabetes – Your Questions Answered*. London: Dorling Kindersley.

Multimedia packages

'Learning Diabetes (Insulin Treated)' and 'Learning Diabetes (Non-insulin Treated)' are multimedia patient education programmes produced as a package called 'Managing Your Health' by Interactive Eurohealth. For information, go to www.interactiveeurohealth.com/index.html.

Useful books for the primary care team

Andrews M, Boyle J (2002). *Transcultural Concepts in Nursing Care*, 4th edn. Philadelphia: Lippincott Williams & Wilkins.

Campbell IW, Lebovitz H (2000). *Fast Facts – Diabetes Mellitus*. Oxford: Health Press.

Chambers R, Stead J, Wakley G (2001). *Diabetes Matters in Primary Care.* Oxford: Radcliffe Medical Press.

Edmonds M, Foster A. (2005). *Managing the Diabetic Foot.* Oxford: Blackwell Publishing.

Fox C, MacKinnon M (2007). *Vital Diabetes*, 4th edn. London: Class Publishing.

Gadsby R (2005). *Delivering Quality Diabetes Care in General Practice.* London: RCGP.

Marso SP (ed.) (2003). *The Handbook of Diabetes Mellitus and Cardiovascular Disease.* London: Remidica.

Patroe L (2001). *An Executive Summary of the Diabetes Development Fund for Black and Minority Ethnic Communities in the North West of England.* London: Diabetes UK.

Pickup J, Williams G (2004). *The Handbook of Diabetes*, 3rd edn. Oxford: Blackwell Publishing.

Watkins PJ, Amiel S, Howell S, Turner E (2003). *Diabetes and its Management*, 6th edn. Oxford: Blackwell Science.

Useful reports/papers

Audit Commission (2000). *Testing Times: A Review of Diabetes Services in England and Wales.* London: Audit Commission.

British Diabetic Association (now Diabetes UK) (1996). *Diabetes and Cognitive Function: The Evidence So Far.* London: BDA.

Burlace S (2001). Reducing stroke risk in ethnic minorities. *Best Practice* 18 July: 14–15.

Campbell H, Hotchkiss R, Bradshaw N, Porteous M (1998). Integrated care pathways. *British Medical Journal* **316**: 133–137.

Department of Health (2000). *National Service Frameworks. Coronary Heart Disease. Modern Standards and Service Models.* London: DoH.

Department of Health (2001). *National Service Framework for Diabetes: Standards.* London: DoH.

Department of Health (2001). *The Expert Patient. A New Approach to Chronic Disease Management for the 21st Century.* London: DoH.

Department of Health (2002). *National Service Framework for Diabetes: Delivery Strategy.* London: DoH.

Diabetes Control and Complications Trial (DCCT) Research Group (1993). The effect of intensive treatment of diabetes on the development and progression of long-term complications in insulin-dependent diabetes mellitus. *New England Journal of Medicine* **329**: 977–986.

Diabetes Control and Complications Trial (DCCT) Research Group (1995). Effect of intensive diabetes management on macrovascular event and risk factors in the diabetes control and complications trial. *American Journal of Cardiology* **75**: 894–903.

Donnan PT, MacDonald TM, Morris AD (2000). Adherence to prescribed medication for patients with type 2 diabetes: a population study. *Diabetic Medicine* **17** (Suppl. 1): 2.

Gray A, Clarke P, Farmer A, Holman R (2002). Implementing intensive control of blood glucose concentration and blood pressure in type 2 diabetes in England: cost analysis. UKPDS 63. *British Medical Journal* **325**: 860–863.

Greenhalgh PM (1997). Diabetes in British South Asians: nature, nurture and culture. *Diabetic Medicine* **14**: 10–18.

Greenhalgh T (ed) (1998). Diabetes care: a primary care perspective. *Diabetic Medicine* **15** (Suppl 3): S1–S64.

Groop LC (1999). Insulin resistance: the fundamental trigger of type 2 diabetes. *Diabetes, Obesity and Metabolism* **1**: S1–S7.

Hansson L et al. (1998). The Hypertension Optimal Treatment (HOT) Study: 24 month data on blood pressure and tolerability. *Lancet* **351**: 1755–1762.

Hippisley-Cox J, Pringle M (2004). Prevalence, care and outcomes for patients with diet controlled diabetes in primary care: cross sectional survey. *Lancet* **364**: 423–425.

House of Commons (2004). *Health, Third Report. Obesity.* London: House of Commons Publications.

Kings Fund (1996). *Counting the Cost of Type 2 Diabetes.* London: Kings Fund/British Diabetic Association (now Diabetes UK).

Medical Devices Agency (now MHRA) (2000). Device Bulletin. Blood Pressure Measurement Devices – Mercury and Non-mercury. MDA DB2000(03). London: MDA.

Modernisation Agency/NICE (2004). *Protocol-based Care: A Step By Step Guide To Developing Protocols.* London: DoH.

Munro N, Rich N, McIntosh C, Foster A, Edmonds M (2003). Infections in the diabetic foot. *British Journal of Diabetes and Vascular Disease* **3**: 132–136.

National Institute for Health and Clinical Excellence (2002). *Management of Type 2 Diabetes: Retinopathy – Screening and Early Management.* Inherited Guideline E. London: DoH.

National Institute for Health and Clinical Excellence (2002). *Management of Type 2 Diabetes. Renal Disease – Prevention and Early Management.* Inherited Guideline F. London: NICE.

National Institute for Health and Clinical Excellence (2002). *Management of Type 2 Diabetes: Management of Blood Glucose.* Inherited Guideline G. London: NICE.

National Institute for Health and Clinical Excellence (2002). *Management of Type 2 Diabetes. Management of Blood Pressure and Blood Lipids.* Inherited Guideline H. London: NICE.

National Institute for Health and Clinical Excellence (2003). *Guidance on the Use of Patient-education Models for Diabetes.* Technology Appraisal 60. London: DoH.

National Institute for Health and Clinical Excellence (2004). *Management of Type 2 Diabetes. Prevention and Management of Foot Problems*. London: NICE.

National Prescribing Centre (2002). When and how should patients with diabetes mellitus test blood glucose? *MeReC Bulletin* **13**: 1–4.

NHS Modernisation Agency (2002). *Workforce Matters. A Guide to Role Redesign in Diabetes Care*. London DoH.

Nutrition Subcommittee of the Diabetes Care Advisory Committee of Diabetes UK (2003). The implementation of nutritional advice for people with diabetes. *Diabetic Medicine* **20**: 786–807.

O'Brien E, Waeber B, Parati G, Staessen J, Myers MG (2001). Blood pressure measuring devices: recommendations of the European Society of Hypertension. *British Medical Journal* **322**: 531–536.

Pierce M, Agarwal G, Ridout D (2000). A survey of diabetes care in general practice in England and Wales. *British Journal of General Practice* **50**: 542–545.

Pinar R (2002). Management of people with diabetes during Ramadan. *British Journal of Nursing* **11**: 1300–1303.

Reasner CA, Burkhard G (2002). Overcoming the barriers to effective glycaemic control for type 2 diabetes. *British Journal of Diabetes and Vascular Disease* **2**: 290–295.

Scott P (2001). Caribbean people's health beliefs about the body and their implications for diabetes management: a South London study. *Practical Diabetes International* **18**: 94–98.

Scottish Intercollegiate Guidelines Network (1997). *Management of Diabetic Cardiovascular Disease. National Clinical Guideline for Scotland*. Edinburgh: SIGN.

Scottish Intercollegiate Guidelines Network (1997). *Management of Diabetic Foot Disease. National Clinical Guideline for Scotland*. Edinburgh: SIGN.

Scottish Intercollegiate Guidelines Network (1997). *Management of Diabetic Renal Disease. National Clinical Guideline for Scotland*. SIGN, Edinburgh.

Scottish Intercollegiate Guidelines Network (1998). *Prevention of Visual Impairment. National Clinical Guideline for Scotland*. Edinburgh: SIGN.

Sinclair A, Turnbull C, Croxson S (1996). Document of care for older people with diabetes. *Postgraduate Medical Journal* **72**: 334–338.

Turner RC, Millns H, Neil H, Stratton I, Manley S, Matthews E, Holman R (1998). UKPDS study group. Risk factors for coronary artery disease in non-insulin dependent diabetes mellitus. UKPDS 23. *British Medical Journal* **416**: 823–828.

UK Prospective Diabetes Study Group (1998). Intensive blood-glucose control with sulphonylureas or insulin compared with conventional treatment and risk of complications in patients with type 2 diabetes. UKPDS 33. *Lancet* **352**: 837–853.

UK Prospective Diabetes Study Group (1998). Effect of intensive blood-glucose control with metformin on complications in overweight patients with type 2 diabetes. UKPDS 34. *Lancet* **352**: 854–865.

UK Prospective Diabetes Study Group (1998). Tight blood pressure control and risk of macrovascular and microvascular complications in type 2 diabetes. UKPDS 38. *British Medical Journal* 317: 703–713.

Williams B, Poulter NR, Brown MJ et al (2004). Guidelines for management of hypertension: report of the fourth working party of the British Hypertension Society. *Journal of Human Hypertension* 18: 139–85.

Wood D, Durrington P, Poulter N, McInnes G, Rees A, Wray R (1998). British Recommendations on Prevention of Coronary Heart Disease in Clinical Practice. *Heart* 80 (Suppl. II). S1–S29.

World Health Organization (1999). *Definition, Diagnosis and Classification of Diabetes Mellitus and its Complications. Part 1. Diagnosis and Classification of Diabetes Mellitus.* Geneva: WHO.

Useful websites

If you cannot find information, you can 'Google' it. Log onto the Internet and type www.google.co.uk into the address box. Then type the topic you want to find into the search box and Google will provide you with a list of the most relevant links to websites on the Internet. Be selective how you search – typing 'diabetes' will bring up thousands of websites, whereas 'diabetes structured education UK' will identify only websites concerned with structured education in diabetes in the UK. When you see the result nearest to what you want, click on the link provided. For an interactive tutorial, go to www.googleguide.com.

British Medical Association – www.bma.org,uk
British Medical Journal – www.bmj.com
British National Formulary – www.bnf.org.uk
Confidential Enquiry into Maternal and Child Health – www.cemach.org.uk
Department of Health – www.dh.gov.uk; for diabetes –
    www.dh.gov.uk/PolicyAndGuidance/HealthAndSocialCareTopics/Diabetes/fs/en
Diabetes Education and Self Management for Ongoing and Newly
    Diagnosed (DESMOND) – www.desmond-project.org.uk
Diabetes UK – www.diabetes.org.uk
Diabetic foot (foot care leaflets in 31 languages) – www.diabeticfoot.org.uk
Dose Adjustment for Normal Eating (DAFNE) – www.dafne.uk.com
Driver and Vehicle Licensing Agency (DVLA) – www.dvla.gov.uk
Epsom and St Helier University Hospitals NHS Trust, Chronic Kidney
    Disease – www.epsom-sthelier.nhs.uk and enter CKD in the search box.
Expert Patient programme – www.expertpatients.nhs.uk
Health Service Ombudsman – www.ombudsman.org.uk
International Diabetes Federation – www.idf.org

Joslin Diabetes Centre (educational website) –
www.joslin.harvard.edu/education
Medicines and Healthcare products Regulatory Agency –
www.mhra.gov.uk
Medscape (an excellent free resource with a section on diabetes) –
www.medscape.com
National Diabetes Support Team – www.diabetes.nhs.uk
National electronic Library for Health, diabetes – www.nelh.nhs.uk/diabetes
National Institute for Health and Clinical Excellence (NICE) –
www.nice.org.uk
National Screening Committee – www.nsc.nhs.uk
NHS Modernisation Agency – www.wise.nhs.uk/cmswise/default.htm
NSC retinopathy – www.nscretinopathy.org.uk
Patient UK (comprehensive, free and up-to-date health information
as provided by GPs to patients during consultations) –
www.patient.co.uk
Quality Assurance Agency – www.qaa.ac.uk
Quality Management and Analysis System –
www.connectingforhealth.nhs.uk/delivery/programmes/qmas
The Information Centre, National Diabetes Audit – www.ic.nhs.uk
UK government – www.publications.parliament.uk
Warwick Diabetes Care – www.diabetescare.warwick.ac.uk
X-PERT Diabetes – www.xpert-diabetes.org.uk

Diabetes UK publications

Diabetes UK publishes a comprehensive catalogue of leaflets, books and
videos. You can access the catalogue online (www.diabetes.org.uk) or request
a free copy from the distribution centre. To order from the wide range
of books, magazines and booklets included in the catalogue, contact
Diabetes UK Distribution:

- ■ *By telephone*: order with Access/Visa/Switch/Delta card by
  calling free on 0800 585 088, quoting the relevant publication
  code.

- ■ *By post*: download a catalogue order form from the website
  (you'll need Adobe Acrobat Reader to view the form), complete
  it and return it to Diabetes UK Distribution, PO Box 1057,
  Bedford MK42 7XQ, with payment by Access/Visa/Switch/
  Delta card or a cheque made payable to Diabetes UK Services
  Limited.

Balance for Beginners

This is a range of magazines for people newly diagnosed with diabetes, or those who would like to update their knowledge:

- *Diabetes Type 1* – also available as an audiotape.
- *Diabetes for Beginners Type 2* – also available as an audiotape.
- *Just for You* – for children.
- *Tots to Teens* – for parents.
- *Pregnancy and Diabetes.*

Booklets

Only a selection is given here; many more are available online or in the catalogue:

- *Understanding Diabetes* (free; downloadable).
- *What Care To Expect* (free; downloadable) – also produced in audiotape format in Bengali, Gujarati, Urdu, Hindi and Punjabi.
- *Coping With Diabetes When You Are Ill.*
- *What is Diabetes?* (free) – in English, Bengali, Gujarati, Urdu, Hindi, Punjabi and Chinese.
- *Diabetes: A Guide for African-Caribbean People.*
- *Diabetes: A Guide for South Asian People.*
- *Healthy Lifestyle, Fasting and Diabetes.*
- *Ramadan and Diabetes* (free) – in Bengali, Gujarati, Urdu, Hindi and Punjabi.
- *Eating Well with Diabetes* (free).
- *Sex and Diabetes – A Guide to Erection Problems.*

Reports

Again, only a selection is given here; many more reports and recommendations are available online:

- *Diabetes Blindness: A Focus on Action* (2005).
- *Structured Patient Education in Diabetes* (2005).
- *Diabetes in the United Kingdom* (2004).
- *Guidelines of Practice for Residents with Diabetes in Care Homes* (1999).

- *Diabetic Medicine* is issued 12 times per year. This can be purchased through professional membership of Diabetes UK.

- *Diabetes Update* is a periodic magazine (free to members) for healthcare professionals interested in diabetes. It is available from Diabetes UK.

- *Diabetes and Primary Care* is published four times a year. It can be obtained from:
      SB Communications Group,
      15 Manderville Courtyard,
      142 Battersea Park Road,
      London SW11 4NB
      Tel: 020 7627 1510
      Fax: 020 7627 1570
      Website: www.diabetesprimarycare.com

- *Journal of Diabetes Nursing* has six issues a year. Subscriptions are available from the SB Communications Group (see above).

- *Practical Diabetes International* is published nine times a year and is available from:
      John Wiley & Sons,
      The Atrium,
      Southern Gate,
      Chichester,
      West Sussex PO19 8SQ
      Tel: 01243 770520
      Fax: 01243 770144

   To subscribe, contact:
      Journals Subscriptions Department,
      John Wiley & Sons Ltd,
      1 Oldlands Way,
      Bognor Regis,
      West Sussex PO22 9SA
      Tel: 01243 779777
      Fax: 01243 843232
      Email: cs-journals@wiley.co.uk

■ *Practice Nurse Journal* is a fortnightly journal for nurses in general practice that is published by:
   Reed Business Information,
   Quadrant House,
   The Quadrant,
   Sutton,
   Surrey SM2 5AS

Subscriptions can be obtained from:
   Practice Nurse Subscriptions,
   Freepost RCCC 2619,
   Reed Business Information,
   Haywards Heath,
   West Sussex RH16 3DH
   Tel: 0845 077 7722
   Fax: 0845 676 0030

Companies

General products

The following companies provide drugs, equipment, booklets, leaflets, posters, videos, identification cards, monitoring diaries, GP information, training, clinic packs, etc. (local representatives will have specific details of what is available). Contact the companies at the addresses or telephone numbers given to ascertain exactly what they do provide.

3M United Kingdom PLC
3M Centre,
Cain Road,
Bracknell,
Berkshire RG12 8HT
Tel: 08705 360036
Website: www.3mhealthcare.co.uk

Abbott Laboratories Ltd
Abbott House,
Norden Road,
Maidenhead,
Berkshire SL6 4XE
Tel: 01628 773355
Fax: 01628 644305
Websites: www.abbottuk.com
www.diabetesnow.co.uk

Bayer plc
Diagnostics Division,
Bayer House,
Strawberry Hill,
Newbury,
Berkshire RG14 1JA
Tel: 01635 563000
Fax: 01635 563393
Email: diagnosticsuk@bayer.co.uk
Website: www.bayerdiag.com

Becton Dickinson UK Ltd
Diabetes Health Care Division,
21 Between Towns Road,
Cowley,
Oxford OX4 3LY
Tel: 01865 748844
Fax: 01865 717313
Website: www.bd.com

CP Pharmaceuticals
(See Wockhardt)

Eli Lilly & Co Ltd
Lilly House,
Priestley Road,
Basingstoke,
Hampshire RG24 9NL
Tel: 01256 315999
Website: www.lilly.co.uk

GSK – GlaxoSmithKline
Stockley Park West,
Uxbridge,
Middlesex UB11 1BT
Tel: 0800 221441
Fax: 020 8990 4328
Email: customercontactuk@gsk.com
Website: www.gsk.com

GSK Consumer Healthcare
GlaxoSmithKline
Consumer Healthcare,
GSK House,
980 Great West Road,
Brentford,
Middlesex TW8 9GS
Tel: 0500 888 878
Fax: 020 8047 6860
Email: Consumer.relations@gsk.com
Website: www.gsk.com

Hypoguard UK Ltd
Dock Lane,
Melton,
Woodridge,
Suffolk IP12 1PE
Tel: 01394 387333/4
Fax: 01394 380152

LifeScan
50–100 Holmers Farm Way,
High Wycombe,
Buckinghamshire HP12 4DP
Tel: 01494 658750
Fax: 01494 658751
Website: www.lifescan.co.uk

Medisense
Abbott Laboratories Ltd,
Mallory House,
Vanwall Business Park,
Maidenhead,
Berkshire SL6 4UD
Tel: 01628 678 900
Fax: 01628 678 805

A. Menarini Diagnostics
Wharfedale Road,
Winnersh,
Wokingham,
Berkshire RG41 5RA
Tel: 0118 944 4100
Fax: 0118 944 4111
Website: www.menarinidiag.co.uk

Merck Pharmaceuticals
Harrier House,
High Street,
Yiewsley,
West Drayton,
Middlesex UB7 7QG
Tel: 01895 452 200
Fax: 01895 452 274
Website:
www.merck-pharmaceuticals.co.uk

**Novartis Pharmaceuticals
UK Ltd**
Frimley Business Park,
Frimley,
Camberley,
Surrey GU16 7SR
Tel: 01276 692255
Fax: 01276 692508
Website: www.novartis.co.uk

Novo Nordisk Ltd
Broadfield Park,
Brighton Road,
Pease Pottage,
Crawley,
West Sussex RH11 9RT
Tel: 01293 613555
Fax: 01293 613535
Website: www.novonordisk.co.uk

Omron Healthcare (UK) Ltd
Opal Drive,
Fox Milne,
Milton Keynes MK15 0DG
Tel: 01908 258258
Fax: 01908 258158
Website:
www.omron-industrial.com/uk/home

Owen Mumford Ltd
Brook Hill,
Woodstock,
Oxford OX20 1TU
Tel: 01993 812021
Fax: 01993 813466
Website: www.owenmumford.com

Pfizer Ltd
Walton Oaks,
Dorking Road,
Tadworth,
Surrey KT20 7NS
Tel: 01304 616161
Fax: 01304 656221
Website: www.pfizer.co.uk

Roche Diagnostics Ltd
Charles Avenue,
Burgess Hill,
West Sussex RH15 9RY
Tel: 01444 256000
Email: lewes.info-uk@roche.com
Website: www.rocheuk.com
and click on 'Health'

Sanofi-Aventis
1 Onslow Street,
Guildford,
Surrey GU1 4YS
Tel: 01483 505515
Fax: 01483 535432
Website: www.sanofi-aventis.co.uk

Servier Laboratories Ltd
Gallions,
Wexham Springs,
Framewood Road,
Wexham,
Slough,
Berks SL3 6RJ
Tel: 01753 662744
Fax: 01753 663456
Website: www.servier.co.uk

Takeda UK Ltd
Takeda House,
Mercury Park,
Wycombe Lane,
Wooburn Green,
High Wycombe,
Buckinghamshire HP10 0HH
Tel: 01628 537900
Fax: 01628 526615
Website: www.takeda.co.uk

Wockhardt UK
(Previously CP Pharmaceuticals)
Ash Road North,
Wrexham Industrial Estate,
Wrexham,
Clwyd LL13 9UF
Tel: 01978 661261
Fax: 01978 660130
Website: www.wockhardt.co.uk

Specific products

Diabetes identity bracelets

Golden Key Co.
1 Hare Street,
Sheerness,
Kent ME12 1AH
Tel: 01795 663403

Medi-tag
Medi-Tag Dept,
Hoopers,
37 Northampton Street,
Hockley,
Birmingham B18 6DU
Tel: 0121 200 1616
Email: Customercare@hoopers.org
Website: www.medi-tag.co.uk

MedicAlert
1 Bridge Wharf,
156 Caledonian Road,
London N1 9UU
Freephone: 0800 581420
Tel: 020 7833 3034
Fax: 020 7278 0647
Email: info@medicalert.org.uk
Website: www.medicalert.org.uk

Insulin travel cool wallets

Frio Cooling Products
PO Box 10,
Haverfordwest,
Dyfed, SA62 5YG
Tel: 01437 741700
Fax: 01437 741781
Website: www.friouk.com

Medical Shop

Freepost OF1727,
Woodstock,
Oxfordshire OX20 1BR
Freephone: 0800 731 6959
Website: www.medicalshop.co.uk

Diabetes-focused organisations for professionals

Blood Pressure Association
60 Cranmer Terrace,
London SW17 0QS
Tel: 020 8772 4994
Membership line:
020 8772 4983
Fax: 020 8772 4999
Website: www.bpassoc.org.uk

British Dietetic Association
5th Floor,
Charles House,
148/9 Great Charles Street,
Queensway,
Birmingham B3 3HT
Tel: 0121 200 8080
Fax: 0121 200 8081
Email: info@bda.uk.com
Website: www.bda.uk.com

British Heart Foundation
14 Fitzhardinge Street,
London W1H 6DH
Tel: 020 7935 0185
Heart Information Line:
08450 70 80 70
Website: www.bhf.org.uk

Diabetes UK
(See page 397)

British Hypertension Society
BHS Administrative Officer,
Clinical Sciences Building,
Level 5,
Leicester Royal Infirmary,
PO Box 65,
Leicester LE2 7LX
Tel: 07717 467 973
Email: bhs@le.ac.uk
Website: www.bhsoc.org
A list of acceptable blood pressure
devices can be found at:
www.bhsoc.org/blood_pressure_list.stm

Institute of Chiropodists
and Podiatrists
27 Wright Street,
Southport,
Lancashire PR9 0TL
Tel: 01704 546141
Website: www.inst-chiropodist.org.uk
A professional body whose aim is to
further the awareness of foot health
issues by the general public.

Podiatry pages
Website: www.podiatrypages.co.uk
A website to enable individuals to
find local chiropodists/podiatrists.

Royal College
of General Practitioners
14 Princes Gate,
Hyde Park,
London SW7 1PU
Tel: 020 7581 3232
Fax: 020 7225 3047
Email: info@rcgp.org.uk
Website: www.rcgp.org.uk

Royal Pharmaceutical Society of
Great Britain
1 Lambeth High Street,
London SE1 7JN
Tel: 020 7735 9141
Fax: 020 7735 7629
Email: enquiries@rpsgb.org.uk
Website: www.rpsgb.org.uk/index.html
A professional society of over
43 000 members working in all
sectors of the profession, both in
Britain and overseas.

Society of Chiropodists
and Podiatrists
1 Fellmonger's Path,
Tower Bridge Road,
London SE1 3LY
Tel: 020 7234 8620
Fax: 0845 450 3721
Website: www.feetforlife.org

Patient support organisations

Diabetes UK
Central Office,
Macleod House,
10 Parkway,
London NW1 7AA
Tel: 020 7424 1000
Fax: 020 7424 1001
Email: info@diabetes.org.uk
Website: www.diabetes.org.uk

Careline
Tel: 0845 120 2960
*(Mon–Fri 9 am–5 pm; the site
operates a translation service, and
recorded information is available
24 hours a day)*
Email: careline@diabetes.org.uk
*A translation service is also
available on the Diabetes UK
website. The Careline provides
information and support on any
aspect of diabetes.*

Regional offices

**Diabetes UK
Northern Ireland**
Bridgewood House,
Newforge Business Park,
Newforge Lane,
Belfast BT9 5NW
Tel: 028 9066 6646
Email: n.ireland@diabetes.org.uk

Diabetes UK Scotland
Savoy House,
140 Sauciehall Street,
Glasgow G2 3DH
Tel: 0141 332 2700
Email: scotland@diabetes .org.uk

Diabetes UK Cymru
Quebec House,
Castlebridge,
Cowbridge Road East,
Cardiff CF11 9AB
Tel: 029 2066 8276
Email: wales@diabetes.org.uk

Diabetes UK Eastern
10 Parkway,
London NW1 7AA
Tel: 01268 272 104
Email: eastern@diabetes.org.uk

Diabetes UK East Midlands
10 Parkway,
London NW1 7AA
Tel: 0115 931 2724
Email: east.midlands@diabetes.org.uk

Diabetes London
10 Parkway,
London NW1 7AA
Tel: 020 7424 1116
Email: London@diabetes.org.uk

Diabetes UK North West
First Floor,
The Boultings,
Winwick Street,
Warrington,
Cheshire WA2 7TT
Tel: 01925 653 281
Email: n.west@diabetes.org.uk

**Diabetes UK
Northern and Yorkshire**
Sterling House,
22 St Cuthbert's Way,
Darlington DL1 1GB
Tel: 01325 488 606
Email: north&yorks@diabetes.org.uk

Diabetes UK South East
10 Parkway,
London NW1 7AA
Tel: 020 8549 5418
Email: south.east@diabetes.org.uk

Diabetes UK South West
10 Parkway,
London NW1 7AA
Tel: 0117 973 2904
Email: south.west@diabetes.org.uk

Diabetes UK West Midlands
1 Eldon Court,
Eldon Street,
Wallsall WS1 2JP
Tel: 01922 614 500
Email: w.midlands@diabetes.org.uk

Other Diabetes UK resources

Information team
Tel: 020 7424 1020
Email: scienceinfo@diabetes.org.uk

Professional Advisory Council
Professional Relations Team
Tel: 020 7424 1130
Email: healthcare@diabetes.org.uk

Research
Website: www.diabetes.org.uk/research

Diabetes Insight
c/o 15 Ravenhill Avenue,
Knowle,
Bristol BS3 5DU
Website: www.diabetes-insight.org.uk
*Information and an online discussion
forum for people with diabetes to learn
from and support each other.*

Sight

Action for Blind People
14–16 Verney Road,
London SE16 3DZ
Tel: 020 7635 4800
Helpline: 0800 915 4666
Fax: 020 7635 4900
Email: info@actionforblindpeople.org.uk
Website: www.afbp.org/homepage.htm
*A national charity that aims to
enable blind and partially sighted
people to enjoy equal opportunities
in every aspect of their lives.*

**Guide Dogs for the Blind
Association**
Burghfield Common,
Reading RG7 3YG
Tel: 0118 983 5555
Email: guidedogs@guidedogs.org.uk
Website: www.gdba.org.uk
*Provides guide dogs and other
rehabilitation services that meet
the needs of blind and partially
sighted people.*

Partially Sighted Society
Queens Road,
Doncaster DN1 2NX
Tel: 01302 323132
Fax: 01302 368998
Email: doncaster@partsight.org.uk
*Emphasis is placed on making
the most of vision through
information, advice, publications
and leaflets, as well as providing
information on local support
groups.*

Royal National Institute for the Blind
105 Judd Street,
London WC1H 9NE
Tel: 020 7388 1266
Helpline: 0845 766 9999
Fax: 020 7388 2034
Website: www.rnib.org.uk

Travel

Department of Health Travel Information
Website: www.dh.gov.uk/travellers
You can apply here for your European Health Insurance Card.

Foreign and Commonwealth Office
Travel Advice Unit,
Consular Directorate,
Foreign and Commonwealth Office,
Old Admiralty Building,
London SW1A 2PA
Tel (not visa enquiries):
0870 850 2829
Fax: 020 7008 0155
Email: consular.fco@gtnet.gov.uk
(travel advice only)
Website: www.fco.gov.uk

Health Protection Scotland
Clifton House,
Clifton Place,
Glasgow G3 7LN
Tel: 0141 300 1100
Fax: 0131 300 1170
Email: hpsenquiries:hps.scot.nhs.uk
Website: www.fitfortravel.scot.nhs.uk

Masta Travel Health
Website: www.masta.org
A shop, library and the ability to compile a health brief for specific countries online.
Travel Health Information Services
20 Oaklands Way,
Hildenborough,
Kent TN11 9DA
Email: mail@travelhealth.co.uk
Website: www.travelhealth.co.uk

Language

Language Line
Swallow House,
11–21 Northdown Street,
London N1 9BN
Tel: 0800 169 2879
Email: enquiries@languageline.co.uk
Website: www.languageline.co.uk

Multifaith calendars

Swindon Borough Council:
http.//193.113.179.211/faith

Equity Challenge:
www.ecu.ac.uk/guidance/religionandbelief/
religionandbelieffaithcalender.html

SHAP:
www.shap.org

Associated problems

British Heart Foundation
14 Fitzhardinge Street,
London W1H 6DH
Tel: 020 7935 0185
Heart Information Line:
08450 70 80 70
(available Mon–Fri 9 am–5 pm;
*a free service for those seeking
information on heart health issues)*
Fax: 020 7486 5820
Email: internet@bhf.org.uk
Website: www.bhf.org.uk
*Aims to play a leading role in the
fight against heart disease.*

HEART UK
7 North Road,
Maidenhead,
Berkshire SL6 1PE
Tel: 01628 628 638
Fax: 01628 628 698
Email: ask@heartuk.org.uk
Website: www.heartuk.org.uk
*The Family Heart Association
merged with the British
Hyperlipidaemia Association in
2002 to form HEART UK.*

National Kidney Federation
6 Stanley Street
Worksop
Notts S81 7HX
Tel: 01909 487 795
Fax: 01909 481 723
Helpline: 0845 601 0209
Website: www.kidney.org.uk
*Aims to promote the welfare of
people suffering from kidney disease
or renal failure and their relatives
and friends.*

QUIT
Tel: 0800 00 22 00
Website: www.quit.org.uk
*The independent charity whose aim
is to save lives by helping smokers
to stop smoking.*

Sexual Dysfunction Association
Windmill Place
Business Centre,
2–4 Windmill Lane,
Southall,
Middlesex UB2 4NJ
Helpline: 0870 7743571
Website: www.sda.uk.net
*A non-profit-making organisation
that puts sufferers in contact with
specialists around the country.*

Stroke Association
Stroke Information Service,
The Stroke Association,
240 City Road,
London EC1V 2PR
Tel (Switchboard):
020 7566 0300
National Stroke Helpline:
0845 3033 100
(open Mon–Fri 9 am–5 pm)
Fax: 020 7490 2686
Email: info@stroke.org.uk
Website: www.stroke.org.uk
*Provides support for people affected
by stroke and their families.*

Weight Watchers
Website: www.WeightWatchers.co.uk
*Helps people to lose weight in the
company of others.*

Appendix 5

Diabetic emergencies: guidelines for health professionals

People with diabetes mellitus are at risk of developing three specific medical (metabolic) emergencies: hypoglycaemia, diabetic ketoacidosis and, in adults, hyperglycaemic hyperosmolar non-ketotic (HONK) coma. A key component of all three is deterioration in mental function, which, if left untreated, leads to coma and ultimately death. Individuals with diabetes taking metformin can develop lactic acidosis, which is also life-threatening.

The text below is adapted from information supplied to the National Patients' Access Team (*Guidelines for the Management of Common Medical Emergencies in General Practice*, September 2001) by a multidisciplinary team led by Professor David Russell-Jones, Royal Surrey County Hospital, UK.

Hypoglycaemia

Hypoglycaemia (a blood sugar level below 4.0 mmol/l) is most commonly the result of the glucose-lowering effect of oral hypoglycaemic drugs or insulin. In a person taking insulin, symptoms usually develop rapidly. In someone taking an oral hypoglycaemic agent, the onset is often more insidious and may even be intermittent, presenting as personality change, focal neurological signs, hunger or dizzy spells. Some non-diabetic people may take insulin or other hypoglycaemic drugs as a form of self-abuse.

Clinical features

Features of hypoglycaemia include sweating, tachycardia, tremor, visual disturbance, focal neurological signs, changes in mental state (confusion, uncooperative behaviour), headache, convulsions and, ultimately, coma and death.

Initial management

Although the blood glucose level at which symptoms develop varies, in principle anyone with a level below 4.0 mmol/l should be considered to be in danger. If possible, check the blood glucose by a finger-prick test (remembering to wash and dry the prick site before taking the blood). If you are unable to measure the blood glucose concentration but you suspect severe hypoglycaemia, give glucose anyway – it will not harm the individual. If hypoglycaemia is confirmed or suspected, the treatment depends on whether or not the person is cooperative.

If the individual is *cooperative*, give approximately 10–20 g glucose orally as either:

■ glucose tablets (3–4 should be sufficient);

■ a sugary (non-diet) drink: one can be made by adding approximately three teaspoons of sugar per 100 ml fluid;

■ GlucoGel (previously known as Hypostop);

■ honey (approximately one tablespoon) held in the buccal cavity.

If necessary the dose should be repeated in 10–15 minutes. The person should then take some complex carbohydrate, such as bread, biscuits or a meal if one is due.

If the person is *uncooperative* but still conscious, try giving oral glucose or glucose gel into the buccal cavity. If the person is semi-conscious or comatose, give glucose or glucagon.

Glucose must be given intravenously (Table A5.1), recovery usually following within 5 minutes of injection. Repeat the dose after 5 minutes if there has been no effect. High-concentration glucose is very irritant (especially if extravasation occurs) and should be given into a large vein through a large-gauge needle. If possible, flush with sodium chloride 0.9% after administration.

Table A5.1 Glucose dosage in hypoglycaemia

Glucose	Strength	Dose	Route
Child	10%*	5 ml/kg	Intravenous
Adult	20%*	50 ml	Intravenous
	50%	25 ml	Intravenous

*This strength will need to be diluted down from 50% glucose

Glucagon can be given intravenously, intramuscularly or subcutaneously (Table A5.2). By intramuscular injection, it takes around 10 minutes to work. Individuals who are starved or have been hypoglycaemic for a long time may not respond. If the person has not responded within 10 minutes of giving glucagon, give intravenous glucose.

If there is no recovery, or there are residual symptoms despite raising the blood glucose level to normal, the person should be transferred to hospital immediately.

Subsequent management

As soon as feasible, start oral glucose and complex carbohydrates. If a long-acting hypoglycaemic has been taken, hypoglycaemia may recur; to avoid this, the person should continue taking a high carbohydrate intake for 24 hours. If the person has recovered fully, ensure that he or she eats high-calorie (sugar) confectionery, sweet biscuits and more sweet drinks followed by complex carbohydrates.

Diabetic control following hypoglycaemia may be poor for a few days. Advise the person to discuss the episode with the diabetes team. The general practitioner (GP), or diabetes clinic responsible for the person's long-term management, should try to establish why hypoglycaemia occurred in order to develop strategies to prevent it happening again. Hypoglycaemia can often be anticipated or promptly reversed by good patient education. The families or companions of those with diabetes who are at risk of hypoglycaemia should be taught how to inject glucagon.

Table A5.2 Glucagon dosage in hypoglycaemia

	Dose	Route	
Glucagon	Child Birth – 1 month 1 month – 2 years 2–18 years	20 µg/kg 500 µg If <20 kg, give 500 µg If >30 kg, give 1 mg	Intramuscular intravenous or subcutaneous
	Adult	1 mg	

Referral advice

Individuals should be transferred to hospital immediately if:

- they do not respond to glucose/glucagon;
- there is residual neurological deficit.

The threshold for referral should be lowered if the person:

- is unable to manage alone;
- gives rise to additional clinical concerns;
- is a child;
- is older and taking an oral hypoglycaemic agent.

Diabetic ketoacidosis

The blood glucose is usually over 25 mmol/l but may be lower). Diabetic ketoacidosis can occur in any patient with type 1 (insulin-dependent) diabetes. It is most commonly precipitated by minor illnesses such as urinary tract infections, gastroenteritis or upper respiratory tract infections.

The rate of development of ketoacidosis varies. If it is the presenting feature in a person newly diagnosed with diabetes, it may have taken days to become established. In otherwise well-controlled diabetes, some symptoms may begin within a few hours of the glucose level rising.

Clinical features

These include polydipsia and polyuria, malaise and weakness, nausea and vomiting, abdominal pain, confusion, disturbance of consciousness and, ultimately, coma and death. The symptoms may initially be masked by those of the precipitating illness. Physical examination may reveal dehydration with tachycardia and postural hypotension, fast, laboured breathing (Kussmaul breathing) and a smell of acetone on the breath.

The diagnosis is based on:

- the clinical history;
- the physical examination;
- the presence of glucose and ketones in the urine;
- a high blood sugar level after a finger or ear lobe prick test.

Referral advice

People with diabetic ketoacidosis should be transferred to hospital immediately. If transfer is delayed, it may be appropriate to start intravenous fluid replacement (e.g. with sodium chloride 0.9%) and to give insulin, but this should be done only after discussion with the hospital medical or paediatric team. Do not delay treatment of a life-threatening precipitating cause if it can be identified.

Hyperglycaemic hyperosmolar non-ketotic coma

HONK-associated coma carries a high mortality. It is characterised by profound dehydration, coma and hyperglycaemia, coupled with absent or low detectable ketones. These individuals:

- usually have an underlying illness such as infection, myocardial infarction or cerebrovascular accident;

- often are middle-aged or older;

- usually have type 2 (non-insulin-dependent) diabetes.

The clinical features may develop over days or weeks and may be the first presentation of diabetes. The person may present finally with focal neurological signs, seizures or coma. The risk of coma is increased in patients taking drugs such as phenytoin, propranolol, cimetidine, thiazide or loop diuretics, corticosteroids or chlorpromazine.

Referral advice

Individuals should be transferred to hospital immediately for rehydration, correction of a grossly disordered metabolic state and treatment of any precipitating factors.

If transfer is delayed, it may be appropriate to start intravenous fluid replacement (e.g. with sodium chloride 0.9%) and to give insulin, but this should be done only after discussion with the hospital medical or paediatric team. Do not delay treatment of a life-threatening precipitating cause if one can be identified.

Table A5.3 Adjustment of insulin dose

Blood glucose level	Ketones present	Action
Less than 13 mmol/l	No	Continue insulin dose as normal
	Yes	Increase the dose of each insulin injection by 2 units and continue until ketones have cleared*
Between 13–22 mmol/l	No	Increase the dose of each insulin injection by 2 units and continue until blood glucose control has been re-established
	Yes	Increase the dose of each insulin injection by 4 units and continue until ketones have cleared*
More than 22 mmol/l	No	Increase the dose of each insulin injection by 4 units and continue until blood glucose control has been re-established
	Yes	Increase the dose of each insulin injection by 6 units and continue until ketones have cleared*

*Individuals with ketones who develop a low blood sugar level (less than 8 mmol/l) should supplement their diet with milk or fruit juice to raise this

Lactic acidosis

Metformin can cause lactic acidosis, especially in those with renal impairment and severe dehydration or sepsis. The most obvious clinical feature is stimulation of respiration, with hyperventilation. If lactic acidosis is suspected, the individual should be transferred to hospital immediately.

General advice ('sick day rules')

It is important to advise those with diabetes (as well as their carers or relatives as appropriate) how to anticipate and prevent a serious deterioration in metabolic control, learning to recognise features and respond to them should they arise. Below is advice designed to reduce the likelihood of a person's diabetes going out of control when he or she becomes otherwise unwell. Further information can be obtained from Diabetes UK (see Appendix 4 for details).

Adults with type 1 diabetes who develop concomitant illness should:

- continue with insulin;
- measure their blood glucose level at least four times a day;
- test for ketones;
- aim to drink just under 3 litres (around 5 pints) of unsweetened fluids each day;
- adjust the dose of insulin according to the blood glucose measurement and the presence, or otherwise, of urinary ketones (see Table A5.3 for suggested advice, but seek local guidance).

Anyone who is vomiting and has persistent ketones should be referred urgently to hospital.

People with type 2 diabetes who develop concomitant illness should:

- continue taking their normal dose of oral hypoglycaemic agent or insulin as prescribed by the diabetes team;
- keep testing their urine and blood glucose level. If the person is on insulin and has a blood glucose level greater than 13 mmol/l, the advice above for patients with type 1 diabetes should be followed;
- if vomiting, be urgently referred to hospital.

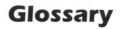

Glossary

ACE inhibitors	angiotensin-converting enzyme inhibitors. Medications that slow the activity of the angiotensin-converting enzyme. Used to treat hypertension
alpha-cells	cells that produce glucagon in the islets of Langerhans in the pancreas
analogue insulins	a new generation of insulins in which the structure of the insulin molecule has been changed to allow it to be absorbed at a different rate
ARB	angiotensin II AT-1 receptor blocker; medication used to treat hypertension
autonomic neuropathy	damage to the nervous system regulating the autonomic functions of the body
beef insulin	*see* bovine insulin
beta-blockers	drugs that are used to treat angina and to lower blood pressure; they can change the warning signs of hypoglycaemia
beta-cells (β cells)	cells that produce insulin in the islets of Langerhans in the pancreas
biguanides	drugs used in treatment of diabetes; they lower blood glucose levels through an increase in uptake of glucose by muscle, and a reduction in absorption of glucose by the intestines and the amount of glucose produced by the liver
bovine insulin	insulin extracted from the pancreas of cattle
calcium channel blocker	medication used to treat hypertension. May be non-dihydropyridine (reno-protective)
chiropodist	a practitioner of chiropody; also called a podiatrist
chiropody	specialty concerned with diagnosis and/or medical, surgical, mechanical, physical and adjunctive treatment of diseases, injuries and defects of the human foot; also called podiatry
DCCT	Diabetes Control and Complications Trial
diabetes insipidus	a disorder of the pituitary gland accompanied by excessive urination and thirst. These symptoms, although similar to those of diabetes mellitus, are **not** accompanied by hypoglycaemia

diabetes mellitus	a disorder of the pancreas characterised by high blood glucose levels, excessive urination and thirst, in addition to other signs and symptoms
diabetic amyotrophy	rare condition causing pain and/or weakness of the legs as a result of damage to certain nerves
diabetic coma	unconscious state characterised by severe hyperglycaemia, ketoacidosis and extreme biochemical imbalance
diabetic maculopathy	pathological disease of the eye caused by diabetes
diabetic nephropathy	renal damage caused by diabetes
diabetic neuropathy	nerve damage caused by diabetes
diabetic retinopathy	eye damage caused by diabetes
diuretics	agents that increase the flow of urine and reduce blood pressure
exchanges	portions of carbohydrate foods that can be exchanged for one another. One exchange = 10 g of carbohydrate
fructosamine	measurement of this indicates diabetes control, reflecting the average blood glucose level over the previous 2–3 weeks. *See* glycated haemoglobin
gestational diabetes	diabetes occurring during pregnancy but usually temporary
glaucoma	disease of the eye causing increased pressure inside the eye
GlucoGel gel	glucose/dextrose gel that can be rubbed on the gums of a diabetic person undergoing a hypoglycaemic episode, and is particularly useful if the patient is uncooperative; available on prescription (FP10)
glycated haemoglobin (HbA_{1c})	this is the part of the haemoglobin that has glucose attached to it; measurement of HbA_{1c} is a test of diabetes control, the amount depending on the average blood glucose level over the previous 2–3 months. *See* fructosamine
glycosuria	presence of glucose in the urine
honeymoon period	occurring from weeks to months after the diagnosis of type 1 diabetes; less insulin is required during this period as a result of the partial recovery of insulin secretion by the pancreas
human insulin	insulin produced by recombinant technology which is close to and has a purity similar to the human species
hyperglycaemia	high blood glucose level
hypo	abbreviation for hypoglycaemia
hypoglycaemia	low blood glucose level

IDDM	insulin-dependent diabetes mellitus – *see* type 1 diabetes. This term is no longer used
IFG	impaired fasting glycaemia
IGT	impaired glucose tolerance
impaired fasting glycaemia	this is a new category, which includes people with fasting glucose levels above normal, but not enough to diagnose diabetes, i.e. between 6.1 and 7.0 mmol/l
impaired glucose tolerance	indicated by a fasting venous glucose value of 6.1–6.9 mmol/l. Confirmed by a 2-hour OGGT of 7.8–11.0 mmol/l
incidence	the number of new cases of a disease occurring during a given time period, usually expressed as new cases per 100 000 of the population per year
inhaled insulin	a way of administering insulin so that it can be taken in the same way that people with asthma take their drugs. Currently in development
insulin coma	severe hypoglycaemia causing the unconscious state and sometimes convulsions
insulin pen	device that resembles a large fountain pen that takes a cartridge of insulin. Injection of insulin occurs after dialling the dose and pressing a button. Some are disposable
insulin resistance	decreased insulin sensitivity, meaning that a higher level of insulin than normal is needed to obtain the same blood glucose-lowering effect
intermediate-acting insulin	insulin preparation with action lasting 12–18 hours
islets of Langerhans	specialised cells within the pancreas that produce insulin and glucagon
isophane	a form of intermediate-acting insulin that has protamine added to slow its absorption
juvenile-onset diabetes	most people with this type of diabetes develop it before the age of 40. This term is no longer in use
ketoacidosis	a serious condition resulting from lack of insulin which, in turn, results in body fat being used to produce energy, forming ketones and acids; it is characterised by high blood glucose levels, ketones in the urine, vomiting, drowsiness, heavy laboured breathing and a smell of acetone on the breath
ketonuria	presence of acetone and other ketones in the urine; detected by testing with Ketostix. Occurs in association with severe hyperglycaemia or in the starving state

lente insulin	a form of intermediate-acting insulin that has zinc added to slow its absorption
lipoatrophy	loss of fat from injection sites; used to occur before the use of highly purified insulins
lipohypertrophy	fatty swelling usually caused by repeated injections of insulin into the same site
maculopathy	pathological disease of the eye
maturity-onset diabetes	outdated term for type 2 diabetes, most commonly occurring in people who are middle-aged and overweight
metabolic syndrome	a cluster of medical problems – diabetes, hypertension, central obesity, abnormal lipids, coronary heart disease
microalbuminuria	excretion of minute traces of protein in the urine; an indicator of early, possibly treatable, renal disease
nephropathy	kidney damage; initially this causes the kidney to 'leak' so that albumin appears in the urine. Later it may affect kidney function and in severe cases lead to kidney failure
neuropathy	damage to the nerves, which may be peripheral or autonomic neuropathy
NIDDM	non-insulin-dependent diabetes mellitus – *see* type 2 diabetes. This term is no longer used
oral glucose tolerance test (OGTT)	test used in the diagnosis of diabetes mellitus; glucose in the blood is measured at intervals before and after the person has drunk a measured amount of glucose after a high-carbohydrate load and fasting before the test. Also used to screen for IGT
PCDS	Primary Care Diabetes Society (see Appendix IV)
peripheral neuropathy	damage to the nerves supplying the muscles and skin; can result in diminished sensation and vibration perception, particularly feet and legs. Muscle weakness may also follow
podiatrist	*see* chiropodist
podiatry	*see* chiropody
polyuria	passing of large quantities of urine as a result of excess glucose in the bloodstream; a symptom of untreated diabetes mellitus (and diabetes insipidus)
porcine insulin	insulin extracted from the pancreas of pigs
PPGRs	postprandial glucose regulators, e.g. repaglinide: drugs that reduce blood glucose levels. They have a similar mode of action to sulphonylureas, but with a faster onset and shorter duration of action

prevalence	the number of cases of a disease at a given point in time, expressed as a proportion of the population
proteinuria	protein or albumin in the urine
RCGP	Royal College of General Practitioners
RCN	Royal College of Nursing
RCP	Royal College of Physicians
renal threshold	the level of glucose in the blood above which it will start to spill into the urine, causing glycosuria; the threshold in normal subjects is 10 mmol/l (blood glucose level). In all subjects, the renal threshold rises with age
retinopathy	damage to the retina
short-acting insulin	insulin preparations with action lasting 6–12 hours
Snellen chart	chart used to assess visual acuity
structured education programme	patient information in a form defined by NICE (2003) as 'a planned and graded programme that is comprehensive in scope, flexible in content, responsive to an individual's clinical and psychological needs, and adaptable to his or her educational and cultural background'
sulphonylureas	drugs that lower the blood glucose levels by stimulating the pancreatic beta-cells to produce more insulin, e.g. tolbutamide, gliclazide
thiazolidinediones	drugs (also called PPAR-gamma agonists and glitazones) that reduce blood glucose and insulin levels. This is achieved by a reduction in insulin resistance, resulting in increased effectiveness of available insulin in liver, fat and muscle
type 1 diabetes	type of diabetes that must be treated with insulin; previously known as insulin-dependent diabetes mellitus (IDDM)
type 2 diabetes	type of diabetes characterised by insulin resistance. It used to be called maturity-onset diabetes but is becoming more frequent in the young. It is much more prevalent in the overweight and obese
UKPDS	UK Prospective Diabetes Study

Index

Page numbers followed by an italic *g* denote glossary entries

borderline diabetes 315
bovine insulin 408*g*
breast screening 282
British Diabetic Association *see*
    Diabetes UK
Buddhists 235
bumetanide, drug interactions 154

calcium channel blockers 341, 408*g*
    betel nut and 232
    in hypertension 339
call and recall 46, 65
    see also recall and follow-up
capsaicin, for neuropathic pain 216
carbohydrates 100, 129, 139, 306
cardiovascular complications, type 2
    diabetes 311
cardiovascular disease 9
    risk in type 2 diabetes 350
    see also heart disease
CARDS (Collaborative Atorvastatin
    Diabetes Study) 353
care in diabetes
    aims 13, 370–2
    auditing 293–300
    coordination of 33
    in general practice *see* general
        practice diabetes service
    indicator points 43–50
    key elements 374–5
    organisation of 14–15
    provision of 372–4
    shared (integrated) 72
    skills necessary for providing
        374–6
    team approach 34–5
    see also care teams
care plans 264, 265–7, 277–8,
    279–80
care processes, rates 299
care teams
    care expected from 359–63,
        372–3
    complaints 363
    education and training *see*
        education and training for
        health professionals

healthcare staff responsibilities
    373
    members of 28–39, 360, 374–5
    specialist team role 15–22
    training for 375–6
cataracts 202
    definition 276
cervical screening 282
children and young people 286,
    298
    paediatric team 16
    prevalence and incidence of
        diabetes 3–4, 6
    referral to specialist paediatric
        team 97
    suspected diabetes 94
chiropodists (podiatrists) 224, 408*g*
    criteria for referral to 223–4
    in planning general practice care
        system 67
    range of expertise 20–1
    role 20–1
chiropody (podiatry) 408*g*
    priority groups 20
    services, links with 84–5
chloramphenicol, drug interactions
    154
chlorpropamide 146–7
cholesterol
    audit results 297
    care process rates 299
    cholesterol-lowering drugs, betel
        nut and 233
    definition 276
    quality indicators 46, 49
    targets for patients 109
    tests 364
    treatment targets 299
cholinergic drugs, betel nut and 232
Christian Scientists 235–6
Christians 236
Cialis 335
cigarettes *see* smoking
cimetidine, drug interactions 154
circulation, abnormal 213–14
clerical staff 37–8
clinical examination 99

detemir 159
diabetes
  borderline 315
  impact on individual 11–13
  management of 280–1
  mild 15
  nature of 280
  newly diagnosed 98, 100–4
  quality indicators for 45–50
diabetes centres/clinics 14, 21–2,
    79–83
Diabetes Control and Complications
    Trial (DCCT) 13, 345
diabetes delivery strategy, National
    Service Framework 73, 264–5
Diabetes Education and Self
    Management for Ongoing and
    Newly Diagnosed see DESMOND
Diabetes Industry Group 367
diabetes insipidus 304, 408*g*
Diabetes Management in Primary
    Care course 382
diabetes mellitus 409*g*
  classification 303–4
  history 304–6
  identification of people with 96
diabetes registers 80–3
  advantages of 80
  setting up 82–3
Diabetes Research and Wellness
    Foundation 367–8
diabetes specialist nurse (DSN), role
    17–19
Diabetes UK 22–4, 378–9, 397–8
  Careline 23, 397
  diagnostic criteria 94
  events 23
  membership benefits for
    healthcare professionals 379
  membership benefits for patients
    and carers 378
  Professional Advisory Council 24
  publications 129, 245, 388–9
  research 23
  Science Information Team 22
  website 23
diabetic amyotrophy 409*g*

diabetic coma 409*g*
diabetic foods 126, 135, 139
diabetic hyperosmolar non-ketotic
    syndrome 97
diabetic ketoacidosis 97, 401
  clinical features 404
  emergencies 404–5
  referral advice 405
  see also ketoacidosis
diabetic kidney disease see diabetic
    nephropathy
diabetic maculopathy 409*g*
diabetic nephropathy (renal disease)
    8, 327–32, 409*g*
  definition 329–30
  summary 328
  see also nephropathy
diabetic neuropathy 213–16,
    333–6, 409*g*
  autonomic 213–14, 334
  peripheral 213–14, 335–6
  summary 334
  symptoms 333
  treatment of pain 214–16
  see also neuropathy
diabetic pregnancy, self-monitoring
    of blood glucose (SMBG)
    188–9
diabetic retinopathy 409*g*
  screening targets 7
  see also eye screening; retinopathy
diabetologists see physicians
diagnosis 92–6
  confirming 94
  Diabetes UK criteria 94
  insulin requirements at 99, 100
  newly diagnosed diabetes 98,
    100–4
  patient education after
    confirmation of 279–92
  training for primary healthcare
    team 376
  type 1 diabetes 308
  type 2 diabetes 312
diagnostic criteria, ADA/WHO
    comparison 351–2
Diamicron 147

foot care teams 8
foot pulses and sensation, definition
  276
foot ulcers 8, 20
  care of 212
  diabetic complications causing
    213–16
  management plans for different
    levels of risk 208–9
  treatment by primary care team
    221–2
fructosamine 409*g*
  serum fructosamine 177, 178
fructose 135
fruit and vegetables 127, 139
frusemide *see* furosemide
funding 43
  GMS contract 29, 42, 43, 65
fundoscopy 73, 197, 199, 201, 364
  dilatation of pupils 203
furosemide, drug interactions 154

gabapentin, for neuropathic pain
  216
gender, and diabetes 4, 5, 6
General Medical Services (GMS)
    contract 29, 41–3
  care system in general practice
    65–6
  clinical quality indicator points
    43–50
  clinical standards 44
  depression in 283
  enhanced services 42
  funding 29, 42, 43, 65
  key principles 41–3
  nurses in 50
  practice-based 41
  revisions (2006) 42–3
  service categories 42–3
  see also Quality and Outcomes
    Framework (QOF)
general practice
  awareness of diabetes 89
  practice-based commissioning 51
  staff *see* general practice staff
  see also primary care

general practice diabetes service
  advertising 79, 80
  aims 63
  diabetes clinics 80, 81
  equipment 74–6
  facilities 72–3
  flexibility 68–9
  frequency of clinics 72
  General Medical Services contract
    65–6
  initial treatment 99–104
  links with specialist services 83–5
  non-attenders 82
  objectives 64
  organisation 68–9
  organisation and resource
    implications 67–8
  patients identified as suitable for
    69
  planning 66–8
  protocol development 65, 66
  registers 80–3
  role redesign 70–1
  setting up 63–5
  shared (integrated) care 72
  staff involved in provision of 69,
    70–1
  time needed to provide care 66, 68
  see also care teams
general practice staff
  maximising contribution of 42
  practice educator 71
  practice manager 37–8
  practice nurse role 30–1
general practitioners (GPs)
  funding 29
  resources and support for 12
  role and responsibilities 28–30
  with special interests (GPwSI),
    role 17
gestational diabetes 92, 188,
    316–19, 409*g*
  diagnosis 317
  management 318–19
  postpartum 318
GI (glycaemic index) 129, 137–40
glargine 159

motivational interviewing 254–5
multifactorial intervention, in type 2
    diabetes 350
multifaith calendars 244, 399
multimedia packages 383
Muslims 238–40
mydriatic eye drops 202

nateglinide 148, 149
    drug interactions 154
National Diabetes Audit 297–9
    care process rates 299
    key findings 297
    key recommendations 298–9
    treatment targets 299
National Health Service *see* NHS
National Institute for Health and
    Clinical Excellence (NICE)
    guidelines
    audit 295–6
    depression 282–3
    lipid control 323–5
    patient education 33, 34
    structured education 246–7
National Service Frameworks 371–2
    for Coronary Heart Disease 323
    for Diabetes: Delivery Strategy 31,
        73, 264–5
    for Diabetes: Standards 7
nausea 180
nephropathy 7–8, 411*g*
    incipient *see* microalbuminuria
    overt *see* proteinuria
    (macroalbuminuria)
    see also diabetic nephropathy
neuropathic pain 206, 214–16
    treatment 216
neuropathy 8–9, 411*g*
    autonomic 213–14, 334, 408*g*
    monofilament testing 207–8
    peripheral 213–14, 336, 411*g*
    testing, quality indicators 45, 48
    see also diabetic neuropathy
NHS
    complaints 363
    health services expected from 359
    regional boards (Scotland) 377

NICE *see* National Institute for
    Health and Clinical Excellence
non-insulin-dependent diabetes
    mellitus (NIDDM) 411*g*
    see also type 2 diabetes
non-steroidal anti-inflammatory
    drugs (NSAIDS), drug
    interactions 154
Northern Ireland, health and social
    care boards 377–8
NovoMix 160–1
NovoNorm 149
NovoRapid 160–1, 164, 180
NSAIDS (non-steroidal anti-
    inflammatory drugs), drug
    interactions 154
nurse prescribing 33–4, 113–21
    background 113–14
    diabetes-related prescriptions 115
    extended formulary 114
    nurse independent prescribers
        114, 115
    principles of 116
    supplementary prescribing 114,
        115, 116, 116–20
    training 120
nurses, in GMS contract 50
Nursing and Midwifery Council,
    Code of Professional Conduct
    30, 32

obesity 47, 127–8, 370–1
    in African/Caribbean community
        242
    prevention, diet and 311
    see also overweight patients;
        weight
obesity register, QOF indicator points
    47
OGTTs *see* oral glucose tolerance
    tests
Ombudsman, Health Service 363
ophthalmic medical practitioners
    201
ophthalmic opticians (optometrists)
    201, 202
opioids, for neuropathic pain 216

opticians
   dispensing 201
   in planning general practice care
      system 68
   types 201
optometrists (ophthalmic opticians)
   201, 202
oral contraceptives 284–5
   drug interactions 154
oral glucose tolerance tests (OGTTs)
   74–5, 92, 94–5, 96, 317, 411*g*
oral medication 141–53
   hypoglycaemic agents 142–53
   patient information 142
osteomyelitis 224
overweight patients
   asymptomatic 99–100
   blood glucose control 347
   metformin and 347
   with type 2 diabetes 103
   see also obesity; weight

paediatric team *see* children and
      young people
pain, neuropathic 206, 214–16
   treatment 216
pain relief, Christian Scientists 235–6
patient education 12
   assessment for 256–63
   checklist of topics 272
   after confirmation of diagnosis
      279–92
   expert patients' help in 71
   group education 258–63
   Internet and 258
   NICE guidelines 33, 34
   in the practice 258–63
   practice educator 71
   primary healthcare team training
      in the provision of 375–6
   reasons for 252–5
   resources for 76–7, 257–8
   structured *see* structured patient
      education
   see also DAFNE; DESMOND;
      X-PERT
patient group directions 120–1

Patient Health Questionnaire
   (PHQ-9) 284
patient information 32
   oral medication 142
patient register 45, 46
patient support organisations
   397–400
Patient UK 368
patients
   asymptomatic 99–100
   interview models 255
   newly diagnosed 98, 100–4, 252
   not remembering advice 256
   participating in own care 31–2
   psychological support for 33, 98–9
   responsibilities 373–4
peer support programmes 350
perindopril 353
peripheral neuropathy 213–14,
   336, 411*g*
peripheral pulses, quality indicators
   45, 48
peripheral vascular disease 8–9,
   206, 327
pharmacists
   independent prescribers 115
   role 375
   supplementary prescribing 120
   see also community pharmacists
phenothiazines
   betel nut and 233
   drug interactions 154
physical activity 3, 100, 136–7,
   138, 370–1
   monitoring 176
   in prevention of type 2 diabetes
      311, 318
   sport 287
physical examinations 364
physicians (diabetologists), role of
   16–17
PIANO analysis toolkit 298
pioglitazone 144, 145
   drug interactions 154
   during Ramadan 240
   side effects 146
planning mechanisms 376–8

Have you found *Providing Diabetes Care in General Practice* useful and practical? If so, you may be interested in other books from Class Publishing:

Coming Soon!

Type 1 Diabetes: Answers at your fingertips   £14.99
Type 2 Diabetes: Answers at your fingertips   £14.99
Both by Dr Charles Fox and Dr Anne Kilvert

The latest edition of our bestselling reference guide on diabetes has now been split into two books covering the two distinct forms of the disease. These books maintain the popular question and answer format to provide practical advice for patients on every aspect of living with the condition.

Available mid 2007

Vital Diabetes   £14.99
Charles Fox and Mary MacKinnon

This handy reference guide gives you all the backup you need for best practice in diabetes care, and includes the vital facts and figures about diabetes for your information and regular use, as well as providing patient and carer information sheets that you can photocopy for patients to take away with them.

> *"Full of the kind of essential and up-to-date information you need to deliver the best practice in diabetes care."*
>
> M. Carpenter,
> Diabetes Grapevine

Vital Asthma   £14.99
Sue Cross and Dave Burns

This book contains the essential information you need if you are part of the community asthma care team, whether you are a practice nurse, specialist nurse, GP, community pharmacist, physiotherapist.

> *'. . . will be welcomed as a concise learning resource by those currently in asthma training, and as an update and a source of reference information by those in practice.'*
>
> Dr Mike Thomas, FRCP, GPIAG
> Research Fellow, Department of General Practice,
> University of Aberdeen

Chronic Obstructive Pulmonary Disease in Primary Care £29.99
Dr David Bellamy and Rachel Booker

This clear and helpful resource manual addresses the management requirements of GPs and practice nurses. In this book, you will find guidance, protocols, plans and tests – all appropriate to the primary care situation – that will streamline your diagnosis and management of COPD.

> *'I am sure it will become a classic in the history of COPD Care.'*
> Duncan Geddes, Professor of Respiratory Medicine and Consultant Physician, Royal Brompton Hospital

Heart Health: Answers at your fingertips £14.99
Dr Graham Jackson

This practical handbook, written by a leading cardiologist, answers the questions your patients may ask about heart conditions. It advises them what they should do to keep their heart healthy, or – if it has been affected by heart disease – how to make it as strong as possible.

> *'Those readers who want to know more about the various treatments for heart disease will be much enlightened.'*
> Dr James Le Fanu,
> *The Daily Telegraph*

Beating Depression £17.99
Dr Stefan Cembrowicz and Dr Dorcas Kingham

Depression is one of most common illnesses in the world – affecting up to one in four people at some time in their lives. *Beating Depression* shows sufferers and their families that they are not alone, and offers tried and tested techniques for overcoming depression.

> *'All you need to know about depression, presented in a clear, concise and readable way.'*
> Ann Dawson, World Health Organization

PRIORITY ORDER FORM

Cut out or photocopy this form and send it (post free in the UK) to:

Class Publishing Priority Service,
FREEPOST 16705   **Tel: 01256 302 699**
Macmillan Distribution   **Fax: 01256 812 558**
Basingstoke, RG 21 6ZZ

Please send me urgently *(tick below)*	Post included price per copy (*UK only*)
☐ **Providing Diabetes Care in General Practice** (ISBN 978 1 85959 154 3)	£32.99
☐ **Type 1 Diabetes: Answers at your fingertips** (ISBN 978 1 85959 175 8)	£17.99
☐ **Type 2 Diabetes: Answers at your fingertips** (ISBN 978 1 85959 176 5)	£17.99
☐ **Vital Diabetes** (ISBN 978 1 85959 174 1)	£17.99
☐ **Vital Asthma** (ISBN 978 1 85959 107 9)	£17.99
☐ **COPD in Primary Care** (ISBN 978 1 85959 140 8)	£??.99
☐ **Heart Health: the 'at your fingertips' guide** (ISBN 978 1 85959 097 3)	£17.99
☐ **Beating Depression: the 'at your fingertips' guide** (ISBN 978 1 85959 150 5)	£20.99
	TOTAL _____

Easy ways to pay

Cheque: I enclose a cheque payable to Class Publishing for _____

Credit card: Please debit my   ☐ Mastercard   ☐ Visa   ☐ Amex

Number .... Expiry date ....

Name ....

My address for delivery is ....

Town .... County .... Postcode ....

Telephone number (*in case of query*) ....

Credit card billing address if different from above ....

....

Town .... County .... Postcode ....

Class Publishing's guarantee: remember that if, for any reason, you are not satisfied with these books, we will refund all your money, without any questions asked. Prices and VAT rates may be altered for reasons beyond our control.